Psychiatry and Its Discontents

Psychiatry and
Its Discontents

Andrew Scull

UNIVERSITY OF CALIFORNIA PRESS

University of California Press, one of the most distinguished university presses in the United States, enriches lives around the world by advancing scholarship in the humanities, social sciences, and natural sciences. Its activities are supported by the UC Press Foundation and by philanthropic contributions from individuals and institutions. For more information, visit www.ucpress.edu.

University of California Press
Oakland, California

Library of Congress Cataloging-in-Publication Data

Names: Scull, Andrew, 1947– author.
Title: Psychiatry and its discontents / Andrew Scull.
Description: Oakland, California : University of California Press, [2019] |
    Includes bibliographical references and index. |
Identifiers: LCCN 2018055944 (print) | LCCN 2018058799 (ebook) |
    ISBN 9780520973572 (Ebook) | ISBN 9780520305496
    (cloth : alk. paper)
Subjects: LCSH: Psychiatry.
Classification: LCC RC454 (ebook) | LCC RC454 .S3567 2019 (print) |
    DDC 616.89—dc23
LC record available at https://lccn.loc.gov/2018055944

Manufactured in the United States of America

27 26 25 24 23 22 21 20 19
10 9 8 7 6 5 4 3 2

For those who have suffered and even now suffer from serious mental troubles:

> I should like to call you all by name,
> But they have lost the lists.

Anna Akhmatova, *Requiem and Poem without a Hero,* translated by D. M. Thomas

And for my friends Amy Forrest and Stephen Cox with gratitude for kindness I cannot adequately repay

Contents

Illustrations

Acknowledgments

Except for the introduction, versions of each of the chapters that follow have appeared previously in a variety of settings, though I have revised most of them for this book. Formal acknowledgments to the journals and periodicals where these pieces first appeared follow, but here I would particularly like to thank Maren Meinhardt at the *Times Literary Supplement,* who has commissioned essay reviews from me on a variety of topics over the years and has tolerated my repeated violation of agreed-upon word limits with grace and good humor; and Louisa Lyon, commissioning editor of *Brain,* who has invited me, an outsider, to reflect periodically on the neuroscientific world—a world of increasing importance to the understanding of contemporary psychiatry.

Alongside a series of reflections and assessments of the work of other scholars, this book includes a number of essays based on my own researches into twentieth- and twenty-first-century materials. The archival work on which these chapters are based owes much to the generosity of the Academic Senate at my longtime employer, the University of California at San Diego, whose research committee has provided vital funds to support my visits to a variety of archives. I could not have written chapter 9 without an extended period of research in the Rockefeller Foundation Archives, and I am grateful to the foundation for a grant-in-aid that made this possible. In that connection, I would particularly like to thank the estimable Tom Rosenbaum, one of the foundation's archivists. Tom helped me many years ago when I was working on my book *Madhouse* (2005), and on this occasion I am once again in his debt for putting his great knowledge and enthusiasm at my disposal. Thank you, too, to D. M. Thomas, for allowing me to quote from his wonderful translation of the poet Anna Akhmatova.

I would also like to express my gratitude to Naomi Schneider, my editor at the University of California Press, with whom I published a previous book nearly thirty years ago. It has been a pleasure to work with her again. Her enthusiasm for this project and the critical suggestions she offered as she read the manuscript have improved both the organization and content of this book. Naomi's assistant, Benjy Malings, has been enormously helpful with the nuts and bolts of preparing the manuscript for publication, and my copy editor, Genevieve Thurston, has done a wonderful job combing the manuscript for errors and omissions. My thanks as well to Tim Sullivan, the director of the press, to Kim Robinson, its editorial director, and to the many others who work behind the scenes. My appreciation goes to all of you for all you do to keep the University of California Press at the forefront of academic publishing.

That recital scarcely exhausts my obligations to those who have helped me so generously over the years. But there are two more individuals to whom I owe a debt I must acknowledge and cannot hope to repay, save with some inadequate thanks here. Although it gives me enormous pleasure, writing is a solitary affliction. Inevitably, despite my best efforts, initial drafts fall short, and even the best of them benefit from sympathetic readings by those with skilled and critical editorial eyes. I am blessed with two friends who have repeatedly set aside their own work to provide detailed responses of this sort, often at short notice, and always in ways that have improved my prose and my arguments. Amy Forrest and Stephen Cox have spared my blushes on numerous occasions, and though my stubbornness means that I have not always taken their sage advice, whatever merit my writing possesses owes much to their editorial skills and labor. It gives me great pleasure to dedicate this collection of essays to the two of them—a small gesture of thanks for their kindness over so many years; and I dedicate this book as well to the millions of those who have suffered, or now suffer, from what too often is the most solitary of afflictions and yet the most social of maladies.

Andrew Scull
La Jolla

1 Introduction

I must be a masochist. Almost a half century ago, I embarked on a study of lunacy reform in Victorian England. I have remained obsessed with madness ever since—as unsavory as many find the subject, and as stigmatized and marginalized as those who suffer from mental disturbances almost universally seem to be. Or perhaps I am simply one of Isaiah Berlin's hedgehogs, fascinated by one big thing.[1] If so, it is a thing that haunts all of our imaginations, one that all our efforts at repression cannot succeed in entirely dismissing from consciousness. Madness reminds us of how tenuous our own hold over reality may prove to be. It challenges our very sense of what it means to be human. Madness continues to tease and bewilder us, to frighten and fascinate, to challenge us to probe its ambiguities and depredations. Reason and unreason coexist uneasily in our everyday lives, their boundaries fraught and contested. And, like every society before it, twenty-first-century America finds its efforts to confront and solve the problems posed by serious forms of mental disturbance largely unavailing and frequently counterproductive.

This volume is a collection of some reflections on various aspects of the psychiatric enterprise that I have written over the past decade or so, many of which I revised extensively as I set about bringing them together for this publication. The essays reflect a lifetime of thinking and writing about mental illness and about those who have made it their professional business to attempt to understand and perhaps ameliorate the sufferings that flow from disturbances of this sort. It is not a history, I'm afraid, of very much in the way of progress, but nor is it one that revels in that sad situation or claims that no advances have been made over the past two centuries.

Madness remains, in my judgment, an enigma. The etiology of the various disturbances psychiatrists have claimed jurisdiction over remains obscure, and the best the profession has been able to offer are palliative measures. For some patients, those interventions have mitigated suffering, and that is something we should not lose sight of and ought to be grateful for. But for many, the weapons at psychiatry's disposal remain ineffective, and sometimes harmful. At times, exceedingly harmful. So, mine is a critical and skeptical view of the psychiatric enterprise. But it is not one that minimizes or denies the reality of mental disturbance and the immense suffering it often brings in its train—not just for its victims but also for those around them. Serious forms of mental illness remain, as they have always been, the most solitary of afflictions and the most social of maladies.

I have made my career in sociology departments, save for a year spent in Princeton's excellent history department, and in an odd way, that has served me well. Historians tend to be hired to plough down a narrower furrow than I would ever be comfortable with, sticking to a particular period and a particular national historiography. The sociology departments I have been fortunate to work in, however, were willing to tolerate someone who spent a good deal of his time working on the distant past and imposed no limits on my scholarship—the University of Pennsylvania, to be sure, because its senior faculty paid little mind to the junior faculty so long as they carried the teaching load; and the University of California at San Diego because its founding figures deliberately distanced themselves from the disciplinary mainstream, and during my time on the faculty, the department has continued to take seriously the idea that sociology can be a historical and comparative discipline.

My first book, as it happens, dealt with the pressing contemporary issue of deinstitutionalization.[2] Its genesis was my experience during my first time on the job market, seeking to persuade North American sociologists that they should hire someone with a bizarre interest in social reform in

Victorian England. I did so in a handful of departments by persuading them that I had something original to say about the origins of the total institutions Goffman had written about just a few years before[3] and by drawing attention to the medicalization of madness that had taken place in the nineteenth century.

Wherever I spoke, however, in those peculiar hiring rituals scholars undergo where they present a canned version of their research, my audience wanted to know what I thought about contemporary developments, and more specifically the abandonment of the asylum. It seemed an odd development to one aware of how much capital, physical and intellectual, Western societies had invested in the institutional solution to mental illness. But it also seemed well worth investigating and trying to understand. So I gave it a shot.

"Community care" was the slogan of the moment, and the consensus appeared to be that abandoning the asylum was a grand reform that would usher the mad back into our welcoming midst, or so the ideologues of the movement would have it. The drugs made it all possible, so the psychiatrists assured us, on the basis of no more than temporal coincidence and their own overweening confidence in chemical cures. It was in part the product of the critical "anti-psychiatry" of people like Goffman and Szasz, claimed their followers. My book rejected or was sharply critical of all these claims, pointing to the limits of antipsychotics and to their many adverse effects, the nonexistence of community care, and the hostility and neglect that were the fate of discharged patients. It argued that deinstitutionalization was driven in great measure by fiscal concerns, and in the United States by the ability to transfer costs between levels of government. And it suggested that the rhetoric of reform masked what was an emerging policy of malign neglect. I think those criticisms have held up rather well, though some of my attempts to link all this to the then-fashionable arguments about the fiscal crisis of the state now strike me as jejune.

Dividing most of my time between two cities in California, I am reminded daily of the consequences of deinstitutionalization as I walk their streets. Visits to New York or London demonstrate that the challenge of the sidewalk psychotic is not uniquely a problem of La-La Land. Though not solely the product of our abandonment of the mentally ill to their fate, the homelessness crisis is most assuredly exacerbated by that decision, made by our political masters. And it is only one dimension of a problem that extends, of course, to the reinstitutionalization of those who would once have been confined in asylums in our massively overcrowded prisons and jails—the very policy asylums were supposed to supplant.

It didn't take much to justify that line of research to my sociological colleagues, which was fortunate for me in my untenured state, but I swiftly returned to my doctoral researches on lunacy reform and spent much of the next two decades on nineteenth-century matters (though I worked on American as well as European themes).[4] Unlike many who claim to produce historical sociology, I do not shy away from the archives—indeed, I love playing historical detective and am continually seduced by the pleasures of encountering the raw materials that any historical analysis and narrative worth its salt must depend on.

Tenure gave me the freedom to follow my intellectual interests wherever I chose to take them, and I have subsequently ranged across an ever-wider historical canvass. I extended my researches on the emergence of psychiatry as a profession.[5] I worked on the mad trade in eighteenth-century England and on the complex relations between doctors, patients, and families in eighteenth-century London.[6] In the mid-1980s, I was one of the first scholars to engage with the history of psychiatric therapeutics,[7] and that led in turn to a detailed examination of experimentation on vulnerable mental patients in twentieth-century America.[8] Then Oxford University Press invited me to write a book on the protean disorder of hysteria, forcing me to pay attention to the *longue durée*.[9]

On finishing this project on the history of hysteria, I decided that before I declined into my dotage I might indulge in a larger fit of scholarly chutzpah. So, I wrote a book I had long fantasized about producing: an extended examination of madness in civilization that started by ranging from ancient Greece and Palestine to China and the Islamic world before focusing on the history of madness in the West from what we used to call the Dark Ages to what purports to be the enlightened present. What is more, I sought to attack this subject as broadly as possible, moving beyond the relations of madness and medicine and madness and confinement to examine insanity's place in religion and in popular and high culture: in music, in the plastic arts, in literature, on the stage, and even in movies.[10]

Over the course of my career, American psychiatry has undergone a transformation as dramatic and fundamental as can readily be imagined. When I began to explore its past, psychiatry, at least in its American guise, was dominated by psychoanalysis. The Freudian movement had first risen to prominence during World War II with the treatment of "war neurosis." Through the 1960s, its hold over the profession and the public imagination steadily grew. With scarcely an exception, the departments of psychiatry at the major medical schools were headed by psychoanalysts or psychoanalytic fellow travelers. The "refrigerator mother" was blamed for the seeming epidemic of schizophrenia. Although Freud himself had questioned the relevance of psychoanalysis in the treatment of psychosis, his more optimistic American epigones were undeterred. Those who reluctantly began to use the first generation of antipsychotic drugs saw them merely as useful therapeutic adjuncts to calm down florid symptomatology so that the "real" work of psychotherapy could proceed. Hollywood dramatized the miracles of the talk cure in movies like *Suddenly, Last Summer* (1959) and *I Never Promised You a Rose Garden* (1977). Anxious American parents turned to Dr. Benjamin Spock for enlightenment and were rewarded with a bowdlerized version of Freud's theory of child development. Bestseller lists saw the appearance of potboilers such as Robert Lindner's *The Fifty-Minute Hour* (1955), titillating the masses with tales of the secrets of the couch. Psychoanalysis ruled the roost.

And then it didn't. More swiftly and silently than the Cheshire cat, psychoanalytic hegemony vanished, leaving behind not a smile but a fractious group of Freudians and neo-Freudians who squabbled among themselves. Professors of literature and anthropology tried feverishly to fend off the notion that Freud had turned into an intellectual corpse, but cruel realities suggested otherwise. Psychoanalysts were rapidly defenestrated, lost their hold over academic departments of psychiatry, and were replaced by laboratory-based neuroscientists and psychopharmacologists. Psychoanalytic institutes found themselves bereft of recruits and forced to abandon their policy of admitting only the medically qualified. The very term "neurosis" was expunged from the official nomenclature of mental disorder, along with the hypothetical Freudian etiologies for various mental disorders. The "surface" manifestations of mental diseases that psychoanalysts had long dismissed as merely symptoms of underlying psychodynamic disorders of the personality became instead scientific markers, the very elements that defined different forms of mental disorder. And the control of such symptoms, preferably by chemical means, became the new Holy Grail of the profession. For a historian of psychiatry, living through such revolutionary times has been remarkable indeed.

This rapidly shifting landscape was the context within which my own scholarship has been conducted, and a number of the essays in the third and fourth parts of this book reflect my efforts to grapple with and come to terms with these emergent realities. But our contemporary travails form part of a much larger history that also deserves our attention, and it is those earlier aspects of our encounter with madness on which the first chapters in this book are focused. As a now infamous social theorist once remarked, "The tradition of all dead generations weighs like a nightmare on the brains of the living."[11] We may be experiencing our own nightmares to add to the ones our cultural inheritance brings in its train. But interpreting the dreams of earlier generations may help us to cope with and comprehend a bit better the novel ones we have since conjured up. Or so the historian must hope.

Much of my work on the history of psychiatry has appeared in book form, including the various studies I have mentioned here. But I have also written many essays, which have appeared in a wide range of journals and periodicals. Academically speaking, these span a great number of disciplines, from law to literature, and from a variety of subfields in history (social history, cultural history, and medical history) to general medical and psychiatric and neurological journals. I have also been invited on a number of occasions to review the contributions of other scholars working on psychiatry (which increasingly extends to the territory of the neurosciences), and to do so for a broad audience of general readers.

The chapters that follow constitute my attempt to grapple with the psychiatric enterprise from a variety of perspectives, and in the remainder of this introduction, I suggest that this kaleidoscopic line of attack can provide a valuable portrait of the complexities and contradictions that mark the Western encounter with madness. That portrait is, of course, refracted through a single sensibility, and I hope this gives some semblance of unity to what is otherwise a deliberately fragmentary approach to the protean history of madness.

I have chosen to divide this book into four separate sections that largely follow chronological lines. However, this has proved possible only to a degree, for some of the issues I have sought to address refuse to confine themselves neatly to a single historical epoch, demanding instead a less chronologically constrained approach. Still, the basic principle applies and informs my organization of the chapters that follow.

Part 1 thus deals from a variety of perspectives with the rise of the asylum era, which was essentially a nineteenth-century phenomenon. Those who have grown up in the past four decades can have little notion of the immense sway the idea of confining the mentally ill once enjoyed. In this opening section, I look at where this idea came from and discuss how we are to understand the near-universal embrace of a segregative response to madness in the Western world two centuries ago. It was on these nineteenth-century museums of madness (and their immediate antecedents) that social historians of psychiatry first concentrated their attention when they sought to provide a more critical and nuanced history of psychiatry than superannuated psychiatrists had previously offered in their own reconstructions of their past.

The mentally ill were not always willingly shut up, in the many senses of that term. Protests about their confinement, accusations that alienists (and family members) had corrupt motives for confining them and that asylums were a form of imprisonment or even a kind of living death—all these objections emerged very quickly once madhouses appeared on the scene. The culture of complaint (which allows us a glimpse of mental illness from the perspective of some of those defined and confined as such) is virtually coextensive with the asylum era. It thus forms a vital part of any sustained attempt to come to terms with the meaning and impact of the Victorian asylum. Likewise, as the utopian expectations that accompanied the discovery of the asylum foundered on the recalcitrant realities of unreason, so too some sufferers looked beyond the newly consolidating psychiatric profession for solutions to the problems posed by mental troubles.

Part 2 looks in turn at how this nineteenth-century legacy played out in the first half of the twentieth century. Freud and psychoanalysis provided a challenge to the understandings and practices of institutional psychiatry and helped to broaden the territory within which the profession of psychiatry began to move. Despite Freud's disdain (to put it mildly) for the

United States, his ideas would later enjoy greater resonance there than anywhere else besides Buenos Aires. But that popularity has now waned, save in some humanities departments in academia. For more than a quarter of a century, these lingering traces of psychoanalysis have provoked wrath among a group of critics, who have launched a war on Freud's ideas and reputation. Paradoxically, I suggest, the very vehemence of Freud's detractors has had the perverse effect of keeping his ideas alive. And perhaps that is not entirely a bad thing.

If psychoanalysis formed the basis for one type of extra-institutional psychiatry, university-based psychiatry was another development that altered the professional landscape. How did an academic psychiatry emerge, and how, more broadly, were careers built and mental illness understood and approached once this extra-institutional psychiatry emerged on the scene? What was it like for a woman to try to build a career in what had hitherto been an all-male profession? And as there began to be some experimentation with forms of noninstitutional practice and psychologically based theories and interventions, what became of therapies within the walls of the asylum? These are issues I examine in part 2.

Part 3 provides a systematic examination of the second half of the twentieth century and the impact of World War II and its aftermath on the fate of psychiatry, most especially in the United States. This was the era that saw a variety of attempts by scholars to place contemporary developments in a larger and longer historical context, and so in this section of the book I tend to range more frequently beyond the temporal boundaries of the postwar era. But I also seek to highlight the growing complexity of the psychiatric landscape and to flag what I take to be some major transformations that mark the period between the outbreak of total war and the end of the twentieth century.

In the last quarter of that century, as we will see, mainstream psychiatry embraced a turn back to biology, and much of academic psychiatry embarked on a romance with neuroscience as a unique source of insight into madness. For many, the very idea of *mental* illnesses came to seem like a category mistake. Schizophrenia, bipolar disorder, and a host of other forms of mental disturbance were surely brain diseases. Their visible manifestations in cognitive, behavioral, and emotional disturbances were epiphenomena, and the real essence of mental illness was to be explained by biology. Psychiatrists, therefore, believed the mentally ill were to be treated with an array of treatments aimed at the body, principally those delivered by the modern pharmaceutical industry. The profession was convinced that the way forward lay in innovations and discoveries made in the laboratory, not those vouchsafed on the couch.

Part 4 contains a series of my essays that confront and critique these developments, and it concludes with my assessment of where psychiatry stands at the end of the second decade of the new millennium. Our ancestors wrestled in various ways with the suffering and turmoil that mental illness brings in its wake. Where has our embrace of contemporary psychiatry as the solution to these troubles left us?

.   .   .   .   .

The title of my most recent book, *Madness in Civilization*, deliberately evoked the English title of perhaps the most famous (or in some quarters infamous) book on the history of psychiatry to appear since 1960. That was no accident. Michel Foucault's work on madness was one of the first serious works on the subject that I encountered in the late 1960s, originally in the abbreviated English translation that appeared under the title *Madness and Civilization* and then in the much longer French original. It was not, I think, at least in Anglophone countries, a famous book when I first read it—as a shoddily produced little paperback on cheap paper published by Mentor Books—but within a decade, the cult of Foucault was in full swing, and his influence across a huge range of scholarly disciplines was undeniable. It is fair to say that Foucault's book helped to persuade me (as it did others) that here was a subject worthy of serious historical attention. However, my reading of the French original had already caused me to be very skeptical of the evidentiary foundation of many of Foucault's claims, and as my own researches in the field proceeded, those doubts only grew. Chapter 2 of this book reflects on Foucault's magnum opus.

From the outset, I welcomed the provocation *Madness and Civilization* provided, and I shared (and still share) some of Foucault's skepticism about the vision of psychiatry as an unambiguously liberating enterprise. But I share only *some* of his stance. Foucault was fundamentally a foe of the Enlightenment and its values. I am fundamentally one of its disciples and defenders. As I have already indicated, I have written extensively about the complexities of psychiatry's past and the uncertainties of its present. If not quite an emperor with no clothes, it is certainly one in a state of advanced *déshabillé*. There is much in its past and present deserving of critical attention. But that is very different from dismissing the whole enterprise *tout court*. Likewise, Foucault seems to me to ignore or misrepresent the disruptions and the suffering madness brings in its train, and more seriously still, to misconstrue many of the complexities that mark the tortured relationship between madness and civilization.

Some may object to that last criticism (or indeed all of the criticisms I have advanced of Foucault's work in this field) because he did not set out to write a history of madness and civilization. Foucault's own encapsulation of what he was about is *Folie et deraison: Histoire de la folie à l'âge classique* (Madness and unreason: The history of madness in the age of reason). That his work was presented to English-speaking audiences as *Madness and Civilization* was not Foucault's idea or even that of his original translator, Richard Howard. Rather, it was a brilliant marketing concept dreamed up by someone at his English-language publisher in charge of publicizing the book. As a marketing ploy, it was an extraordinary success. And as long as Anglophone readers had access only to a highly abridged version of Foucault's text, the grounding of the grand generalizations that marked the book had to be taken on trust.

Eventually, though, and despite copyright disputes that seemed to drag on endlessly, a complete English translation of the original did finally appear. Some greeted it with hosannas: a masterpiece had finally been revealed in its full glory to a linguistically handicapped Anglo-American audience. As chapter 2 of this book will quickly reveal to the reader, I had a decidedly less sanguine reaction.

Psychiatry was born of the asylum, of the decision, embraced across Western Europe and North America in the first half of the nineteenth century, to lock up the seriously mad in what purported to be a therapeutic isolation. Utopian expectations (which, like all Utopian ideologies, were doomed to end in disappointment), accompanied the mass confinement of the insane, and it was within this vast network of reformed madhouses that a collective consciousness formed among those charged with administering them—a collective consciousness that pronounced madness a uniquely medical problem and rapidly created professional organizations, journals, and monographs that gave seeming substance to alienists' self-proclaimed expertise in its identification, management, and cure. These nineteenth-century museums of madness were built on earlier foundations, though these antecedents were small and scattered madhouses, scarcely the Great Confinement conjured up by Michel Foucault.

Within less than a century, some alienists and medical psychologists (or, as they increasingly called themselves, psychiatrists) were seeking to escape the confines of asylum life and to embrace new sites within which to practice their art. Relabeling asylums "mental hospitals" fooled no one, least of all psychiatrists, and though the bulk of the profession remained trapped inside the walls of these places as surely as their patients, the more ambitious and entrepreneurial had already begun to embrace the alternatives of the clinic and the consulting room. Yet it was only after World War II that the profession's center of gravity shifted decisively away from the asylum (a phenomenon I examine in more depth in chapters 10, 11, and 12), and only from the 1960s onward that the Victorian bins began to vanish from the scene (something I analyze further in chapter 3).

The legitimacy of the psychiatric enterprise has been almost perpetually under siege, as Charles Rosenberg once sagely remarked.[12] Mainstream medicine may have its critics, and even in the twenty-first century, some stubborn souls still resist its blandishments, sometimes opting for the snake oil salesmen who peddle alternative medicines. But the troubles of physicians on this front, justified as some of them may be, are as nothing when set alongside those of their psychiatric brethren, if brethren they be. The fierce criticisms of psychiatry sometimes (and perhaps most painfully) emerge from within its own ranks, but more often from some of those whose welfare it claims to be advancing. Psychiatry's claims to expertise and its protestations that its interventions are benevolent and beneficent are mocked and excoriated by the very people it proclaims itself in business to help. The profession exists, and has almost continually existed, as chapter 4 makes plain, within a culture of complaint.

At times, dissatisfaction with the medical remedies on offer has prompted some to seek alternative pathways to resolve their mental troubles. In the United States, where religiosity, if not religion, has retained a hold over the popular mind that is unparalleled elsewhere in an increasingly secularized

West, these alternatives have sometimes involved an embrace of religiously based accounts of the origins of mental turmoil and even theologically based attempts at therapy. Given Americans' willingness to accept variants of the forms of Christian belief that originated in the Old World, some of these alternative therapies have tied themselves closely to novel kinds of Christianity, like Seventh Day Adventism and Christian Science. More recently, those have been joined by what I regard as an even more bizarre cult, Scientology, which has made psychiatry its sworn enemy, set up a museum in Tinseltown devoted to exposing the field's horrors and depredations, and denounced the whole psychiatric enterprise as an "Industry of Death." With its vast financial resources and ruthlessness, and its Hollywood connections, Scientology's critique of psychiatry has drawn as much attention and publicity as the teachings of Mary Baker Eddy, the founder of Christian Science, once did. Chapter 5 examines this uniquely American phenomenon.

Part 2 brings together four essays that bear on the question of where a psychiatry hitherto largely confined to institutional settings and isolated from the rest of medicine might move its base of operations (and in the process create a new geography of madness). The flirtation many Americans engaged in with a religiously based psychotherapy, whether embodied in the doctrines of Christian Science or in the more "respectable," upmarket guise of the Emmanuel Movement, led by the Reverend Elwood Worcester in Boston, prompted some disenchanted psychiatrists and neurologists to claim psychotherapy for medicine. There were indigenous moves along these lines, as Eric Caplan has documented.[13] But, beginning in the early twentieth century, there were also flirtations with various forms of psychotherapy being developed in Europe.

The French psychologist Pierre Janet, who had trained under Jean-Martin Charcot in Paris, visited the United States in 1904 and in 1906, and on the latter occasion he delivered a course of lectures on dissociation, fixed ideas, and the subconscious at Harvard. Janet had attracted the New England neurologist Morton Prince, among others, to his theories. Paul Dubois, the Swiss psychologist, had his book *The Psychic Treatment of Nervous Disorder* translated by William Alanson White and Smith Ely Jelliffe in 1904,[14] and his "persuasive therapy" enjoyed a brief vogue in some circles. But in the long run, it was another European physician, who visited the United States only once, in 1909, who had the greatest impact on American psychiatry. Indeed, for a quarter-century after World War II, his doctrines dominated the commanding heights, such as they were, of American psychiatry and had an enormous impact on American culture, both popular and highbrow. That man, of course, was Freud, and the spread and influence of psychoanalysis is something I will have occasion to recur to several times in the chapters that follow. The irony that psychoanalysis enjoyed its greatest influence in the New World, not the Old, is magnified by Freud's visceral hatred of America and Americans.

Freud has been a long time a-dying. *Time* magazine may have announced his demise in 1993, but like a figure from the world of the undead, he displays an uncanny ability to resurrect himself. Or rather, neither his lingering band of disciples nor his severest critics have been able to leave him alone, instead repeatedly disinterring his life and his work and parsing every exquisite detail. The Freud Wars, as they have come to be called, have now lasted as long as the Thirty Years' War, which devastated seventeenth-century Europe, and alas no resolution is in sight. One of the doughtiest warriors on the death-to-Freud side is the former Freudian Frederick Crews, and his latest salvo prompted me to write my own assessment of the state of hostilities and of whether anything Freudian survives or deserves to do so. It is the first essay in part 2.

Phyllis Greenacre, one of the three central figures in chapter 7, became arguably the most prominent American-born psychoanalyst in the 1940s and 1950s. She was a powerful figure at the New York Psychoanalytic Institute, who, as the psychoanalyst's analyst, knew more than most about the profession's dirty laundry but was a model of discretion. Before her move from Baltimore to New York, however, Greenacre had served as Adolf Meyer's assistant at Johns Hopkins University in its newly established department of psychiatry.

It was Meyer and Meyerian psychiatry, not Freud and psychoanalysis, that dominated American psychiatry in the first four decades of the twentieth century, in substantial measure because, as the first professor of psychiatry at Johns Hopkins, then America's preeminent medical school, he occupied the most powerful institutional position in the country and trained many of those who moved into academic chairs once other medical schools began to find room for the subspecialty that they had hitherto scorned. Meyer was an eclectic who hid the barrenness of his doctrines behind a fog of verbal obscurantism that he summed up as "psychobiology." The man who became Greenacre's husband, Curt Richter, was, it could be argued, the person who gave the most seeming substance to this nebulous concept, not least by discovering the circadian rhythm, something that quite possibly should have won him a Nobel Prize.[15]

The intersecting and overlapping careers of Greenacre, Meyer, and Richter allow us to witness the appeal and the limits of Meyer's approach to the management of mental illness and the interplay between biological, social, and psychological approaches to mental illness. Simultaneously, the involvement of Meyer and Greenacre in one of the earliest examples of the radical experimentation that was visited on the bodies of mental patients in the first half of the twentieth century helps us to grasp the extraordinary vulnerability of the institutionalized insane. In the face of unambiguous evidence that focal sepsis and "surgical bacteriology"—the removal of teeth, tonsils, spleens, stomachs, uteruses, and colons—were not only therapeutically useless but also killing and maiming patients, Meyer's actions and inaction provide a vivid example and reminder of the recurrent failures of professions to police themselves. Simultaneously, the episode throws into stark relief the choices that confront a potential whistle-blower and how these were exacerbated in this case by Greenacre's gendered vulnerability. Meyer's suppression of her work foreshadowed the failures of the profession to rein in the extraordinary wave of damaging somatic treatments that characterized the 1930s and 1940s.

The most reviled of these in the contemporary world is the lobotomy, which is now almost universally excoriated and viewed as the most signal example of psychiatry run amok. Yet Egas Moniz's decision to excise portions of the frontal lobes of a handful of Portuguese mental patients and the subsequent "refinement" and popularization of psychosurgery by the Washington, DC, neurologist Walter Freeman and his neurosurgical partner James Watts, was hailed in many quarters as an extraordinary breakthrough—"surgery for sick souls," as the *New York Times* science reporter William Laurence informed his readers.[16] Nearly a decade and a half after the first operation, the innovation won Moniz the 1949 Nobel Prize in Medicine.

In 1946, at the height of the procedure's popularity, a version of it was performed on a once-anonymous patient who we now know was an unfortunate man named Henry Molaison. H. M., as he was referred to in the scientific literature for decades, was the pet subject of a whole host of psychologists. The operation destroyed his ability to remember, and he became a prize specimen for those who would build a science of memory. Chapter 8 explores this remarkable story and again raises disturbing questions about professional ethics.

Psychiatry had long occupied the status of the stepchild of medicine. Even as the fortunes of general medicine soared with the advent of the bacteriological revolution and the reforms of medical education that constrained the oversupply of doctors that had characterized the nineteenth century, psychiatry's marginalization seemed to worsen. Adolf Meyer's appointment to a chair at Johns Hopkins gave some small semblance of academic respectability to an isolated, ill-paid, and despised group that seemed increasingly distant from the rest of the medical profession. But so long as most psychiatrists were recruited to the profession by apprenticing in one of the vast bins, where hopelessness and routine were the order of the day, their physical and intellectual isolation was self-perpetuating, and the profession's prospects correspondingly dim.

The Rockefeller Foundation had played a major role in the transformation of American medical schools and medical education during the first three decades of the twentieth century. Its influence was felt everywhere. Its largesse and its prompting underwrote the growing links between the basic sciences and clinical medicine, and between the laboratory and the bedside. It also helped to eliminate the proprietary and second-tier medical schools and thus, intentionally or not, diminished the problem of the oversupply of MDs.

The foundation's decision, at the very outset of the Great Depression, to switch its focus elsewhere and to place the primary emphasis of its medical division on the support and development of psychiatry was thus a momentous one. Chapter 9 explores the factors that led to this paradoxical decision and the way its foundation officers then proceeded. Whole academic departments were created ex nihilo, and the token psychiatric course or two on other faculties were reworked to create some semblance of a place for psychiatry in the university. And alongside this institution building came some eclectic investments in psychiatric research. One consequence of all this money and activity was the creation of a new psychiatry, one that was for the first time distant from the asylum and even, for the most part, from routine clinical encounters with patients, save as research subjects. Although the postwar period saw the foundation souring on the initiative and beginning to doubt its payoffs, the academic psychiatry it had brought into being now had a new and even more powerful paymaster, the federal government in Washington. Divided between the Old Guard, who ministered to the more than half million inmates in traditional asylums; the academic psychiatrists, who were trying to cement their place in the emerging knowledge factories that universities were fast becoming; and a growing cadre of psychiatrists who had found a way to make a living from office-based practices, American psychiatry was in the process of becoming a very different sort of animal.

.   .   .   .   .

Part 3 of this book consists of a series of interrogations of the transformations that overtook the profession of psychiatry in the second half of the twentieth century. The essays attempt to assess what prompted these changes and what they tell us about the current state of the profession. Psychiatrists have their own versions of these developments, and I begin by critiquing two recent examples of the genre.

Over the years, psychiatrists seem to have been more disposed than most of their fellow medics to dabble in history. Often, but not always, they emulate politicians who try to use their memoirs to establish their favorite version of events before historians cast a critical eye over the scene. That is far from universally the case, and indeed one of the more welcome developments in the history of psychiatry over the past quarter-century or so has been the emergence of clinician-historians who take the history side of the equation seriously and who bring a uniquely valuable perspective to the topics they choose to address. Regrettably, the synoptic in-house versions of portions of the history of psychiatry that I examine in chapters 10 and 11 are not written by authors who belong in their company.

The most wide-ranging of the two accounts I look at in those two chapters was a book written by the chair of the Columbia University Department of Psychiatry, Jeffrey Lieberman, shortly after he stepped down as president of the American Psychiatric Association. Lieberman claims that the history of his specialty has hitherto been ignored, and he announces that his goal is to set the record straight. It is an entirely false claim, matched only by the falsity of the history of heroes and villains he then proceeds to invent for his readers. For him, history is a morality tale, a movement from darkness to enlightenment: a history whose most distinguishing features are how lately psychiatry was riddled with superstition and error and how fortunate mental patients are to now live in a world where we finally understand mental illness is brain disease and minister to it with a range of extraordinarily effective therapies. The only thing standing in the way of psychiatric nirvana, it would appear, is the public's ignorance of just how much progress has been made—and hence its reluctance to volunteer for treatment.

Lieberman peddles one sort of fairy tale. His British colleague Michael Trimble offers another. During the last third of the nineteenth century, a new medical specialty appeared and laid claim to jurisdiction over nervous and mental disorders. Neurology (which in the American case was born out of the slaughter and carnage of the Civil War) defined itself as the curator of diseases of the brain and the nervous system. Its primary initial targets were those with organic lesions of the brain, the spinal cord, and the peripheral nervous system, and the American branch initially treated those with traumatic war-related injuries. But neurologists everywhere soon found their waiting rooms flooded with another kind of patient, those with "functional" nervous illness—disorders whose etiological roots were mysterious and obscure.

Some of these "nervous" patients were suffering from a controversial condition with an ancient pedigree that some were disposed to dismiss as a form of malingering: hysteria. Others, the neurologists decided, were victims of an alternative pathology they dubbed "neurasthenia," or weakness of the nerves. Either way, neurologists found themselves ministering to cases of mental disease. In their eyes, this was not inappropriate, since their shared assumption was that insanity was a brain disease, and who better to treat and understand these patients than the people who made the scientific study of the brain their calling?

The stage was set for a savage jurisdictional fight with the alienists, who ran the asylums and had long claimed mental illness as their exclusive fiefdom. For a quarter-century, the argument raged, until a truce was called. Each specialty retreated to its own heartland, but there were always a few souls who lingered in the borderlands and a portion of the neurological fraternity who began to entertain the heretical idea that functional mental illnesses might have psychological roots. Freud, who had trained as a conventional neurologist first in Vienna and then in Paris under Jean-Martin Charcot, was one of their number, though many associate him only with the talking cure.

Mainstream neurologists have fared only a little better than their psychiatric counterparts when it comes to curing the awful maladies with which they are often confronted. Where they have become more accomplished is in tracing the pathological roots of many of the disorders they have identified, separating them into different syndromes, and providing a prognosis for those unfortunate enough to be stricken with them. If psychiatry was seen for much of history as suffering from a deadly mixture of etiological ignorance and therapeutic impotence, the perception of neurology was that it was only afflicted with the latter. The ability to reliably name and predict the course of its disorders, offer some form of palliative care in certain cases, and demonstrate postmortem findings to support its diagnoses somehow made neurology a high-status specialty and not the medical pariah psychiatry has often seemed to be.

As I will discuss in subsequent chapters, one of the more notable features of the dominant strand of psychiatry in the last quarter-century and more has been its determined embrace of what one leading psychiatrist, Steven Sharfstein, has called a bio-bio-bio model of mental illness. The (re)embrace of the brain (and in some quarters, the genome) has prompted an alliance, in academic psychiatry at least, with neuroscience and to some degree with neurology. Hence the attraction in some circles of relabeling the psychiatric enterprise "neuropsychiatry." And hence the temptation to construct a historical genealogy for a subspecialty with that name, however artificial and unconvincing the result.

Professions traffic in ideas as well as in attempting to connect those ideas to the realm of practice. Abstraction, as the Chicago sociologist Andrew Abbott has argued, plays a vital role in the life of a profession and its ability to sustain its social legitimacy.[17] Chapter 12 examines the sets of ideas that have prevailed in psychiatry (and to a lesser extent psychology) since the birth of the profession in the mid-nineteenth century. While no ideology is ever completely dominant, I suggest that it makes sense to regard the ruling ideas in the psy-complex (as some have called it) as marked by three major periods and patterns: the dominance of ideas rooted in and justifying asylumdom, the institutional complex that gave birth to the profession; the partial eclipse of that institutionally based ideology by psychoanalysis in the quarter-century following World War II, a period that also saw the rise of a different set of ideas and practices linked to the laboratory and to the rival academic discipline of psychology; and the marginalization of psychoanalytic perspectives that has taken place since 1980 and the concomitant triumph of the notion that mental illnesses are nothing more and nothing less than diseases of the brain.

Ideas do not develop and perpetuate themselves in a vacuum. World War II, the Cold War, and the associated growth of the federal government brought about striking changes in American society. Science and medicine were transformed by massive infusions of federal funding, and the American system of higher education saw an extraordinary expansion. The changes wrought by the Rockefeller Foundation's two decades of support for academic psychiatry were soon eclipsed by the impact of Washington. The prohibition against the involvement of the federal government in the direct provision of psychiatric services that had existed since President Franklin Pierce vetoed legislation to provide such support in 1854 remained firmly in place, but the influx of ever-larger sums of money to underwrite new programs of research and training, and the growing affluence of the postwar era, expanded the number of psychiatrists to an unprecedented extent.

·   ·   ·   ·   ·

Part 4 looks at a world where mainstream psychiatry has eviscerated madness of meaning. Murdered memories, according to Freud, refuse to remain buried, and the troubles they foment in the unconscious create all manner of mischief. The traumas of war—specifically the shell shock of the Great War and the combat neurosis that afflicted the greatest generation—did not conform precisely to the sexual etiology Freud had constructed to explain neurosis, but these epidemics of mental breakdown struck many as rooted in another kind of trauma and were considered to be prima facie evidence of the psychogenesis of at least some forms of mental disorder. Mental illness, on this account, was deeply connected to questions of meaning and repression.

That industrialized warfare and the maintenance of sanity are often at odds with one another is a painful lesson that apparently needs to be relearned periodically. The Vietnam War—when the military forces of the most powerful nation on the planet were defeated by Third World peasants, and when the lies and obfuscations of American politicians exacerbated the fallout from drafting young men to fight a deeply unpopular war—was no exception to the rule. Though initially denied by the military brass, the incidence of long-term psychiatric casualties eventually became a major issue. Angry veterans allied themselves with sympathetic psychiatrists, and the upshot, after much political maneuvering, was the creation of a new diagnostic category that was entered into the American Psychiatric Association's *Diagnostic and Statistical Manual of Mental Disorders (DSM)*: post-traumatic stress disorder, or PTSD. But when Robert Spitzer, the editor of the *DSM*, was persuaded to include this stress-related disorder, he did so by widening the diagnosis to include other forms of traumatic breakdown, not just those incurred in the course of military hostilities. The seemingly endless series of wars the United States has waged has nonetheless ensured an ongoing parade of psychiatric casualties among the troops, a phenomenon I consider in chapter 13.

Psychiatry's embrace of neuroscience and the associated claim that mental illness could be reduced to disorders of the brain has had major consequences both within and outside the profession. Internally, it has decisively changed the focus of much psychiatric research. But in bowdlerized form, it has also had a profound impact on many people's view of mental disorders. Helped along by marketing copy produced by Big Pharma to increase the sales of its magic potions, the public has been encouraged to view depression, bipolar disorder, and schizophrenia as problems of biochemical imbalances and malfunctioning brains. Perhaps the Holy Grail of uniting diagnosis and underlying pathology can finally be realized with the help of another remarkable tool of modern medicine, developed during the same decades? Can modern imaging technology, with its CAT and PET scans and MRIs, at last give us the means to view the inner workings of the brain and allow us to visualize the physical pathologies psychiatrists assure us lie behind the social and psychological manifestations of mental illness?

The Cambridge University professor of developmental psychopathology Simon Baron-Cohen heads the school's Autism Research Centre and has been at the forefront of making such claims. His series of books aimed at a general audience has spread these claims widely and attracted a considerable following among politicians and the chattering classes.[18] He has been particularly aggressive in promoting the idea that functional MRIs can provide a reliable window into our consciousness. He claims to be able to use fMRIs to distinguish male from female brains and to identify the physiological differences that explain autism and lack of empathy.[19] Such assertions have prompted lay disciples to write popular science treatises that embrace these ideas and attempt to disseminate them to a still broader audience, pronouncing them to be the latest findings of esoteric brain science. All this is, I suggest, nothing more than pseudoscience, a modern version of phrenology, but the sense that it is rooted in the unquestionable authority of the laboratory, and the seductive qualities of the carefully constructed color images of the brain that are mobilized in its support, have given it an undeserved authority. Chapter 14 gives some of the reasons why we should resist its charms.

Empathy and autism are not the only fronts on which the neuroscientists have been advancing their claims. As early as the nineteenth century, some psychiatrists had demonstrated a fascination with the intersection of crime and mental illness. Symbolically, the question of how to distinguish between madness and badness rapidly acquired enormous significance for the fledging profession as it sought—often unsuccessfully—to be recognized as the arbiter of the dividing line between the two.[20] In the mid-twentieth century, some psychoanalysts sought to erase the distinction entirely, asserting that criminality was simply an expression of underlying mental illness and that it thus required treatment, not punishment.[21] Not many bought these Freudian arguments. Indeed, many dismissed them as a classic instance of psychiatric overreach. But armed with their images of the brain, neuroscientists have now entered the fray. They argue, like their psychoanalytic predecessors, that their science can supersede the messy "commonsense" on which the legal system rests and finally deliver an unchallengeable basis for distinguishing the sheep from the goats, determining with scientific certainty guilt and innocence, and much else besides. A legal system based on weighing testimony and relying on the intuitions of lay jurors can at last give way to the certainties of the laboratory. Or perhaps not, as chapter 15 argues.

The human brain is a simply remarkable object. That its structure and functioning might have some relevance to our behavior, our social selves, and the ways in which we construct and respond to the cultures that surround us is surely a truism. But to move beyond crude generalizations and recognize when we are being sold a bill of goods under the guise of science are difficult tasks. Humans, like other mammals, possess double brains—brains that are composed of two hemispheres. Many other organs are also duplicated, of course: eyes, lungs, kidneys, testicles, and ovaries immediately come to mind. But the duality of the brain seems a particularly fascinating aspect of our physical nature, and where once it was thought that the two halves of the divided brain were identical and simply replicated each other, we have for a long time known that this is not so. It is not just the obvious fact of contralaterality, made manifest when a left hemispheric stroke paralyzes activity on the right-hand side of the body, and vice versa; there seem to be broad functional differences between the two hemispheres, and the question is what to make of these differences and their implications. Chapter 16 examines the ambitious attempts of one highly unusual psychiatrist and neuroscientist, who began his professional life as an English don at Oxford, to connect the wiring of the two halves of the brain to central characteristics of the historical evolution of Western culture. The ambition is far-reaching, the erudition remarkable, and the conclusions largely speculative—and the claimed alternation in the dominance of one hemisphere or the other in different historical eras is asserted but not explained.

Contemporary psychiatry often seems bent on robbing mental illness of its meanings. If Freud and his followers once sought to explain mental illness on the level of meaning, to probe its roots by searching for hidden meanings, and to substitute consciousness for the tangles that lay hidden in the depths of the unconscious, modern biological psychiatry has no time for such fairy tales. Madness, orthodox psychiatry asserts, has no meaning.

It represents the epiphenomenal manifestations of an underlying, purely physical pathology and is worthy of no more attention than is merited by its status as the trigger that brings mental pathology to our attention.

This crude biological reductionism is a viewpoint that came to dominate American psychiatry in the 1980s, and it persists as the orthodox psychiatric viewpoint to this day. That epistemology, and the practices that flow from it, can be traced quite precisely to the publication of the third edition of the *DSM* in 1980.

It is true that this document was not American psychiatry's last word on the subject. There have been four revisions since, the most recent materializing—after years of delay and controversy—in May 2013. But all of these versions have hewed to the same basic approach to mental illness: establishing a classificatory system that relies on a mechanized method of diagnosis. It is a line of attack that quite deliberately ignores problems of validity (that is, whether the various labels correspond in any defensible way to differences in underlying pathology). As was true of all of medicine in the eighteenth century (but is no longer the case in other medical specialties), psychiatry continues to rely solely on symptoms and behaviors to render its judgments. Supposedly, the conditions it diagnoses will ultimately be grounded in biology, for the assertion that mental illnesses are brain diseases has become dogma. But that remains a speculation largely ungrounded in evidence, save in the cases of organic conditions like Alzheimer's and Huntington's disease.

Any portrait of twenty-first-century American psychiatry must, of necessity, come to grips with the *DSM* phenomenon. My concluding chapter attempts precisely that task and asks what we are to make of a profession whose identity and legitimacy are closely tied to what increasingly is seen, sometimes even at the very highest levels of the profession, as an approach on the brink of collapse.

PART I

The Asylum and Its
Discontents

2 The Fictions of Foucault's Scholarship

MADNESS AND CIVILIZATION REVISITED

History of Madness is the book that launched Michel Foucault's career as one of the most prominent intellectuals of the second half of the twentieth century. It was not his first book. That was a much briefer volume on *Maladie mentale et personalité* that had appeared seven years earlier, in 1954, in the aftermath of a bout of depression and a suicide attempt. (A translation of the second edition of that treatise would appear in English in 1976, over Foucault's vociferous objections.) But *History of Madness* was the first of his works to attract major attention, to begin with in France, and a few years afterward in the English-speaking world. Still later, of course, would come the swarm of books devoted to the "archeology" of the human sciences, the place of punishment in the modern world, the new medical "gaze" of Paris hospital medicine, the history of sex—the whole vast oeuvre that constituted his deconstruction of the Enlightenment and its values, and that served to launch the Foucault industry, influencing and sometimes capturing whole realms of philosophical, literary, historical, and sociological inquiry.

But in the beginning was *Madness*. It was a book introduced to the anglophone world by a figure who then had an iconic status of his own, the renegade Scottish psychiatrist R. D. Laing. For it was Laing, fascinated by existentialism and other things French, who recommended the project to the Tavistock Press. He pronounced it "an exceptional book, . . . brilliantly written, intellectually rigorous, and with a thesis that thoroughly shakes the assumptions of traditional psychiatry." In those days, his imprimatur counted for much.

In its English guise, at least, Foucault's history of madness had one great merit for a book introducing a difficult and then unknown author—someone working in an intellectual "tradition" that was not just foreign to the intellectual idioms of most English-speaking people but also remote from their interest or sympathy. That merit was brevity, a delightful quality little valued by most academics. Short yet sweeping, spanning the whole of the Western encounter with unreason from the High Middle Ages to the advent of psychoanalysis, the book in its first English incarnation also possessed a wonderful title. *Madness and Civilization* advertised its wares far more effectively than its plodding French counterpart: *Folie et déraison: Histoire de la folie à l'âge classique.* Where the new label came from—from Foucault himself, from Laing, from the publisher, from the first translator, Richard Howard?—I was for many years unable to discover. Even some of Foucault's most faithful followers were unable to enlighten me. But without question, it was a remarkable piece of packaging, arresting and provocative, and calculated to pique the interest of almost anyone who came across it. I finally thought to contact Richard Howard, and he solved the mystery: a marketing person at the publishing house (which had refused Howard's request to be allowed to translate the full text of the original, thinking it unsalable) was the one who came up with the marvelous idea for the new title.

Madness and Civilization was not just short. It was not weighed down by any of the apparatus of modern scholarship. For what appeared in 1965 was a truncated text, stripped not only of several chapters but also of the thousand and more footnotes that decorated the first French edition. Foucault himself had abbreviated the lengthy volume that constituted his doctoral thesis to produce a small French pocket edition, and it was this version (which contented itself with a small handful of references) that appeared in translation. (To be more precise, it was this pocket edition, plus about fifteen pages of the original text, added back by Foucault, that was now presented to an English-speaking audience.) The translation could be read in a few hours, and if its extraordinarily large claims rested on a shaky empirical foundation, this was perhaps not immediately evident. The pleasures of a radical reinterpretation of the place of psychiatry in the modern world (and, by implication, of the whole Enlightenment project to glorify Reason) could be absorbed in very little time. Any doubts that might surface about the book's claims could always be dismissed by gestures toward the far weightier and more solemn French edition—a massive tome that monoglot English readers were highly unlikely, indeed unable, to consult for themselves, even supposing that they could have laid their hands on a copy.

None of this seems to have rendered the book's claims implausible, at least to a complaisant audience. Here, indeed, is a world turned upside down. Foucault rejects psychiatry's vaunted connections with progress. He rejects the received wisdom about madness and the modern world. Generation after generation had sung paeans to the twin movement that took mad people from our midst and consigned them to the new world of the asylum, and captured madness itself for the science of medical men. Science and humanity were jointly in evidence here. Foucault advanced the reverse interpretation. The "liberation" of the insane from the shackles of superstition and neglect was, he proclaimed, something quite other—"a gigantic moral imprisonment."

The phrase still echoes. Since the highly skeptical, not to say hostile, stance it encapsulates came to dominate four decades of revisionist historiography of psychiatry, there is a natural temptation to attribute the changed intellectual climate, whatever one thinks of it, to the influence of the charismatic Frenchman. But is it so? There were, after all, myriad indigenous sources of skepticism in the sixties, all quite separately weakening the vision of psychiatry as an unambiguously liberating scientific enterprise.

It is not as though such a perspective had ever gone unchallenged, after all. Psychiatrists' pretensions have seldom been given a free pass. Their medical "brethren" have always been tempted to view them as witch doctors and pseudoscientists, seldom demonstrating much respect for their abilities or much willingness to admit them to full-fledged membership in the field of medicine. And the public at large has likewise displayed few illusions about their performance and competence, dismissing them as mad-doctors, shrinks, bughouse doctors, and worse. The crisis of psychiatric legitimacy, as Charles Rosenberg once shrewdly remarked, has been endemic throughout the profession's history.

But the years when Foucault came to prominence were a particularly troubling time for defenders of the psychiatric enterprise. There was the work of Erving Goffman, the brilliant if idiosyncratic American sociologist whose loosely linked essay collection *Asylums* lent academic luster to the previously polemical equation of the mental hospital and the concentration camp. Goffman dismissed psychiatry as a "tinkering trade" whose object was the collection of unfortunates who were the victims of nothing more than "contingencies." Then there was the renegade New York psychiatrist Thomas Szasz, who declared that the very existence of mental illness was a myth and savaged his fellow professionals as oppressors of those they purported to help, calling them self-serving creatures who were nothing more than prison guards in disguise. And there was R. D. Laing himself, now dismissed in most quarters as a yesterday's man but at that time welcomed, in the feverish atmosphere of the sixties, as the guru who had shown the adolescent mental patient as the fall girl, the designated victim of the double bind of family life, and who had, yet more daringly, launched the notion of schizophrenia as a form of super sanity. More prosaically, a new generation of historians, abandoning their discipline's traditional focus on diplomacy and high politics, were in these years embracing social history and "history from below," and doing so in an intellectual climate of hostility to anything that smacked of Whig history and its emphasis on progress. The birth of the revisionist historiography of psychiatry was thus attended by many midwives and had a more complex genealogy than the oracular utterances of a French intellectual.

Still, Foucault's growing stature in both serious intellectual circles and among the luminaries of café society was not without significance. He undoubtedly helped to establish the centrality of his subject and to rescue the history of psychiatry from the clutches of a combination of drearily dull administrative historians and psychiatrists in their dotage. For that, at least, he deserves our gratitude.

It is curious, particularly in light of Foucault's prominence in the Anglo-American as well as the Francophone world, that it took almost a half-century for the full text of the French original to appear in translation. Certainly, the delay does not reflect any increase in the ranks of French-speaking scholars in Britain and the United States. To the contrary, linguistic incompetence and insularity even among humanists seem to have grown, not shrunk, in these years. So, one must welcome the decision of Routledge (the heirs of Tavistock) to issue a complete translation. The publishers even included the prefaces to both the first and second full French editions (Foucault had suppressed the former on the book's republication in 1972). And they added the text of Foucault's side of an exchange with Jacques Derrida over the book's thesis, originally a lecture Foucault had given at the Collège Philosophique in March 1963. But the warmth of the welcome one accords to the belated appearance of the unabridged *History of Madness* depends on a variety of factors: the nature of the new material now made available to anglophones; the quality of the new translation; the facts that the complete text reveals about the foundations of Foucault's scholarship on the subject of madness; and—an issue I will flag but not expand on here—one's stance vis-à-vis his whole anti-Enlightenment project.

As to the first of these, the full version of *Madness* is more than twice as long as the text that originally appeared in English and contains almost ten times as many footnotes, not to mention an extended list of Foucault's sources. To the footnotes and sources I will return. Substantively, the major additions are whole chapters that were omitted from the first English edition: a chapter examining "the correctional world . . . on the threshold of modern times" and its associated "economy of evil"—a survey that claims to uncover the abrupt creation of "grids of exclusion" all over Europe and of "a common denominator of unreason among experiences that had long remained separate from each other"; a chapter discussing "how polymorphous and varied the experience of madness was in the classical age"; a series of chapters that make up much of the early sections of part 2 of Foucault's original discussion, including a lengthy introduction; a chapter and a half of his examination of how eighteenth-century physicians and savants interrogated and came to understand the phenomenon of madness; and the greater part of a long chapter on "the proper uses of liberty," which examines the bringing together of what Foucault insists were the previously separate worlds of medical thought and of confinement. In place of the few pages on Goya, Sade, and Nietzsche that were labeled "Conclusion" in the Richard Howard translation, there is a much longer set of musings on the nineteenth century that begins with an adjuration that "there is no question here of concluding," not least because "the work of [Philippe] Pinel and [William] Tuke"—with which the substantive portion of Foucault's analysis ends—"is not a destination."

To these formerly untranslated chapters, one must add the restoration in other portions of the text of a number of individual paragraphs and sometimes whole sections of Foucault's argument that were simply eliminated from the abridged version of his book: elaborations, for example, of portions of his famous opening chapter on "the ship of fools"; a long concluding section previously omitted from his chapter on the insane; and passages originally left out of his discussion of doctors and patients.

Even confining ourselves to this brief and cursory summary of what was translated for the first time, the potential interest and importance of *Madness* is clear. How many people will actually plough through the extended text is not so clear. The new translation is not much help in that regard. The words "dreary," "dull," and "dispirited" come to mind, and stay there. Nor is the translation always reliable, leaning often in the direction of inaccurate paraphrase. Howard's version, however incomplete the text from which he worked, sparkles by comparison. Compare, for example, the respective renditions of the book's famous opening lines.

Foucault's text:

A la fin du Moyen Age, la lèpre disparaît du monde occidental. Dans les marges de la communauté, aux portes des villes, s'ouvrent comme de grandes plages que le mal cessé de hanter, mais qu'il a laissées stériles et pour longtemps inhabitables. Des siècles durant, ces étendues appartiendront à l'inhumain. Du XIVe aux XVIIe siècle, elles vont attendre et solliciter par d'étranges incantations une nouvelle incarnation du mal, une autre grimace de la peur, des magies renouvelées de purification et d'exclusion.

Murphy and Khalfa give us:

At the end of the Middle Ages, leprosy disappeared from the Western world. At the edges of the community, at town gates, large, barren, uninhabitable areas appeared, where disease no longer reigned but its ghost still hovered. For centuries, these spaces would belong to the domain of the inhuman. From the fourteenth to the seventeenth century, by means of strange incantations, they conjured up a new incarnation of evil, another grinning mask of fear, home to the constantly renewed magic of purification and exclusion.

Howard's version:

> At the end of the Middle Ages, leprosy disappeared from the Western world. In the margins of the community, at the gates of cities, there stretched wastelands which sickness had ceased to haunt but had left sterile and long uninhabitable. For centuries, these reaches would belong to the non-human. From the fourteenth to the seventeenth century, they would wait, soliciting with strange incantations a new incarnation of disease, another grimace of terror, renewed rites of purification and exclusion.

But what even a weak translation does not hide or disguise is the kind of evidence on which Foucault erected his theory. Those more than a thousand previously untranslated footnotes now stand revealed, and the evidence appears for what it is. It is not, for the most part, a pretty sight.

Foucault's research for *Madness* was largely completed while he was in intellectual exile in Uppsala, Sweden. Perhaps that explains the superficiality and dated quality of much of his information. To be sure, he had access to a wide range of English, French, and German medical texts from the seventeenth and eighteenth centuries as well as the writings of major philosophers like Descartes and Spinoza. A number of the chapters that appeared for the first time in English with the new translation make use of these primary sources to analyze older ideas about madness. One may object to or accept Foucault's reconstructions, but these portions of his argument at least rest on readings of relevant source material.

By contrast, much of his account of the internal workings and logic of the institutions of confinement, an account on which he lavishes attention, is drawn from their printed rules and regulations. But which of us would be so naïve as to assume that such documents bear any close relationship to the mundane realities of life in these places or provide a reliable guide to their quotidian logic? To be sure, there are references to a handful of archival sources, all of them French, which might have provided some check on these published documents, but Foucault never systematically or even sensibly employed such materials so as to examine possible differences between the ideal and the real. Nor does he give us any sense of why these particular archives were chosen for examination, what criteria were employed to mine them for facts, or how representative the examples he provides might be—these are matters passed over in discreet silence.

Of course, by the very ambitions they have set for themselves, comparative historians are often forced to rely to a substantial extent on the work of others, so perhaps this use of highly selective French materials to represent the entire Western world should not be judged too harshly. Perhaps, except the secondary sources on which Foucault repeatedly relies for the most well-known portions of his text are so self-evidently dated and inadequate to the task, and his own reading of them is so often singularly careless and inventive.

Foucault alleges, for example, that the 1815–16 House of Commons inquiry into the state of England's madhouses revealed that Bethlem (often known by its popular nickname, Bedlam) placed its inmates on public display every Sunday and charged a penny a visit to each of the some 96,000 annual sightseers for the privilege of viewing them. In reality, the reports of the inquiry contain no such claims. This is not surprising: public visitation (which had not been confined to Sundays in any event) had been banned by Bethlem's governors in 1770, and even before then the tales of a fixed admission fee turn out to be apocryphal. (The notion of nearly 2,000 visitors crowding the wards on an average Sunday might have been enough to give anyone pause, but why should a little skepticism get in the way of a good story?) Foucault is bedeviled by Bethlem's history. He makes the remarkable claim that "from the day when Bethlem, the hospital for curative lunatics, was opened to hopeless cases in 1733, there was no longer any notable difference between the London hospital and the French *Hôpital Général,* or any other house of correction." And he speaks of Bethlem's "refurbishment" in 1676. In reality, it had moved in that year from its previous location in an old monastery in Bishopsgate to a grandiose new building in Moorfields designed by Robert Hooke.

Monasteries surface elsewhere in his account. We are told with a straight face that "it was in buildings that had previously been both convents and monasteries that the majority of the great asylums of England . . . were set up." A bizarre notion. First, there were no "great asylums" set up in England in the classical age. Vast museums of madness did not emerge until the nineteenth century (when they were purpose-built using taxpayers' funds). And second, of all the asylums and madhouses that existed in the seventeenth and eighteenth centuries, only Bethlem was ever housed in a former convent or monastery, and when it was, its peak patient population amounted to fewer than fifty inmates, hardly the vast throng conjured up by Foucault's image of "grands asiles."

It is odd, to put it mildly, to rely exclusively on nineteenth- and early twentieth-century scholarship to examine the place of leprosy in the medieval world. It is peculiar to base one's discussion of English and Irish Poor Law policy from the sixteenth through the eighteenth century on, in essence, only three sources: the dated and long-superseded work of Sir George Nicholls (1781–1865), E. M. Leonard's 1900 textbook, and an eighteenth-century treatise by Sir Frederick Morton Eden. And for someone purporting to write a history of the Western encounter with madness, it is downright astonishing to rely on a tiny handful of long-dead authors as a reliable guide to English developments: Jacques Tenon's eighteenth-century account of his visit to English hospitals, supplemented by Samuel Tuke's *Description of the Retreat* (1813) and Hack Tuke's *Chapters in the History of the Insane* (1882).

Foucault's sources for his accounts of developments in Germany, Austria, and even France are equally antique and unsatisfactory. The whole of part 1 of *Madness* has a total of 28 footnotes (out of 399) that cite twentieth-century scholars, and the relevant list of sources in the bibliography lists only twenty-five pieces of scholarship written from 1900 onward, only *one* of which was published after World War II.

Things do not improve as the book proceeds. Foucault's bibliography for part 2 lists but a single twentieth-century work, Gregory Zilboorg's *The Medical Man and the Witch During the Renaissance* (1935), scarcely a source on that subject calculated to inspire confidence among present-day historians (and one that he himself criticizes). In part 3, he lists a grand total of eleven books and articles written in his own century.

This is not merely a solipsism of footnote style. Throughout *History of Madness*, we encounter this sort of isolation from the world of facts and scholarship. It is as though nearly a century of scholarly work had produced nothing of interest or value for Foucault's project. What interested him, or shielded him, was selectively mined nineteenth-century sources of dubious provenance. Inevitably, this means that his elaborate intellectual constructions are built on the shakiest of empirical foundations, and, not surprisingly, many turn out to be wrong.

Take his central claim that the Age of Reason was the age of a Great Confinement. Foucault tells us that "a social sensibility, common to

European culture, . . . suddenly began to manifest itself in the second half of the seventeenth century; it was this sensibility that suddenly isolated the category destined to populate the places of confinement. . . . The signs of [confinement] are to be found massively across Europe throughout the seventeenth century." "Confinement," moreover, "had the same meaning throughout Europe, in these early years at least." And its English manifestations, the new workhouses, appeared in such "heavily industrialised" places as seventeenth-century Worcester and Norwich (!).

But the notion of a European-wide Great Confinement in these years is purely mythical. Such massive incarceration quite simply never occurred in England in the seventeenth and eighteenth centuries, whether one focuses one's attention on the mad, who were still mostly left at large, or on the broader category of the poor, the idle, and the morally disreputable. And if Gladys Swain and Marcel Gauchet are correct in the analysis they present in *Le sujet de la folie: Naissance de las psychiatrie* (1997), even Foucault's claims about the confinement of the mad in the classical age in France are grossly exaggerated, if not fanciful—for they conclude that less than five thousand lunatics were locked up even at the end of the eighteenth century, a "tiny minority of the mad who were still scattered throughout the interior of society."

Foucault's account of the medieval period fares no better in the light of modern scholarship. Its central image is of the *Narrenschiff*, "the ship of fools," laden with its cargo of mad souls in search of their reason, floating down the liminal spaces of feudal Europe. It is through the *Narrenschiff* that Foucault seeks to capture the essence of the medieval response to madness, and the practical and symbolic significance of these vessels loom large in his account. *"Le Narrenschiff . . . ait eu une existence réelle,"* he insists. *"Ils ont existé, ces bateaux qui d'une ville à l'autre menaient leur cargaison insensée."* (The ship of fools was real. They existed, these boats that carried their crazed cargo from one town to another.) But it wasn't, and they didn't.

The back jacket of *History of Madness* contains a whole series of hyperbolic hymns of praise to its virtues. Paul Rabinow calls the book "one of the major works of the twentieth century." R. D. Laing hails it as "intellectually rigorous." And Nikolas Rose rejoices that "now, at last, English-speaking readers can have access to the depth of scholarship that underpins Foucault's analysis." Indeed they can, and one hopes that they will read the text attentively and intelligently and will learn some salutary lessons. One of those lessons might be amusing, if it had no effect on people's lives: the ease with which history can be distorted, facts ignored, the claims of human reason disparaged and dismissed, by someone sufficiently cynical and shameless and willing to trust in the ignorance and credulity of his customers.

3 The Asylum, the Hospital, and the Clinic

The asylum, an institutional space devoted exclusively to the management of the mad, has in some respects a much longer history than is commonly realized. Hospitals for the sick and infirm were established in the Byzantine Empire in the fifth century CE, quite soon after the collapse of the Roman Empire in the West. Usually charitable enterprises, hospitals spread into the Near East as Christian foundations well before the rise of Islam. In the years after the Prophet's death in 632, however, Arabs rapidly expanded the Islamic world, and in 750 it stretched from northern India all across North Africa and encompassed most of Spain. Under Islamic rule, hospitals proliferated from the late eighth century onward, until, by the late twelfth century, no large Islamic town was without a hospital. Like Christianity, Islam proclaimed the obligations of the rich to the poor, and Muslims could certainly not be seen to be less charitable than their Christian counterparts. Among those for whom these hospitals made specific provision were the insane, and given the special needs of those who had lost their senses and the difficulty of coping with them in an institution also attempting to cope with physical illness, it was not uncommon to have the mad removed to a separate establishment.[1]

Evidence about what transpired in these asylums is fugitive and fragmentary. Travelers' reports frequently mention barred windows and chains and speak of patients being beaten, something advocated even by the great Arab physician Avicenna (Ibn Sina, 980–1037), who saw it as a way to knock some sense into the wildly irrational. Much, though by no means all, of what we think of as Arab medicine was the creation of non-Muslims—Christians and Jews—and it borrowed liberally from the pagan medicine of Greece and Rome and the texts of the Hippocratics and of Galen. Unsurprisingly, then, besides the repressive measures employed to create some semblance of order, the inmates were also treated, as Galen had recommended, with cooling baths and diets designed to cool and moisten their bodies, therapies that aimed to counteract the heating and drying effects of the burnt black or yellow bile that was presumed to cause their madness. Herbal remedies were also widely employed (including lavender, thyme, pear or pomegranate juice, chamomile, and black hellebore), and Avicenna suggested that milk and ointments applied to the head might be of some use.

Perhaps the largest asylum in the Arab world was the Mansuri Hospital in Cairo, founded in 1284. Its floor plan survives, showing separate cells for male and female patients. Given the great reluctance of Muslim men to expose their womenfolk in public, this suggests that some female patients proved too difficult to manage in a domestic setting. Yet even the Mansuri asylum provided for at most a few dozen lunatics at a time. Arab asylums elsewhere accommodated fewer still and almost certainly were expected to house only the most frantic and unmanageable lunatics. For the most part, as was virtually always the case in Western Europe in this period, the mad were dealt with informally and remained very largely the responsibility of their relations.[2]

In its centuries under Islamic rule, Spain saw the establishment of a number of hospitals, with the Granada hospital perhaps the most notable. Following the Christian *Reconquista*, which was essentially complete by 1492, a whole series of asylums following Arab precedent are known to have existed, seven by the fifteenth century, including Valencia, Zaragoza, Seville, Valladolid, Palma de Mallorca, Toledo, and Barcelona. Greco-Roman medicine began to be reimported to Western Europe from the

Arab world in the Middle Ages, first in the aftermath of the Christianization of Spain, and thereafter as the Crusades brought Europeans into contact both with Arab learning and with hospitals and asylums. The printing press greatly accelerated the cultural impact of first Arab medicine and then the Greek and Roman medical texts that had largely been lost in the West, except for the survival of isolated manuscripts scattered in a handful of monasteries.[3]

Hospitals now began to appear in Western Europe, facilitated by the revival of trade and economic activity. They were often monastic foundations. As the shared root of "hospital" and "hospitality" reveals, they were not specifically medical enterprises to house the sick, but also sheltered pilgrims, the orphaned, the halt, the lame, and the blind. Still, some of these monastic hospitals gradually acquired a reputation for handling the mentally ill. Perhaps the most famous of these was Bethlehem, later better known as Bedlam. The first asylum in the English-speaking world, Bedlam took its name from the monastic order that had founded the Priory of St Mary of Bethlehem in Bishopsgate, London, in 1247. In its early years, Bethlehem took in the usual heterogeneous population of unfortunates that found themselves in medieval hospitals, but by the time of a census taken in 1403, we know that of the nine people then resident, six were *menti capti*, deprived of their wits.[4]

Soon enough, its corrupted name Bedlam had become synonymous with madness itself, a process greatly accelerated by the appearance of mad scenes in Elizabethan and Jacobean drama. It was not just Shakespeare but also Middleton, Fletcher, Dekker, Shirley, Ben Jonson, and Marston, among others, who introduced Bedlam to a wider audience. The asylum itself remained quite small. In 1632, for example, it was reported to contain twenty-seven patients, and in 1642, forty-four. In this respect, it resembled its counterparts elsewhere in Europe. The entrepreneurial Dutch, for example, seeking to house a small number of violent and troublesome madmen, took to using lotteries to raise the necessary funds. The Amsterdam Dolhuis, founded on a small basis by private charity in 1562, was enlarged and rebuilt with the money thus raised. It reopened in 1617, and the city's example was soon followed by Leiden and Harlem. In the aftermath of the restoration of Charles II to the English throne in 1660, the burghers of London took the hint, and Bethlem was rebuilt on a grander scale in 1676, to a design by Robert Hooke, in Moorfields, just outside the city wall. It was an unfortunate choice, since the uncompacted fill that had been used to fill up the old moat proved unstable, and by the second half of the eighteenth century, the asylum's fabric had begun to crumble; roof and walls separated, and rain began to inflict further damage on the structure, not to mention the misery it inflicted on the patients.

Undeniably, these charity asylums gradually grew larger in the seventeenth and eighteenth centuries, and new establishments added to their number: St Luke's and then a number of provincial charity asylums sprang up in Britain; religious foundations opened in France and elsewhere. As England became a steadily more prosperous commercial society in these years, still another type of asylum began to emerge. The private, profit-making madhouses operated in a market free from all regulation, taking some of the more troublesome mad folk off the hands of wealthy families who sought relief from the troubles and scandal that a mad relative in their midst imposed, and soon expanding their services to take the most troublesome paupers who had lost their wits.[5] France, too, began to see some private madhouses founded in the eighteenth century, euphemistically called *maisons de santé*, where the high-born whose antics disturbed their relations could be shut up, in every sense of the term.

Michel Foucault has spoken of the long eighteenth century as witnessing the "Great Confinement" of the insane.[6] His conceit is to conflate the mad with a far larger population of the dissolute, the idle, and the morally disreputable, like prostitutes, petty criminals, beggars, and the physically incapacitated, who began to be swept up into the so-called *hôpitaux généraux*, beginning with the founding of the first such establishment in Paris in 1656, and to pronounce the whole heterogeneous mass the exemplars of Unreason. Now, it is perfectly true that the Salpêtrière, the first of these, housed in an old gunpowder factory that gave it its name, contained perhaps a hundred lunatics when it opened, but these were, and their descendants remained, but a small fraction of the whole (they amounted to perhaps a thousand out of a total population of ten thousand at the time of the French Revolution). The *hôpitaux généraux* were not asylums in the conventional sense, and indeed their mad inmates, far from giving these institutions their identity, were simply an afterthought. Consider, for example, the description of who lurked in the Salpêtrière provided by the French surgeon Jacques Tenon in 1788, the year before the revolution and a hundred and thirty years after its foundation:

> The Salpêtrière is the largest hospital in Paris and possibly in Europe: this hospital is both a house for women and a prison. It received pregnant women and girls, wet nurses and their nurslings; male children from the age of seven or eight months to four and five years of age; young girls of all ages; aged married men and women; raving lunatics, imbeciles, epileptics, paralytics, blind persons, cripples, people suffering from ringworm, incurables of all sorts, children afflicted with scrofula, and so on and so forth. At the center of this hospital is a house of detention for women, comprising four different prisons: *le comun,* for the most dissolute girls; *la correction,* for those who are not considered hopelessly depraved; *la prison,* reserved for persons held by order of the king; and *la grande force,* for women branded by order of the courts.[7]

Even confining our attention to the French case, the exaggerations and distortions of speaking of an eighteenth-century great confinement of the mad are manifest, the more so when we move beyond the French capital and consider the state of affairs in the provinces. In Montpellier, for example, a city of some thirty thousand souls, and home to France's second most prominent medical school at the time, barely twenty mad folk were locked up when the revolution broke out. In Dijon, the numbers were smaller still: a mere nine mad women were confined at the Bon Pasteur.[8] In a wider European perspective, the idea that the eighteenth century saw any systematic incarceration of lunatics in madhouses and asylums becomes even less sustainable. The flourishing trade in lunacy in England, for example, gave birth to a whole series of gothic novels portraying the horrors of the madhouse and the danger of sane women, in particular, being shut up improperly alongside the mad. But the reality was less lurid. By 1800, all the madhouses in England together confined a grand total of no more than 2,500 lunatics.

The massive incarceration of the mad was instead a nineteenth-century phenomenon, and one that came to characterize the whole of Europe, and North America besides. The English, who had locked up fewer than three thousand in asylums in 1800 confined one hundred thousand a century later. A similarly startling increase in the numbers housed in asylums could be seen in France, Germany, the Netherlands, the Austrian Empire, Italy, Ireland, and Russia, not to mention the United States, Canada, and

Mexico. Sending the insane to an asylum came to be seen as one of the hallmarks of a civilized society. Indeed, Sir James Paget, physician to Queen Victoria, was moved to call the asylum "the most blessed manifestation of true civilization the world can present."[9]

Such language reflects the utopian expectations that attended what David Rothman has called "the discovery of the asylum" in the nineteenth century.[10] The new asylum was born of an extraordinary optimism about what a properly organized madhouse could accomplish. A powerful combination of moral architecture—that is, buildings designed as therapeutic instruments—and a moral treatment that mobilized the remnants of reason even the maddest patient still possessed, and encouraged the lunatic gradually to extend their powers of self-control until these allowed the suppression of unruly thoughts and behavior: this, argued the enthusiasts for making the asylum the place of first resort in cases of madness, would restore a very large fraction of the insane to the ranks of the normal.

If eighteenth-century madhouses had acquired the reputation of being human zoos where the sane came to taunt and tease the inmates—recall William Hogarth's canonical image of the naked Tom Rakewell confined in Bedlam, being stared at by tittering society ladies amused by the sight of the crazed—or "moral lazar houses" where the deranged were hidden and hope and humanity abandoned, their nineteenth-century counterparts were everywhere held up to be vastly different. These asylums, their proponents insisted, had been transmuted into the "moral machinery" through which minds could be strengthened and reason restored. Like the Invisible Hand now held to regulate civil society, "the system is at once both beautiful and self-operating. [The] presence [of keepers] is required to regulate the machine, but its motions are spontaneous," serving all but imperceptibly to secure "the tranquilization of the unhealthy mind."[11]

Moral treatment, the key to the reformed asylum, seems to have emerged in quite similar guises in England, France, and Italy,[12] and thence to have underpinned the movement to build whole networks of asylums at state expense. Interesting enough, in its most famous and influential English and French versions, it was initially the work of laymen: William Tuke, a Quaker tea and coffee merchant who had founded the York Retreat in 1796 and developed the approach in a collaboration with the lay couple who administered the asylum, George and Katherine Jepson;[13] and Jean-Baptiste

Pussin and his wife (who was nicknamed the Governess) at the Bicêtre and the Salpêtrière, respectively.[14] But very quickly, the central tenets of moral treatment were absorbed and transformed by medical men and used as the basis for their claims that they were uniquely qualified to run the new asylums. What had begun in Tuke's hands as a critique of the failures of asylum medicine became instead central to the ideology of the medical superintendents who by the middle of the nineteenth century had achieved a medical monopoly of the treatment of the mad. In the nineteenth century, that is, the birth of the asylum simultaneously marked the emergence of a newly self-confident and organized group of specialists in mental medicine. The alienists' claims to expertise and to the capture of this new jurisdiction rested firmly on their management of the reformed asylums.[15]

Across Europe and North America, a veritable mania for building asylums at state expense marked the middle decades of the nineteenth century. France passed a law making the construction of provincial asylums compulsory in 1838, a belated response to an earlier report from Pinel's protégé and successor, J. E. D. Esquirol, documenting what he claimed were the horrors of treatment of the insane in prisons, jails, and the community. In England, permissive legislation passed in 1807, the County Asylums Act, allowed taxes to be collected and spent for the construction of reformed asylums, and two acts of 1845 made asylum construction compulsory and introduced a national inspectorate, the Lunacy Commission, to oversee and police the new establishments, as well as the existing charity asylums and profit-making madhouses. In the United States, there were a handful of private asylums, but the doctrine of the separation of powers was held to preclude federal involvement, so it took state initiatives to create a national network of asylums.[16] That the process was accomplished in only a decade and a half was substantially due to the indefatigable efforts of the Yankee moral entrepreneur Dorothea Dix, who dragooned state legislators in the north, south, and west to do her bidding. Not content with this accomplishment, Dix also took time to browbeat British politicians into imposing tax-supported asylums on a hitherto resistant Scotland.[17] Political fragmentation in Italy and Germany led to more halting progress in those countries, but eventually they too embraced the mantra that for the most serious forms of mental disorder the asylum was the best and perhaps the only solution.

But the extravagant claims that lunacy reformers had made about the asylum rapidly proved an illusion. Cure rates were of the order of a third of patients treated, and the upshot was a steady increase in the fraction of patients who became long-stay patients and a steady rise in the size of the average asylum. The York Retreat, which served as a model for Anglo-American reformers, initially provided for no more than thirty patients. The so-called corporate asylums that brought moral treatment to America and served as the model for the first state hospitals there were scarcely much larger.[18] By the 1860s, asylums containing upward of a thousand patients were not uncommon. By the early twentieth century, there were asylums like Milledgeville, in the state of Georgia, which had a population well in excess of ten thousand. At Epsom, outside London, more than twelve thousand patients were crowded on a single site. It was the hordes of the hopeless, the legions of chronic patients, that constituted the public image of the asylum. The optimism that had marked the early part of the century was replaced by an equally profound pessimism. And the asylum's reputation once more sank until it was viewed as "the Bluebeard's cupboard of the neighbourhood."[19]

Over the past two decades, scholars have sought to complicate the picture of the late nineteenth-century asylum as little more than a warehouse for the unwanted. They have stressed the ways families used the asylum for their own purposes, to secure some temporary relief from the burdens of caring for a mentally ill family member. And they have pointed out that even in this era, there remained a not-insignificant movement of patients out of the asylum and back into the community.[20] The public image of the asylum as a cemetery for the still breathing is thus clearly somewhat at odds with reality.[21]

Still, modern scholarship notwithstanding, the silting up of asylums with chronic patients is what dominated late nineteenth-century perceptions of these places. The effects were felt on many levels. Psychiatry as a profession had to account for its manifold failures as a therapeutic enterprise, a particularly acute problem given the utopian expectations that had accompanied the birth of the asylum, and to which the profession had contributed. Those who had choice in the matter—and that was not, of course, the poor and those with limited resources—redoubled their efforts to avoid the stigma and the sense of hopelessness that enveloped the asylum. And public authorities grew steadily less willing to expend what they perceived to be extravagant sums of money on a population whose prospects of reclamation seemed poor at best.

Psychiatrists increasingly argued that the inmates thronging the wards of the asylum were degenerates, evolutionary throwbacks whose biological defects were engraved on their bodies and brains, visible in their physiognomy, and incapable of being cured. Indeed, the risk of releasing these defectives into the community was that, lacking the restraints of the more sensible and civilized, they would recklessly multiply their kind, overwhelming the healthy stock that constituted the bulk of the population. It was an account that simultaneously explained away the profession's failures and provided a new rationale for building and maintaining asylums as places to quarantine the biologically unfit and prevent a further increase in the numbers of defectives. It brought into being a new emphasis on eugenics—the purported science of encouraging the better sort to breed while precluding the defective classes from doing so, either through preventive detention in asylums or via involuntary sterilization. The Nazis would later take the logic of this position a step further and order the extermination of these "useless eaters," as their propaganda proclaimed mental patients to be.

Mental illness has always carried with it enormous stigma. The language of biological degeneration and inferiority served only to strengthen those age-old prejudices, and the extraordinarily negative perceptions of the late nineteenth-century asylum encouraged the well-to-do to seek any possible alternative—including treatments at spa towns in Germany and France, an array of sanatoria and homes for the nervous, and quack remedies of all sorts. In the United States, for example, the Kellogg brothers took over a failing sanatorium in Battle Creek, Michigan, run by the Seventh Day Adventist Church, and turned it into a lucrative business patronized by presidents and captains of industry, Hollywood stars, and legions of the great and good, all of whom came to be detoxified and have their mental batteries recharged.

But whatever protection the theory of degeneration offered to those running asylums, it could not completely insulate psychiatry from the perception of failure. American psychiatry came under sustained attack in the 1870s and 1880s from a group of rival specialists who had emerged from the carnage of the American Civil War. The asylum physicians, sneered the New York neurologist Edward Spitzka, were "experts at everything but the diagnosis, treatment and pathology of insanity," and he harshly condemned "the grated windows, crib-beds, bleak walls, gruff attendants, narcotics and insane surroundings of an asylum."[22] Invited to address America's assembled psychiatrists at the fiftieth anniversary of the formation of the professional association of asylum physicians, the Philadelphia neurologist Silas Weir Mitchell was equally savage in his criticisms. Speaking for an hour, he denounced asylums and their doctors in no uncertain terms. He accused them of presiding over an assembly of "living corpses, . . . pathetic patients who have lost even the memory of hope, [and] sit in rows, too dull to know despair, silent, grewsome machines which sleep and eat, eat and sleep." "Asylum life," he concluded, "is deadly to the insane."[23] The leading English alienist, Henry Maudsley, who had gratefully cut his ties with the asylum system for an office-based practice, concurred: "I cannot help feeling, from my experience, that one effect of asylums is to make permanent lunatics."[24] Historians have generally agreed. In Gerald Grob's words, "After 1860, . . . the continuous rise in the number of resident chronic patients had all but obliterated the therapeutic goals of many hospitals. . . . Virtually every hospital in the nation was confronted with a problem whose magnitude was clearly increasing rather than diminishing. . . . Overcrowded conditions and the accumulation of chronic patients" were increasingly the norm, as the transformation of mental hospitals into "strictly welfare institutions as far as their funding and reputation were concerned . . . solidified their custodial character."[25]

In France, the crisis of psychiatric legitimacy had surfaced as early as the 1860s and 1870s. Antipsychiatric sentiments surfaced in the popular press. Many in the medical profession seemed poised to join the chorus of disapproval. The eminent neurologist Jean-Martin Charcot was beginning to experiment with the hypnotic treatment of hysterical patients, but while the scantily dressed women who drew crowds to his weekly demonstrations entertained tout Paris, they did little for the reputation of alienists and their institutions. And eventually, on Charcot's death, his hysterical circus collapsed amid recriminations, accusations that his demonstrations had been faked, and an abandonment of his whole approach.[26] Though the fears expressed by Jules Falret, a prominent asylum doctor, proved overblown, the professional uncertainty his remarks revealed was real enough. "The law of 1838 and the asylums for the insane are being attacked on all sides,"[27] he complained, and in this he was not wrong. But in the final analysis, it turned out that the public had grown used to the mass confinement of the mad and showed little disposition to destroy the institutions that had cost so much to build, so psychiatry's position, while weak and marginal, was never truly threatened.

For the most part, the fate and standing of psychiatry remained very much bound up with that of the asylum. Psychiatrists were trapped in the asylum almost as securely as their patients. Training for neophytes took place on an apprenticeship basis, as doctors were recruited to serve as lowly assistant physicians, a situation made possible in part by the over-crowded state of the medical profession in the closing decades of the nine-teenth century. In essence, the profession had virtually no presence in universities in most countries. There was a lectureship in mental diseases at the University of Edinburgh in Scotland, but not even this sort of posi-tion existed south of the border. In the United States, the first professor-ship of any note would not be filled until the end of the first decade of the twentieth century, and there would not be a second chair until the Rockefeller Foundation started extensively funding psychiatry in the 1930s. There were textbooks, which provided some semblance of formal knowledge, but there was little in the way of sustained research and a general sense of intellectual stasis. Weir Mitchell's critique of psychiatry's failings was all too accurate. In unguarded moments, asylum doctors admitted as much. Bedford Pierce, superintendent of the York Retreat, the asylum that had been so influential in launching the drive to build these places in Britain and the United States, confessed to the "humiliat-ing reflection . . . that it is not possible as yet to make a scientific classifica-tion of mental disorders."[28] And speaking as the newly installed president of the American Medico-Psychological Association, Charles Hill suc-cinctly confessed, "Our therapeutics are simply a pile of rubbish."[29]

By the end of the nineteenth century, asylums were being relabeled as mental hospitals, a piece of reform-by-word magic that did little to disguise an increasingly grim reality. Throughout the first half of the twentieth cen-tury, hospital populations continued to grow, and at least until the out-break of World War II, the profession's center of gravity continued to rest firmly within the walls of the institutions. Freud's psychoanalysis had suggested one pathway for the profession out of asylumdom, and the experiences of World War I added a further stimulus to outpatient practice, as doctors who had been forced to deal with shell shock patients in the field tried to translate the model of extra-institutional practice to civilian life. Child and marriage guidance clinics provided a small number of practitioners with an alternative site for their work, as did the newly emerging juvenile courts,[30] but these employed but a small minority of the profession, which otherwise continued to concentrate its attentions on a burgeoning population of compulsorily certified patients locked up in mental hospitals.

Only in Germany and Austria did a different pattern emerge during the course of the nineteenth century. From midcentury onward, German psychiatry sought to emulate the linking together of clinical practice, the laboratory, and academic research that was bringing the rest of German medicine into international prominence. Politically fragmented until 1870, the congeries of principalities and kingdoms that made up Germany had chosen to compete for visibility and prestige through underwriting science and knowledge production. University-based clinics and institutes brought together teaching and research in novel ways, and it was this approach that German psychiatry adopted as its own. Germany had its barracks-asylums, certainly, but in addition it developed a series of smaller clinics attached to universities, where interesting patients could be studied and laboratory research pursued.[31] As time went on, German psychiatrists developed research programs examining the brain and spinal cord, creating new techniques for fixing and staining cells for microscopic examination, in search of the physical roots of madness. There were a handful of successes, including Alois Alzheimer's identification of the neurofibrillary tangles associated with the disease to which he gave his name and the subsequent discovery by Hideo Noguchi and J. W. Moore of the syphilitic spirochete in the brains of patients suffering from general paralysis of the insane. For the overwhelming bulk of the insane, however, the hypothesized brain lesions proved elusive, as they remain today.

Asylums in this model served largely as a source of pathological material for the dissecting table. German psychiatry evinced little interest in treating patients, who were seen, as elsewhere, as biological degenerates.

By the 1930s, many of the leading lights of the profession were collaborating eagerly with the Nazi regime, first sterilizing the mad and then murdering them en masse. Asylums were temporarily emptied, but not by some grand therapeutic breakthrough.

Elsewhere, there were few attempts to emulate the German model of research-oriented clinics. One exception was the Phipps Clinic at Johns Hopkins, established with funding from a Pittsburgh steel millionaire. Johns Hopkins as a whole had sought to emulate the basic features of the German knowledge factories, and Adolf Meyer, the Swiss immigrant it appointed as its first professor of psychiatry, spoke airily of psychobiology and tried to turn the Phipps into a research enterprise that would solve some of the mysteries of madness.[32] While Meyer went on to train many psychiatrists who occupied chairs across the country as new academic departments were created, his program produced no therapeutic breakthroughs and little by way of significant new research.[33]

Henry Maudsley, the most prominent British alienist of the late Victorian and Edwardian age (he hated the term "psychiatrist"), had grown distant from his professional colleagues and left the fortune he had accumulated from his private practice to fund a hospital he intended to become an alternative and a reproach to the asylum system he had abandoned. The Maudsley Hospital and its associated Institute of Psychiatry sought to combine care of selected patients with academic research and professional training, and eventually, after World War II, it came to be led by one of Meyer's protégés, Aubrey Lewis. But like the Phipps, it was better at producing psychiatrists than at unlocking the keys to madness.

Mental hospitals grew relentlessly in the first half of the twentieth century. In the United States, for example, the number of mental patients quadrupled in this period, while the general population of the country simply doubled, and space had to be found for the rapid rise in the number of inmates. On Long Island, the New York authorities built or expanded three barracks-asylums at Central Islip, Kings Park, and Pilgrim that together at their peak contained nearly thirty-five thousand patients. Desperate to do something to stem the tide, and to reinforce their own sense of professional competence, asylum superintendents had at their disposal large numbers of patients who were legally without rights by virtue of their status, hidden from public view, and seen by most as incapable of making rational choices

THE ASYLUM, THE HOSPITAL, AND THE CLINIC

about their own treatment. Many psychiatrists fell prey to the temptation to experiment on these captive bodies. In Austria, Hungary, Germany, Portugal, Britain, and the United States, an orgy of experimentation ensued. Malarial therapy, deep sleep therapy, surgical excision of focal sepsis, insulin coma therapy, metrazol-induced seizures, electroshock therapy, and lobotomies—all these drastic remedies and more have attracted considerable scholarly attention in recent decades.[34]

Imperial powers had exported the asylum model to deal with mad white colonists as early as the nineteenth century.[35] Despite the deteriorating public image of mental hospitals, their centrality to the provision of mental health services in the first half of the twentieth century saw versions of them exported to the colonies and to other parts of the non-Western world, like China. These asylums, too, have begun to attract their historians. Asylum psychiatry in these settings was transformed in some interesting directions, for while Western-trained psychiatrists looked with condescension on indigenous beliefs and practices, imperial psychiatry in such settings almost universally experienced enormous difficulty in transforming popular local customs.[36] Very occasionally, there was resistance to the expansion of the asylum model in societies where Western influence was limited. Japan, for example, continued to rely largely on home confinement until the mid-twentieth century, and as a late adopter, it has proved equally reluctant to move away from a reliance on the mental hospital.[37]

Though mental hospital populations continued to grow in the 1930s and 1940s, conditions in the asylums were deteriorating even further. The Great Depression meant both more patients, some driven by want, and decreased budgets. Total war, when it came, worsened the situation and in addition created shortages of both psychiatrists and staff. The Nazis were busy "solving" the problem of their institutionalized population by resorting to mass murder. Occupied Vichy France took a different tack, savagely cutting mental hospital budgets to the point where patients starved—death rates tripled in the war years, with an estimated forty-five thousand patients in French mental hospitals dying of starvation and disease—an outcome some historians have called "soft extermination."[38] Elsewhere, conditions were not quite so dire, though they were shocking enough in all conscience. In the immediate aftermath of the war, for example, conscientious objectors who had been forced to serve as mental hospital attendants published memoirs and photographs of scenes that resembled Dante's Inferno, while journalists just back from viewing the horrors of the Final Solution spoke of the conditions they found in their own country's state mental hospitals, calling them "American Death Camps."[39]

This generation of critics sought reform of the mental hospitals, not their demise. The 1950s and 1960s, however, saw the publication of a series of sociological studies of the mental hospital that increasingly argued that the defects were a structural feature of these "total institutions," as the Canadian American sociologist Erving Goffman dubbed them, and thus their flaws were ineradicable.[40] "The abandonment of the state hospitals," said Ivan Belknap, summarizing an emerging consensus, "might be one of the greatest humanitarian reforms and the greatest financial economy ever achieved."[41] Renegade psychiatrists like Thomas Szasz, often labeled anti-psychiatrists, chimed in, equating mental hospitals with concentration camps.[42] And the then British minister of health, Enoch Powell, gave a widely reported speech denouncing mental hospitals as a failed experiment, announcing his government's plan to close them all, and offering to be the first to set the torch to their funeral pyre.[43] The legitimacy of what had been the dominant response to serious mental illness for more than a century reached its nadir.

Powell proved to be a prophet. In Britain, mental hospital populations had reached their peak in 1954. In the United States, the inflection point came a year later, and in both countries the mental hospital population then declined year after year, quite slowly and almost imperceptibly at first, but by the second half of the 1960s, at an accelerating pace. Certainly, the systematic destruction of any sense that the mental hospital provided a therapeutic function, or even valuable sheltered care, was of considerable ideological importance, smoothing the way toward the abandonment of segregative modes of controlling madness. But scholars with a variety of perspectives have demonstrated that neither these shifts in sentiment nor the other factor most often invoked to explain the demise of the mental hospital—that is, the psychopharmacological revolution that began with the introduction of phenothiazine under the trade names Thorazine (in the United States) and Largactil (in Europe)—were the primary factors behind the emptying out of the Victorian bins. Instead, many have argued, what took place was a conscious shift in social policy, much of it driven by fiscal concerns.[44]

Whatever the precise weight one places on the various factors that contributed to deinstitutionalization and the virtual abandonment of the chronically mentally ill that has been a feature of social policy all across the industrialized world, the fate of the mental hospital is beyond doubt. A handful still linger, but in a much-shrunken state. Most have shut their doors. On occasion, they have been reincarnated as upscale housing for the nouveau riche or as luxury hotels, as on the island of San Clemente in the Venice lagoon—in both cases, care is taken to disguise their stigmatizing history. But in most instances, they have just moldered away: dust to dust, ashes to ashes, as the Bible would have it. Mental hospitals have become a fast-vanishing relic of the past, their distinctive moral architecture preserved only through the lenses of some creative photographers who have devoted themselves to recording the last moments of museums of madness that will soon have disappeared from our collective consciousness.[45]

4 A Culture of Complaint

PSYCHIATRY AND ITS CRITICS

I venture to suggest that few branches of the medical profession have been as subject to complaints as psychiatry. The mad (or some of them) were vocal critics of their doctors long before there was such a thing as psychiatry—or at least an organized profession that went by that name. For psychiatry as a term of art only came into broad usage in the English-speaking world a century or so ago. Before the early twentieth century, those purporting to minister to diseased minds called themselves (or were referred to by others) asylum superintendents, medical psychologists, or alienists. Earlier still, in the eighteenth and through the first part of the nineteenth century, they answered to the name "mad-doctor," a label that nicely captures the ambivalence with which society at large has always seemed to regard those who lay claim to expertise in the treatment of the mentally ill. Complaints about psychiatry continue to the present. Indeed, as I will show in the concluding section of this chapter, in the last half century, the voices of the patients have been amplified by still other powerful complainers: by social scientists who have suggested that the psychiatric emperor has no clothes and, more disturbingly still, by critics from within the profession of psychiatry itself—not just renegades like Thomas Szasz and Ronald Laing but mainstream psychiatrists as well.

Complaints have frequently functioned as a motor of change in this arena, as in other fields of medicine. Complaints about the horrors of the ancien régime madhouse and about the confinement of the sane amid the lunatic played a vital role in generating the moral outrage that fueled the Victorian lunacy reform movement and in successive revisions of commitment laws—though it has to be added that the law of unintended consequences operated with particular force in these arenas. The asylums that were one generation's solution to the problems of serious psychosis became the object of complaints and agitation for a later generation seduced by the siren song of "community psychiatry"; and the hedging about of the psychiatric commitments process with legal entanglements likewise became a late twentieth-century bête noir. But complaints have also been directed against particular forms of psychiatric treatment and have played an important role in creating greater circumspection among psychiatrists about the use of treatments like lobotomy and shock therapies, and more recently even in raising concerns about the contemporary reliance on psychopharmacology as the sheet anchor of current psychiatric practice.[1]

Most recently of all, as I will discuss in the concluding sections of this chapter, complaints from the very center of the psychiatric enterprise—the authors of the third and fourth editions of the psychiatric bible, the *DSM;* and the head of the US National Institute of Mental Health, Thomas Insel, who presides over the vital federal presence in basic mental health research, dispensing billions of dollars—have threatened to destabilize the psychiatric profession in its entirety. *DSM 5,* as the fifth edition is called, has been labeled a useless, antiscientific document, a hindrance to progress. Perhaps worse still, Insel has complained openly about the mythical status of such "diseases" as schizophrenia and depression. Complaining about psychiatry scarcely gets more dangerous and delegitimizing than that.

Though medical speculations about the origins of madness have an ancient lineage, the emergence of what ultimately became the modern profession of psychiatry—that is, the routine engagement of some medics in the management of the mad—cannot really be traced back much further than the eighteenth century. As the nineteenth-century term "asylum superintendent" suggests, the emergence of what eventually became a community of practitioners specializing in mental illness was intimately bound up with the parallel creation of a new social space—the madhouse, or the asylum. It was in and through the management of these establishments that doctors developed some claim to skill in the management of the depressed, the demented, and the deranged, and it was their control over the rapidly expanding network of such places in the Victorian era that ultimately helped to constitute and consolidate their position as an organized, well-defined, albeit still suspect, profession.

The eighteenth-century "trade in lunacy" was produced by and responded to the opportunities created by the growth of a consumer society—the emergence of a market for all sorts of goods and services that had traditionally been supplied on a subsistence basis, if they were supplied at all. It must be understood, as the late historian Roy Porter suggested, as part of the same developments that saw the rise of dancing masters, fencing instructors, hairdressers, pottery manufacturers, and other novel service occupations.[2] Those practicing the trade in lunacy took over the burdens of coping with an initially small fraction of those whose disturbed emotions, cognitions, and behaviors rendered them inconvenient, if not positively impossible, to live with—rather as undertakers began to emerge to handle the comparatively unpleasant and stigmatizing task of dealing with and disposing of corpses. The mad had traditionally been a liability that fell primarily on the shoulders of their families. The disruptions they visited on the texture of daily life—the uncertainty, the threat, and the terror they might provoke—were ones their relations bore primary responsibility for dealing with. In the entrepreneurial culture that prevailed in eighteenth-century England, those who could afford it might for the first time relinquish these problems to others, and when poor lunatics were judged sufficiently threatening and disruptive, the creaky mechanism of the Old Poor Law might occasionally pay to confine them in newfangled madhouses.

By no means was the new trade in lunacy a medical monopoly. To the contrary, in its early years, the madhouse business attracted all manner of entrepreneurs willing to speculate in, and earn a living from, trafficking in this particular form of misery. The keepers of madhouses were a heterogeneous lot, for there were no barriers to entry and no oversight of the industry. And though traditional humoral medicine could readily stretch its explanatory schema to account for mania and melancholia, and its bleedings, vomits, purges, and dietary regimens could be easily rational-

ized as remedies for the excesses of bile and blood that supposedly produced mental turmoil, there was no compelling reason, so far as many
potential customers were concerned, to prefer those who professed some
sort of medical expertise to others who promised similar services, especially respite from the travails madness brought in its train and the shutting up of a source of social shame and embarrassment out of public view.
To be sure, the growing number of madhouses and the experience of
attempting to control and manage the mentally disturbed day after day
meant that those running these places perforce developed techniques and
some measure of skill in the handling of such awkward customers. The
very variety of establishments and operators led to experiments with
different approaches, and since claims to provide cure as well as care
could provide a comparative advantage when it came to securing clients,
many were not slow to advance them, and some rather bizarre pieces of
apparatus—swinging chairs, devices to mimic the experience of drowning,
chairs to immobilize the patient and cut him or her off from sources of
sensory stimulation—were invented to assist in the task.[3]

One of the key benefits madhouses could potentially offer families was
the capacity to draw a veil of silence over the existence of a mad relation.
But this shutting up of the mad in what purported to be therapeutic isolation could easily be cast in a more sinister light. Drawing boundaries
between the mad and the sane is scarcely a simple task. At the margin,
ambiguities abound. Madhouses, with their barred windows, high perim-
eter walls, isolation from the community at large, and enforced secrecy,
inevitably invited gothic imaginings about what transpired hidden from
view, and such stories almost immediately began to circulate.

Some were fictional. Pulp fiction was another innovation of the emerging consumer society, and Grub Street hastened to produce melodramas
with madhouse settings. One of the most successful of these, first published in 1726 and passing through myriad editions, staying in print for
more than three-quarters of a century, was Eliza Haywood's novella *The
Distress'd Orphan*. As was customary in such gothic tales, the confinement that structured the story arose from familial conflict over a romantic
liaison and the control of a personal estate: Annilia, the daughter of an
eminent city merchant, who had lost both parents at a young age and was
heiress to a substantial fortune, finds herself nefariously confined as

insane by her uncle and guardian, Giraldo, after falling in love with a foreigner (Colonel Marathon). Her uncle is determined that she should marry his own son, Horatio, which would ensure the passage of her estate as her dowry. The confinement (mimicking what was often the case in reality) was initiated in her own home by the uncle ordering her door locked and "one of the Footmen to bring a Smith, that her Windows may be barr'd," under the pretense of protecting Annilia from her own mischievous and suicidal propensities: "For 'tis not Improbable but when she finds she is restrain'd in her Humour she may offer to throw herself out."[4]

Annilia, however, is not to be so easily intimidated, and her uncle ratchets up the pressure by arranging for her to be carted off to a madhouse, secretly and in the dead of night, her screams silenced by "stopping her mouth."[5] There, she finds herself at the mercy of "inhuman Creatures," "Ruffians," "pityless [sic] Monsters," and "ill-looked fellows" wedded to the terrific mode of instilling "awe" and dread in their patients via lashings, mechanical restraint, and neglect.[6] Heywood's melodrama plays up the symbolic homology between the constraints of the madhouse—its bolts, bars, and chains—and the tyranny of life as a lady, bereft of any semblance of legal and social equality. Only the intervention of her lover, Colonel Marathon, who surreptitiously enters the madhouse and then heroically scales its walls with his "trembling" sweetheart draped across his broad shoulders, allows her to escape back to "freedom" after three months of confinement. Then the evildoers are punished, virtue is rewarded, and the titillating story comes to a satisfying close.

Heywood's portrait of the mad-business as corrupt and cruel, unconcerned with the mental status of those it confined, struck a deep chord with an audience prone to believe the worst about what happened in madhouses. And such complaints were not confined to the realm of fiction. Mrs. Clerke's case came before the courts in 1718, and the testimony at the trial made plain that women with fortunes (in this instance, a rich widow) were genuinely vulnerable to being incarcerated as mad in just the ways that were exploited in the literary narratives of the time—all the more so, given the hazy boundaries of those disorders of mind and body being constituted by doctors and owned by sufferers as vapors, spleen, and nerves.[7] Research by the Cambridge historian Elizabeth Foyster into the records of the King's Bench court has shown that Mrs. Clerke's case was scarcely unique. Women were, indeed, especially liable to false confinement in madhouses, locked away by husbands eager to enforce their authority over the property of wives and to sanction their "reasonable" restraint and correction.[8]

Whereas emotionally and socially susceptible females predominated as the victims and complainants in this partly literary and partly literal construction of the madhouse, there were also a fair number of actual and fictional male equivalents suffering similar fates. A particularly noisy example was the obsessive-compulsive printer, proofreader, and author of a *Concordance to the Holy Bible* (1737), which remains in print to this day, Alexander Cruden. The very obsessiveness that allowed Cruden to compile his monumental work in his garret after work each day translated less well to his picaresque daily life. After losing his job in 1729 as French reader to the Earl of Derby (it turned out that he had never heard spoken French, having learned the language through his work as a proofreader, and thus attempted a Scots-inflected phonetic pronunciation of the text put before him), he rushed off to learn the language at the hands of a family of Huguenot refugees and then rode to Lancashire, nearly killing his horse in the process, to demand his job back—to no avail. When, in 1739, he obsessively stalked ladies above his station, informing them that God had chosen each of them for his spouse, he was imprisoned in a madhouse; years later, in 1753, he was once again confined in a mental institution after getting into a fight with a group of drunken youths who were swearing and blaspheming in the London streets.

Escaping on the first occasion by sawing through the bed leg and gathering up the chain that had bound him to it, he hobbled through the streets of London, one foot shod in a slipper, the other bare, until he reached the Lord Mayor's house. He then brought a lawsuit for £10,000 in damages, which he lost, and in the aftermath he published a series of pamphlets in which he pronounced himself a "London citizen exceedingly injured" by a form of "British Inquisition."[9] In these publications, he denounced James Monro, the mad-doctor who had treated him, as a Jacobite and an adulterer. James's son, John Monro, was called in to treat Cruden on the occasion of this confinement, but he was at least spared from being the target of Cruden's unsuccessful lawsuit, though Cruden lampooned him in the next round of pamphlets he wrote to protest being locked up.[10]

James Newton (1670?-1750), the proprietor of a madhouse in Islington, was one of the few to be convicted for a false confinement, or, as an anonymous 1715 pamphlet put it, for "violently keeping and misusing" William Rogers at the behest of his wife.[11] But many others were lambasted, suspected of following suit. Calling on a growing common knowledge and concern about such abuses, the novelist Tobias Smollett had his mock-heroic English Don Quixote, *Sir Launcelot Greaves* (1762) seized and carried off to a madhouse run by the eponymous Bernard Shackle, giving the him the occasion to warn that "in England, the most innocent person upon earth is liable to be immured for life under the pretext of lunacy, sequestered from his wife, children, and friends, robbed of his fortune, deprived even of necessaries, and subjected to brutal treatment from a low-bred barbarian, who raises an ample fortune on the misery of his fellow-creatures, and may, during his whole life, practice this horrid oppression, without question or control."[12] Daniel Defoe had earlier raised similar fears,[13] which by the 1730s had become sufficiently universal to become the subject of an opera-burlesque.[14] Before the century's end, in the wake of further critiques and protests by pamphleteers and disaffected former patients,[15] the image of these "mansions of misery" could scarcely have been less salubrious.

The mid-eighteenth century thus saw a torrent of criticism of the unregulated state of private madhouses, fed by scandalous tales of alleged false confinement and intermittent, but influential, appeals for legislative intervention—all of which were met initially with official indifference. Eventually, however, the rising tide of complaints of corruption, cruelty, and malfeasance in the mad-trade forced a reluctant House of Commons to launch a half-hearted inquiry into the mad-business in 1763, and the limited testimony it took proved damning. All the instances of false confinement that came to light involved women who had allegedly been falsely confined by their husbands and other family members. Witnesses stressed the use of ruses and trickery to initiate and perpetuate these confinements, and noted the obstruction of contact with the outside world, in particular through being locked up and mechanically restrained night and day, having visitors refused and correspondence barred, and being "treated with Severity" by keepers.[16] The women themselves complained that they received no medicines or medical treatment whatsoever and were never even attended by a medical practitioner, or not, at least, until a habeas corpus had been effected.

Complaints notwithstanding, it was another eleven years before the Act for Regulating Madhouses (14 George III c. 49) was finally passed. Porter has suggested that the prolonged delay in enacting legislation should be seen as a function of the opposition of the College of Physicians, some of whose members "had a large financial stake in metropolitan madhouses."[17] Yet Parliament handed over the power to license and inspect madhouses in the metropolis to the college, which proved as indolent in carrying out the task as the magistrates who were charged with performing these tasks in the provinces. In every respect, the legislation seems to have been little more than a token gesture.

Patient protests against their mad-doctors became even fiercer in the nineteenth century, as lunacy reformers secured legislation compelling the tax-supported construction of mental hospitals, and thousands on thousands of patients flooded into the expanding empire of asylumdom. Perhaps the most socially prominent contributor to this literature was John Perceval, son of the last British prime minister to be assassinated, Spencer Perceval. The younger Perceval patronized a prostitute while a student at Oxford. A pious Evangelical Christian, he feared he had contracted syphilis, so he dosed himself with mercury and soon lapsed into a delusory religious state, which led his family to lock him up, first in Edward Long Fox's madhouse near Bristol, Brislington House, and then in what became the favorite asylum for the English upper classes, Ticehurst House in Sussex. Elaborate as these establishments were, they could not provide accommodations that matched Perceval's expectations. He complained that his attendants were violent and that they failed to display sufficient deference to their distinguished, gentlemanly patient. Shortly after his transfer to Ticehurst in 1832, he considered himself cured. Yet his confinement continued. The angrier he became, the more the Newingtons, in whose establishment he was confined, insisted that he was still unfit for release. Deprived of his privacy and his dignity, Perceval was furious. He was finally released in October 1833 (though his doctors were still not sure of his sanity), and he subsequently penned an anonymous account of his captivity, savaging both Fox and the Newingtons. When that failed to attract much attention, he issued a revised and enlarged edition under his own name, something that permanently alienated him from many of his family members.[18]

Finding his complaints were still largely ignored, Perceval became one of the founders in 1845 of that wonderfully named Victorian organization, the Alleged Lunatics' Friend Society. Perceval and his cohorts (who included Luke Hansard, whose family published the parliamentary proceedings, and who had two mad sisters confined in asylums; Captain [later Admiral] Richard Saumarez, two of whose brothers were locked up as lunatics; and Richard Paternoster, a discharged lunatic who claimed he had always been sane), now made usually fruitless efforts to secure the release of patients whom they claimed were improperly confined. The *Medical Times* spoke scornfully of their activities: "The members of this Society are apt to see things through a hazy and distorted medium. . . . They have wandered about the country, prepared to lend an ear to the idle story of every lunatic they could meet with; they have pestered the Home Secretary, and ever and anon obtruded their opinions and schemes upon such members of the Upper and Lower House as would listen to them." Others had a pithier put-down: they called them "The Lunatics' Society."[19]

Most of those whose cases the society took up were men, but the most famous complainer of the late 1840s was a woman, Louisa Nottidge, whose suit against her brothers for kidnapping and false imprisonment in a madhouse produced a string of newspaper reports that titillated literate Englishmen and a proclamation from the judge who heard the case that cast scorn on the pretensions of the alienists who had confined her. Nottidge was a maiden lady of a certain age, one of several unmarried sisters who had been left considerable sums by their father, and who subsequently became devotees of a defrocked Anglican clergyman, a certain Mr. Prince, who set up a commune in the West of England that he called Agapemone, or the Abode of Love. Prince preached that the Day of Judgment had come and that only his followers would be saved. Later, he appeared to announce (his preaching was convoluted and confusing) that he was the Holy Ghost made flesh. And flesh was something the Abode of Love appeared to worship: there were rumors that female recruits had to present themselves naked or risk damnation. Three of Nottidge's sisters had already married members of the sect, turning over their fortunes to them, and when Nottidge seemed likely to follow suit, her brother and brother-in-law descended at night and abducted her, locking her up in Dr. Arthur Moorcroft's asylum, Moorcroft House in Hillingdon, Middlesex. Learning where she was confined, her coreligionists brought a writ of habeas corpus and secured her release. Hence the lawsuit, which was decided in her favor (though damages were assessed at a mere £50), and the scathing statement from the judge that mad-doctors were a danger to the liberty of free-born Englishmen and that "no lunatic should be confined in an asylum unless a danger to himself or others."[20] (Nottidge, incidentally, fled back to the Abode of Love and handed over all her money to Prince. She would remain there until her death in 1858, and indeed thereafter, for she was buried beneath Agapemone's lawn.)[21]

And other women were perhaps the most famous complainers during the second half of the nineteenth century. The novelist and politician Sir Edward Bulwer-Lytton (he of the infamous opening line, "It was a dark and stormy night") had a sharp-tongued and spendthrift wife, Lady Rosina, of whom he eventually tired. His novels proving hugely successful, he set up a stable of mistresses. The married couple's domestic bliss was by now gone. Bulwer-Lytton on occasion beat Rosina and perhaps sodomized her. They officially separated in 1836, nine years after their marriage. Then Lady Lytton began her own career as a writer; much of what she wrote was barely veiled criticism of her estranged husband, full of her sense of rage and betrayal.[22] He threatened to ruin her if she kept it up. An affair in Dublin cost her custody of her children, and the whole sorry business of a broken Victorian marriage took a further turn for the worse when Lady Lytton discovered that her daughter, dying of typhoid, had been exiled by Bulwer-Lytton to a down-at-heel boarding house.

Lady Rosina began to bombard her well-connected husband and his powerful friends with letters filled with obscenities and libels, and eventually, in 1858, when Bulwer-Lytton stood for re-election at Hertford, she showed up and denounced him before the electors, haranguing them for nearly an hour. The response from her angry spouse was immediate: he cut off her allowance (which, in any event, he had paid only intermittently and with great reluctance) and forbade her any contact with their son. But then he took a further step, which he would live to regret: he obtained the legally required lunacy certificates from two compliant doctors and had Rosina confined in a madhouse run by Robert Gardiner Hill.

Shutting up Lady Rosina was intended to silence her; it had the opposite effect. Bulwer-Lytton evidently thought that his many connections—his close friendship with one of the Lunacy Commissioners, John Forster, for example, and with the editor of the *Times* (who indeed tried to protect him by suppressing all mention of the scandal)—would keep the matter quiet. But the *Times*'s great rival, the *Daily Telegraph* (whose very existence, ironically enough, owed much to Bulwer-Lytton's efforts to reduce the stamp tax that newspapers had to pay), took great delight in pursuing the salacious scandal. Within weeks, Bulwer-Lytton, facing an avalanche of bad publicity, capitulated, releasing his wife on condition that she relocate abroad—something she briefly did, only to return and spend the rest of her life blackening his name, not desisting even after his death from complications following ear surgery.[23]

The enormous suspicion with which many regarded those who ran asylums intensified in the aftermath of a series of other cases calling into question the motives and competence of even the most prominent alienists of the age. John Conolly, previously the superintendent of the first public asylum for London at Hanwell, and famous for his role in abolishing mechanical restraint in his asylum, was held liable for major damages in the case of a Mr. Ruck, whose certificates he had signed at the instigation of Ruck's wife. It turned out that the proprietor of the madhouse to which the alcoholic Ruck had been consigned paid Conolly fees for the referral, not to mention a further £60 a year for so long as Ruck remained confined.[24]

Forbes Winslow, who in 1848 had founded the first English journal on the science and treatment of mental illness, the *Quarterly Journal of Psychological Medicine,* had a different problem. He testified at the lunacy inquisition held in the case of the immensely wealthy William Windham that the gentleman was mad: he openly masturbated; ate voraciously at dinner parties and then vomited at table so he could eat yet more; had impersonated a train guard and nearly caused a train crash; wore servant's clothes; and had contracted syphilis and then married a prostitute. But for whatever reason, many of Winslow's colleagues, Conolly prominent among them, insisted that Windham was eccentric, not mad. The jury agreed. At a staggering cost of some £20,000, Windham had secured his freedom.[25] He drank, spent, and fornicated his way to oblivion in the space of scarce two years, dying at only twenty-five. The jury's verdict in this extraordinary case was just one more sign of how deeply suspicious of madhouses (and those running them) the British public remained, and it was a mistrust that would be nurtured and fed by yet more scandal and evidence of financial corruption on the part of alienists in the remaining years of the nineteenth century.

The cases of Ruck and Windham remind us that a great many of the Victorian causes celèbres revolved around the improper confinement of men, not women—though, like the coverage of the Nottidge affair and the case of Lady Rosina, the newspaper attention to cases featuring men was often intensified by lurid tales of sexual impropriety (Ruck had fathered two children in a long-running affair with his sister-in-law, and Winslow's sexual escapades were legion). Still, perhaps the most determined and in some ways the most effective complainers about psychiatry were two women: Louisa Lowe and Georgina Weldon, both spiritualists, and both major sources of trouble for those claiming expertise in mental medicine.[26]

Some of us might conclude that those who harbor a belief in automatic writing or the ability to commune with spirits in other worlds have a tenuous hold on reality, but in the Victorian era, such notions were seen as plausible even by many highly educated folk—Lunacy Commissioners and alienists included.[27] But the content of the messages Louisa Lowe received from the netherworld had its own complications: her automatic writing included much that was obscene and upsetting, not least the allegation that her husband, Reverend Lowe, was engaged in an incestuous relationship with their seven-year-old daughter and was a serial adulterer besides. (No other evidence existed to support either accusation.) And Georgina Weldon was a real-life Mrs. Jellyby who persuaded her husband to lease the grand Tavistock House and then turned it into a slum: her pet dogs left their excrement everywhere; her children ran wild, dressed in rags and living in filth; and adopted "orphan" children were brought in randomly, given singing lessons, and put up to public performances conducted by the estimable Mrs. Weldon herself. All sorts of dubious adults—including the French opera composer Charles Gounod and his mistress, and a con man and his common-law ex-prostitute wife—added to the mix, until the household grew so unbearable that poor Mr. Weldon moved out, though he continued to pay the bills.[28]

The gentlemen who had made the mistake of marrying these formidable ladies sought to shake themselves loose from the domestic horrors that enveloped them by arranging for their wives to be certified as lunatics and sent to a madhouse: Mrs. Lowe was confined at Brislington House and then Lawn House in Hanwell (John Conolly's old madhouse, by that time being run by his misanthropic and misogynist son-in-law Henry Maudsley), and finally at Lyttleton Forbes Winslow's Sussex House Asylum in Hammersmith. Foreseeing the fate that awaited her, Mrs. Weldon escaped from her would-be captors, waited for her certificates to expire, got a clean bill of health from her own choice of doctors, and then filed a whole series of lawsuits against all comers that occupied and entertained British courtroom onlookers for much of the 1880s.

As with Bulwer-Lytton, Mr. Winslow and Mr. Lowe badly miscalculated. Louisa Lowe wrote harrowing accounts of her captivity and spent nearly two decades attacking the motives and competence of the alienists with whom she had come into contact, most notably in the bestselling critique *The Bastilles of England, or The Lunacy Laws at Work* (1883). Georgina Weldon proved even more resourceful. She launched a string of lawsuits (seventeen in 1884 alone), which delivered her endless publicity and more than a few damage awards. Juries and judges seem to have shared her low opinion of the mad-doctors and their diagnoses, and to have sympathized with the notion that it was odious to lock up the eccentric and the unconventional in asylums. It became her life's work to humiliate her husband and the medics he had employed to try to bring her to heel. "May God give me the means, give me the allies, to ruin them," she wrote in her diary. And God duly obliged, or Mrs. Weldon acted nobly in his place. Reputational ruin was her goal, and her accomplishment—as was changing the lunacy laws. In 1890, a new Lunacy Act required the involvement of a magistrate in all certification of lunatics, and certificates were made valid for only a year at a time. In practice, such legal changes served only to ossify still further the empire of asylumdom.

Nor did these changes choke off the culture of complaint. Consider just the examples of Virginia Woolf, Janet Frame, and Sylvia Plath. Sir William Bradshaw in *Mrs. Dalloway* (1925) is a brutal fictionalized rendition of Woolf's own disastrous encounter with Sir George Savage, whose psychiatric practice centered on the chattering classes. Sylvia Plath's roman à

clef *The Bell Jar* (1963), a novel that became a feminist classic in the aftermath of its author's sad suicide, casts mid-twentieth-century psychiatry,
and particularly its resort to shock treatments, in a distinctly unflattering
light. From the late 1940s onward, the New Zealand novelist Janet Frame
spent years of her life in a series of dire mental hospitals, where, like many
of her contemporaries, she endured life-threatening insulin comas, not to
mention more than two hundred electroshocks, all for naught. At one
point, in 1951, she came within weeks of being lobotomized, only to have
her brain and her talents spared when she won a major literary prize.
These encounters with the horrors of institutional psychiatry are the dominant theme of her novels and her three-volume autobiography,[29] which
was made into the award-winning film *An Angel at My Table* (1990).

And in the twentieth century, as in the one preceding it, complaints
came from pens of men as well. Ken Kesey's *One Flew Over the Cuckoo's
Nest* (1962) was based on its author's experiences in a California mental
hospital. Adapted by Milòs Foreman, the film version featured Jack
Nicholson in the role of a lifetime, as the rebel Randle P. McMurphy. Fairly
or unfairly, the film cemented psychiatry's reputation in many quarters as
an instrument of repression. It ended with the irrepressible McMurphy
reduced to a vegetable by a lobotomy.[30]

Among social scientists, the period between the late 1950s and the 1970s
saw the development of a steadily more elaborate set of complaints about
psychiatry and its pretensions. A series of increasingly critical ethnogra-
phies of the mental hospital in particular culminated in Erving Goffman's
searing 1961 critique of them as "total institutions."[31] Their nearest ana-
logues, he suggested, were such things as prisons and concentration camps.
Far from being places of treatment and cure, they were more properly seen
as engines of degradation, misery, and oppression that worsened, or even
created, the symptoms of chronic mental illness. Within five years, the
California sociologist Thomas Scheff had advanced an even more audacious hypothesis: mental illness, he alleged in his *Being Mentally Ill* (1966),
was not a medical disease at all but a matter of labels. Scheff's arguments
were seriously flawed, conceptually and empirically, and over the years he
steadily retracted his more extreme statements. But the fact that they were
granted credence in some quarters is a measure of how much damage the
culture of complaint had done to psychiatry's public standing.

Besides, in those same years, equally fierce complaints were being launched from within psychiatry itself. Scottish psychiatrist R. D. Laing was voicing the heretical (and in my view absurd) claim that schizophrenia was a voyage of discovery that should be indulged and encouraged, and he was temporarily receiving a respectful hearing among intellectuals. Across the Atlantic, Thomas Szasz published the bestselling *The Myth of Mental Illness* (1960), followed by a host of derivative publications that repeated the theme that mental illness was nothing more than a bad metaphor with no legitimate status as an object of medical science. His fellow psychiatrists, he proclaimed, systematically violated their patients' rights and trust, acting as jailers and agents of social control on behalf of society at large, not as therapists.

Szasz's assaults on his profession were legitimized in part by accumulating evidence of its inability to distinguish the mad from the sane. Throughout the 1960s and 1970s, a series of careful studies had demonstrated that psychiatrists, when confronted with a patient, could not be relied on to reach a consistent conclusion about his or her mental state.[32] A meticulous cross-national comparison had shown that manic depression was diagnosed five times as often in Britain as in the United States, the mirror image of the situation with respect to schizophrenia.[33] In courtrooms and clinics, psychiatrists cast doubt on their clinical competence by routinely failing to agree about what was wrong with a given patient, or whether anything was wrong at all.[34] This embarrassing state of affairs was made far worse in 1973, when *Science* published a paper by the Stanford psychologist David Rosenhan, "On Being Sane in Insane Places," that purported to show how readily psychiatrists were deceived when confronted with sham patients.[35]

Though the American Psychiatric Association had published two editions (in 1952 and 1968) of a *Diagnostic and Statistical Manual,* which purported to list a variety of types of mental disorder, most psychiatrists paid them little mind, and in any event, they proved useless as practical guides to diagnosis.[36] But amid the rising tide of complaints, the unreliability of the diagnostic process had become a major liability for the profession, a threat to its very legitimacy that was far greater than the long-standing culture of complaint among patients, whose grumblings were always vulnerable to the counter-allegation that they came from those of dubious mental competence.[37] Stung into action, mainstream psychiatry urgently sought to address the problem. The upshot, in 1980, was the publication of the third edition of the *DSM*.

What *DSM III* (and its various successors) represent, however, is not an attempt to cut nature at the joints. Unable even at this late date to demonstrate convincing chains of causation for any major form of mental disorder, the task force that produced the manual abandoned any pretense at doing so. Instead, they concentrated on maximizing inter-rater reliability among psychiatrists, developing lists of symptoms that allegedly characterized different forms of mental disturbance and matching those to a tick-the-boxes approach to diagnosis. When faced with new patients, psychiatrists would record the presence or absence of a given set of symptoms, and once a threshold number of these had been reached, the person they were examining was given a particular diagnostic label, and comorbidity was invoked to explain away situations where more than one "illness" could be diagnosed. Disputes about what belonged in the manual were resolved by committee votes, as was the arbitrary decision about where to situate cut-off points—that is, how many of the laundry list of symptoms a patient had to exhibit before they were declared to be suffering from a particular form of illness. Questions of validity—such as whether the new classificatory system corresponded with distinctions in nature so that the listed "diseases" corresponded in some sense with distinctions that made etiological sense— were simply set to one side. If diagnoses could be rendered mechanical and predictable, consistent and replicable, that would suffice.[38]

In the years that have followed, the successive editions of the *DSM* have grown like the Yellow Pages on steroids. Definitions have been broadened, ever-newer forms of pathology have been "discovered" (most neatly helping to create markets for new versions of psychoactive drugs), and more and more of the range of normal human experience has been drawn into psychiatry's net.[39] Bipolar disorder, once rare, has become an epidemic, and psychiatrists have diagnosed it for the first time in children. Depression is now widely called the common cold of psychiatry, so broad its remit and so frequent its diagnosis. The decision in 2013 to treat grief as a mental illness will amplify that trend. There has been a massive increase in children being diagnosed with autism and attention deficit hyperactivity disorder, not to mention things like school phobia.

One might expect this expansion of the psychiatric imperium to encounter some pushback—and so it has in some quarters. In Oregon as early as 1970, complaining patients formed the short-lived Mental Patients Liberation Front. In California, angry patients formed NAPA in 1974 (named after California's largest remaining traditional mental hospital—the initials stand for Network Against Psychiatric Assault). In 1988, patients who called themselves consumer-survivors created Support Coalition International, later renamed MindFreedom International. But there have also been some paradoxical developments. NAMI, the National Alliance on Mental Illness, was formed in 1979, primarily by the families of mental patients, and has acted largely to defend contemporary, somatically orientated psychiatry and to promulgate the notion that mental illness is purely biological, simply a brain disease—a notion so congenial to Big Pharma that they have secretly underwritten NAMI's operations with large sums of money.[40] And efforts by some to tighten the wording of diagnoses like autism—loosened in 1994 in *DSM IV,* with devastating effects—have encountered huge opposition from parents who want the diagnosis and the state assistance it brings in managing their children.[41]

But perhaps the most striking thing about the debates that erupted over the latest edition of the manual, *DSM 5,* was their source. For the most vocal critics of the document that for more than three decades has taken its place at the very heart of contemporary psychiatric practice, and that must be used by health providers in the United States if they expect to receive reimbursement from the medical insurance industry, have turned out to be psychiatrists themselves, and not just any psychiatrists, but the editors of the third and fourth editions of the manual, Robert Spitzer and Allen Frances.[42] Relentlessly, these two men attacked the science (or rather the lack of science) that lay behind the proposed revisions and raised warnings that they would further extend psychiatry's tendency to pathologize normal human behaviors. For orthodox psychiatrists, it was a deeply embarrassing spectacle. It is one thing to be attacked by Tom Cruise and the Scientologists (a group easy to dismiss as a cult), but quite another to come under withering assault from one's own. Wounded, the leaders of American psychiatry struck back with ad hominem attacks, alleging that Spitzer and Frances were clinging to past glories, and going so far as to suggest that Frances, by far the more energetic of the two, was motivated by the potential loss of $10,000 a year in royalties he still collected from *DSM IV*.[43] (Left unmentioned was how dependent their professional association had become on the many millions of dollars in royalties a new edition promised to provide.) The prolonged controversy forced a delay in the issuance of the new manual but seems to have done little to alter its basic structure and contents.

It has sufficed, however, to undermine, perhaps fatally, the legitimacy of *DSM* 5 and perhaps the psychiatric profession's standing more broadly. On May 6, 2013, just two weeks before *DSM* 5 was due to hit the marketplace, Thomas Insel, the director of the National Institute of Mental Health (NIMH), made an announcement. The manual, he proclaimed, suffered from a scientific "lack of validity. . . . As long as the research community takes the *D.S.M.* to be a bible, we'll never make progress. People think everything has to match *D.S.M.* criteria, but you know what? Biology never read that book." The NIMH, he said, would be "reorienting its research away from *D.S.M.* categories [because] mental patients deserve better." In the spirit of piling on, one of the former directors of the institute, Steven Hyman, added his assessment of the whole enterprise. It was, he opined, "totally wrong in a way [its authors] couldn't have imagined. . . . What they produced was an absolute scientific nightmare. Many people who get one diagnosis get five diagnoses, but they don't have five diseases—they have one underlying condition."[44] Just what that condition might be remains startlingly unclear. A few months before his savage dismissal of *DSM* 5, Insel had gone even further, expressing incredulity that most of his psychiatric colleagues "actually believe [that the diseases they diagnose using the *DSM*] are real. But there's no reality. These are just constructs. There is no reality to schizophrenia or depression. . . . We might have to stop using terms like depression and schizophrenia, because they are getting in our way, confusing things."[45]

Some might argue that to hear the head of the NIMH saying such things might itself be construed as being a trifle confusing, or even destabilizing. Surely, if someone in his position keeps uttering such unpalatable truths, the very legitimacy of the psychiatric enterprise will be threatened. A century ago, it was the inmates in the asylum who were complaining about psychiatry. Now the psychiatric piñata is being whacked by the mad-doctors themselves. An extraordinary development, to be sure. Whatever else these developments portend, one thing is certain: the old tradition of complaining about mental medicine shows no sign of withering away, though complaining about psychiatry in its latest incarnation has assumed some newly surprising forms.

5 Promises of Miracles

RELIGION AS SCIENCE, AND SCIENCE AS RELIGION

Illness, Mary Baker Eddy assured her followers, was all in the mind. Prayers could dispel the illusion that one was sick, for illness was purely a matter of belief, and God's power, once acknowledged and accepted, had the capacity to heal, redeem, and restore anyone. All that was necessary was to abandon the false faith in matter and embrace the workings of the Spirit: "The physical healing of Christian Science," she wrote, "results now, as in Jesus' time, from the operation of divine Principle, before which sin and disease lose the reality in human consciousness and disappear as naturally and as necessarily as darkness gives place to light and sin to reformation."[1]

Though only one thousand copies were printed of the first edition (1874) of her *Science and Health,* by 1891 it had appeared in fifty editions. (It remains in print to this day, having sold, its publishers claim, more than ten million copies.) In the closing decades of the nineteenth century, thousands had flocked to join her Church of Christ, Scientist, and many of them paid the princely sum of $300 apiece to learn the practice of spiritual healing at her Massachusetts Metaphysical College. Cancer, tuberculosis, heart disease, diphtheria, blindness, and a host of lesser ailments vanished under her stern gaze, or so her followers testified. By the early twentieth century, the number of those professing Christian Science had grown from the twenty-six followers who had founded the first church in 1879 to more than one hundred thousand souls.

Mother Eddy's teachings had made her rich, and she could well afford to ignore Mark Twain's savage assessment of her qualities and motives: "Grasping, sordid, penurious, famishing for everything she sees—money, power, glory—vain, untruthful, jealous, despotic, arrogant, insolent, pitiless where thinkers and hypnotists are concerned, illiterate, shallow, incapable of reasoning outside of commercial lines, immeasurably selfish."[2] In her writings, he continued, "not a single (material) thing is conceded to be real, except the Dollar." For those seeking her guidance, "the terms are cash; and not only cash, but cash in advance. . . . Not a spiritual Dollar, but a real one." Eddy owned the Church lock, stock, and barrel, and nothing stood in the way of its "hunger . . . for the Dollar, its adoration of the Dollar, its lust after the Dollar, its ecstasy in the mere thought of the Dollar."[3] However apt Twain's evaluation, his words had little effect, and for decades the ranks of Christian Science continued to swell. Indeed, his own daughter became a devotee.

Nineteenth-century America gave birth to a host of new forms of Christianity, and Christian Science was not the only one to link its teachings to the promotion of health. The Seventh Day Adventists, for instance, who trace their origins back to the Second Great Awakening and the expectations of the End of Time and the second coming of Christ that gripped the followers of William Miller in the early 1840s, made wholeness and health (and an emphasis on "pure" food) a central part of their daily lives. Once the church-owned Western Health Reform Institute passed into the hands of the Kellogg brothers, two prominent adherents to the faith, it was quickly transformed into the Battle Creek Sanitarium. The 106 patients it had attracted in 1876 were swamped by the 7,006 who patronized it in 1906 alone. All sorts of affluent patients—"nervous" invalids, those plagued by insomnia and headaches, burdened by the stresses of modern life, or complaining of a multitude of aches and pains—came to recharge their batteries. John Harvey Kellogg introduced them to a regime based on a cleansing, vegetarian diet (he claimed that meat rotted in the gut and poisoned the system), frequent enemas to cleanse the colon, abstinence from alcohol and sex, cold showers, electrotherapy and phototherapy, and plentiful open-air exercise. Clean bowels and defecating several times a day were, it would seem, the route to health and happiness, and an in-house laboratory for fecal analysis provided a scientific check on the patients' progress.[4]

It was a formula that attracted both the great and the not so good. Patients included Lincoln's widow, Mary Todd Lincoln; Amelia Earhart; Alfred Dupont, Henry Ford, and John D. Rockefeller; presidents Warren G. Harding and William Howard Taft; Thomas Edison; and the original Tarzan, Johnny Weissmuller. In the long run, though, it was the Kelloggs' breakfast cereal business—originally a spin-off for those unable to afford a sanitarium visit—that made them multimillionaires.

Unlike the Battle Creek Sanitarium, which retained its respectable status until an ill-advised expansion on the eve of the Great Depression brought it to the brink of bankruptcy, Christian Science was almost immediately attacked as a "mind-healing cult." That the bulk of Mary Baker Eddy's followers were female (72 percent in 1906) probably didn't help the Christian Science cause, given the low opinion most fin-de-siècle males had for the "weaker" sex's powers of reasoning. Nor did its founder's lack of visible qualifications, either theological or medical. (Kellogg, by contrast, was a trained physician.) Still, medical men began to worry about what the medical historian Barbara Sicherman called the "exodus of patients from the doctor's waiting room to the minister's study."[5] It was a concern that led the New York neurologist Charles Dana to suggest to his colleagues, "We must find out the good behind these false methods and organize it into some wise scientific measure which we can prescribe. Until we do this there will be a continual succession of new cults, Christian Science, osteopathy, etc., to the discredit of medicine and more especially of psychiatry."[6]

Another form of religiously based psychotherapy did indeed begin to emerge in Boston, centered around the ultrarespectable Church of Christ Emmanuel and led by two clergymen, Elwood Worcester and Samuel McComb. At first, Worcester and McComb sought allies among leading Boston physicians, who examined some of the many followers who showed up for psychotherapy and lent the Emmanuel Movement their support. Very quickly, however, the movement veered toward an emphasis on religious consolation and psychotherapy, and men like the Harvard professors William James and James Jackson Putnam recoiled from the Frankenstein they belatedly realized they might have helped create.[7] On

Freud's only visit to the United States, in 1909, he took time to reject these "affronts to science and reason," and to caution that "the instrument of the soul is not so easy to play, [and] any amateur attempt may have the most evil consequence."[8] The Emmanuel Movement persisted for perhaps a decade more and then gradually faded from sight, its only lasting legacy being its links to the birth of Alcoholics Anonymous.

The impulse to yoke together the spiritual and the psychological (and in some cases injunctions about diet and regimen), and to connect these doctrines to claims at having discovered the royal road to health and well-being, was not confined to the fin de siècle. To the contrary, the 1950s, 1960s, and 1970s saw a rash of efforts along these lines, and like a handful of their precursors, some of these enterprises proved vastly profitable for those who created them. Among the least organized of these (as befits its counterculture origins) was the Human Potential Movement, an amalgam of vague doctrines derived from humanistic psychology that saw itself as rescuing its followers from the sterility of mainstream psychology and organized religion. Claiming that their methods could enhance psychological health, creativity, and personal growth, a variety of therapists marched under this banner, promising greater mindfulness and a healthier, more productive existence.

Christian Science and the Emmanuel Movement had their origins in the spiritualism and transcendentalism of New England, but it was California that gave birth to most of their latter-day successors. Esalen, Erhard Seminars Training (EST), Arthur Janov's Primal Scream Therapy, and the like all had their origins in La La Land, as did Scientology, arguably the most long-lasting, profitable, and sinister of all these organizations that claimed to contribute in novel ways to health and human happiness. Christian Science had secured a prominent following among celebrities, most especially the Hollywood crowd. Joan Crawford, Cecil DeMille, Mary Pickford, Mickey Rooney, Doris Day, King Vidor, and Ginger Rogers all succumbed to its charms. The 1940s and 1950s saw many of their counterparts embrace psychoanalysis in its place, but the derivatives of the Human Potential Movement proved more attractive in Tinseltown in later decades.

Esalen attracted such disparate figures as Joan Baez, Aldous Huxley, Yoko Ono, and John Denver, among a host of others. Primal Scream Therapy's most famous patient was John Lennon (Yoko Ono also attended sessions). But Scientology has surpassed them all, accruing vast wealth, a legion of followers in the movie business (though a decreasing following elsewhere), and the legal status of a modern religion—which it acquired in the United States and Britain after long legal fights and many murky maneuvers.[9]

Remarkably, of course, its doctrines were the product of L. Ron Hubbard, a hack science fiction writer who proceeded to write a self-help book, *Dianetics* (1950), that recycled the usual bromides that populate the pages of that genre, with an added dash of the Eastern mysticism that so many of its rival pop psychologies also embraced. *Dianetics* promised to increase the intelligence of its readers, eliminate negative and unwanted emotions, and alleviate a host of illnesses. Those who sought "exquisite clarity and mental liberation" had found their man. Within two years, more than a hundred thousand copies of the book had been sold. Four years later, Hubbard decided that the therapeutic techniques he had discovered deserved a different kind of status: that of a religion.

Scientologists are taught that most physical and mental diseases are psychic phenomena rooted in scars called engrams that its audits bring to the surface and thus expel. Their bodies are but a temporary housing for their Thetans, souls that have existed for millions, if not billions, of years and will survive their earthly demise. Getting rid of the problems locked in their reactive minds is the goal of increasingly expensive therapy sessions, which serve to remove the poisonous experiences that otherwise remain trapped in their subconscious, extract ever-greater amounts of money from their pockets, and provide the church with a litany of discrediting information about them that it can deploy as it sees fit.

Mary Baker Eddy's seminars, where she taught acolytes how to become Christian Science therapists, earned her a small fortune. Scientology's far more elaborate series of audits and its years-long pathway to spiritual enlightenment have yielded a vast one. Fiercely critical of psychiatry, which it calls an "industry of death," it has repelled all legal challenges to its existence. To those willing to listen to its siren songs, it promises "the attainment of Man's dreams through the ages of attaining a new and higher state of existence and freedom from the endless cycle of birth, death, birth." At length, one enters the wondrous state of being "clear": "Clear is the total erasure of the reactive mind from which stems all the anxieties and problems the individual has." Pay even more—hundreds of thousands of dollars in some cases—and you can advance still further, to the status of an OT, or Operating Thetan. Indeed, just hand over enough money, set aside your critical faculties, and you too can attain Nirvana.

Human credulity is a wonderful thing.

PART II Whither Twentieth-Century
Psychiatry?

6 Burying Freud

It is a truth universally acknowledged, that Freud is dead. Any number of reference books will confirm that he died in London on September 23, 1939. Most agree that his death was a case of doctor-assisted suicide from a lethal dose of morphine administered by his long-time personal physician, Dr. Max Schur, when the agonies of his decades-long struggle with cancer of the jaw became unbearable. It seems, however, that like a zombie, Freud cannot remain quietly in his grave—or in his case, urn.

For a quarter-century, critics and defenders have sparred over his legacy and its value. One side of the famous Freud wars insists he is an intellectual as well as a literal corpse, while a chorus of epigones indignantly insists that reports of his demise are greatly exaggerated. Freud lives, or at least his great invention, psychoanalysis and its associated theory of mind, lives on as one of the great discoveries of the human race, on a par with Copernicus's heliocentric theory of the universe and Darwin's theory of evolution. Is Dr. Freud Dr. Fraud, as many British psychiatrists of the early twentieth century alleged? Or is he someone whose explorations of the dark corners of our unconscious represent the most daring and successful attempt to date to probe the mysteries of human nature?

Certainly, psychoanalysis has lost most of the luster it once commanded in psychiatric circles. Mainstream British psychiatry, it is true, never warmed to the Viennese doctor. Britain's first professor of psychiatry called his doctrines a "seething mass of foulness" and "insidious poison," and another prominent colleague predicted that Freud's system would soon go "to join pounded toads and sour milk in the limbo of discarded remedies."[1]

In the United States, after some initial hesitations, it was quite otherwise. For at least a quarter-century after World War II, American psychiatry was dominated by psychoanalysis. Virtually all the major academic departments of psychiatry were headed by Freudians or Freudian fellow travelers who professed allegiance to psychodynamic psychiatry. Americans were used to shelling out hard cash for their medical care, and in the affluent times that followed the war, the more well-to-do among them flocked to the analytic couch. The top recruits to the psychiatric profession paid large sums to undergo training analyses to secure access to the most "interesting" (and lucrative) patients, and they were rewarded with incomes far higher than those of the average physician. The dregs among the trainees retreated to the humdrum existence of an institutional psychiatrist, dispensing "directive-organic therapy" (electroshock, lobotomy, and, increasingly, psychotropic drugs) instead of the magic talking cure. In 1954, a state hospital psychiatrist made on average $9,000 a year; his psychoanalytic colleague, $22,000.

The dominance of Freudian ideas was not confined to the formal setting of the analyst's office. The social and geographical mobility that marked the postwar years saw young mothers who were cut off from extended multigenerational families turn for child-rearing advice to books, most especially Benjamin Spock's *Baby and Child Care* (1946), one of the bestselling books of all time (more than fifty million copies sold), where they encountered a perspective on childhood deeply indebted to Freud's ideas. Such world-famous analysts as Bruno Bettelheim taught those unfortunate enough to have children with autism or schizophrenia that these problems were their fault: refrigerator mothers had wreaked emotional and cognitive devastation on their offspring. Often crudely, as is their wont, the moguls of Hollywood wove psychoanalytic themes into many a movie, from Hitchcockian thrillers to dramas and melodramas, and novelists happily embraced the chance to write of sex and repression. Madison Avenue embraced the art of subliminal advertising, led by Freud's nephew, Edward Bernays, and artists sought to treat with the world of the surreal. In universities, would-be philosophers, social scientists, and literary sorts all encountered Freud, and most pronounced themselves enriched by the experience—no one more so than the young professor of literature Frederick Crews, who channeled his enthusiasm for Freud and all things Freudian into well-received work on psychoanalysis and literary criticism.

But beginning in the late 1970s, mainstream American psychiatry repented of its infatuation with Freud. Embracing the magic potions of modern psychopharmacology (and selling their souls to Big Pharma), late twentieth-century psychiatrists opted for a crude biological reductionism. Pills rapidly replaced talk as the dominant response to disturbances of emotion, cognition, and behavior. A resurgent biological psychiatry taught a broader public that mental illness was a disease of the brain, not the mind—a product of a murky mix of unfortunate hereditary endowment and faulty brain biochemistry, such as defects of dopamine or a shortage of serotonin. Biobabble replaced psychobabble. Those still enamored of superegos, egos, and ids and who preferred to wrestle with transference and countertransference found themselves exiled to the margins of the profession.

The defenestration of psychoanalytic psychiatry occurred with remarkable speed. Within less than a decade, academic departments engaged in an Oedipal revolt against their Freudian "fathers" and instead installed neuroscientists as their leaders. The third edition of the *DSM* (1980) dispensed with all reference to Freudian ideas, cast aside such diagnoses as neurosis and hysteria, and treated symptoms as the essence of psychiatric illness, not the surface manifestations of deeper psychological conflicts requiring interminable psychoanalytic inquiries. Trainee professionals deserted the psychoanalytic institutes in droves. In 2010, the American Psychoanalytic Association reported a 50 percent decline over a thirty-year period in the number of applicants for training and what they called "an even more precipitous decline in applications from psychiatrists." Until the 1980s, American psychoanalysis had resolutely rejected the idea of lay analysts. Everyone who sought its imprimatur had to possess a medical degree.

But even the waiving of this requirement, in 1987, could not stem the collapse of the enterprise. The demographic trends are cruel and unmistakable: in 2012, the International Psychoanalytic Association announced that 70 percent of the members of its component societies were aged between fifty and seventy, 50 percent were older than sixty, and as many as 20 percent of the training analysts were over the age of seventy. As for academic psychology, it has never had much truck with Freud. William James, who attended one of Freud's 1909 lectures at Clark University, was scornful about the theories, attacking symbolism as "a most dangerous method" and dismissing Freud as "a man obsessed with fixed ideas" and someone who appeared to be "a regular *halluciné*."[2] University departments of psychology, then and now, responded to psychoanalysis by simply ignoring it, treating it as beneath mention.

Yet if Freud is dead, the news has taken an inordinately long time reaching the publishing industry. Indeed, those bent on selling books still seem endlessly fascinated by the man, and every publishing season produces a new crop of books on psychoanalysis and its founder. In 2016 alone, for example, Harvard University Press and Cambridge University Press issued two huge new biographies, by Elisabeth Roudinesco and Joel Whitebook, respectively, and there must be at least three dozen other accounts of Freud's life out there, all competing for attention and all presumably finding some sort of audience.

Most of these biographies ought more properly to be labeled hagiographies, stretching all the way from Ernest Jones's three volume sanitized version of his master to Peter Gay's notoriously varnished account of the heroic Freud single-handedly wrestling with and subduing the daemons of the unconscious. The Princeton philosopher Richard Wollheim even ventured the opinion that Freud did "as much for [humanity] as any other human being who has ever lived."[3] Not to be outdone, the prolific psychoanalyst Christopher Bollas announced that "the Freudian Moment . . . had changed man forever" and had arrived in the nick of time, "at the moment when its implementation might rescue humanity from self-destruction."[4]

Biographies, of course, are but the tip of the iceberg. There is a host of volumes of varying degrees of sophistication, masticating and regurgitating Freudian ideas and often providing incestuous accounts of the psychoanalytic enterprise, their utility as a defense of this form of psychiatry marred only by the notorious factionalism that has gripped the movement from its very earliest years. Then again, anyone inclined to doubt that Freud still has a massive following need only publish something even faintly disapproving about him or his work. An army of defenders will rise up at once to accuse the critic of intellectual sloppiness, misunderstanding, or, worse, faults reflecting the author's unconscious hostility or unresolved resistance to the truth.

For over a quarter-century, however, an increasing number of Freud's critics have been anything but just faintly disapproving. There have been, it is true, sober, dense, and dull monographs, such as Adolf Grunbaum's examination of the philosophical foundations of psychoanalysis (or the lack thereof), but by design those rarely find a broad public audience.[5] Other writers have been much less restrained, and the ferocity of their assaults, couched (if I may be permitted a bad pun) in much fiercer and more polemical language, have sparked wide-ranging intellectual fights that erupt with great frequency and passion on both sides. There is a profound irony here. Freud's most severe critics want to insist that he is a dead parrot, a charlatan whose ideas can be safely and properly ignored. Yet to (mis)quote a leading anti-Freudian, Frank Cioffi, "Freudian apologists [have every reason to] welcome [their] objections as the Undead welcome nightfall,"[6] for the very fervor of the critics' objections helps to sustain the notion that there is something profoundly important at stake here. For an intellectual or an intellectual edifice, to be ignored is far worse than to be attacked as misguided or wrong.

At this point, the Freud bashers (as their opponents have dubbed them) might do well to learn this lesson and let the sectarian members of what they regard as a hopeless cult argue with one another in a hermetically sealed, ever-diminishing circle. That is a tactic that seems beyond their grasp or capacity though. Instead, as night follows day, the issuance of still another paean of praise to the alleged discoverer of the unconscious provokes an equally predictable counterblast from the opposition.

On cue, Frederick Crews, who has been one of the most savage combatants since the early 1990s, has now issued another assault on the psychoanalytic redoubt. As its title signals, *Freud: The Making of an Illusion* is directed principally at the character of the founding father. By destroying the reputation of the man, Crews evidently seeks to drive a stake through the heart of the undead (or perhaps to scatter Freud's ashes to the wind, beyond retrieval). He is relentless in the pursuit of his target, utterly unsparing, not scrupling to use any weapon that comes to hand. Freud, as he emerges from these pages, is a revolting and quite deplorable human being, the complete opposite of the Olympian, near-immortal figure of flawless integrity Peter Gay once presented to us.

In life and in death, a Praetorian Guard sought to protect Freud's reputation. His Secret Committee, with gold rings to signal their loyalty, was a cabal that surrounded him and sought to ward off debate and excommunicate and punish heretics. Later, Ernest Jones and Freud's daughter Anna worked alongside such powerful analysts as Kurt Eissler, the director of the Freud Archives, to sanitize Freud's papers and letters, to embargo many of them for decades (some until 2113), and to publish bowdlerized and misleading versions of crucial materials. Jeffrey Masson, the renegade analyst who succeeded Eissler as director of the Freud Archives, began to break down this wall of silence and obfuscation in the 1980s by publishing Freud's complete correspondence with a friend he once adored, Wilhelm Fliess, and in our own century, Freud's huge correspondence with his fiancée Martha Bernays has been made available at the Library of Congress.

These documents are some of the most vital resources Crews draws on in constructing his case for the prosecution, and there is much in them that is deeply damaging to Freud's reputation. But Crews is scarcely unique in subjecting Freud's life to close scrutiny. Crews may be said to have behaved like Captain Ahab pursuing his whale for more than a quarter-century, but others have exhibited a still greater obsessiveness, and no one more so than Peter Swales. A high school dropout and the former publicist for the Rolling Stones, Swales subsequently became fixated on Freud and has devoted decades of his life to a minute examination of the Viennese doctor's every move. Despite his lack of formal academic training, Swales has proved to be an extraordinary sleuth, finding all sorts of new source material, hunting down obscure details, uncovering the identities of many of Freud's pseudonymous patients, exposing the depths of Freud's involvement with cocaine, and much more besides. Swales has inspired many more conventional academic figures to follow in his footsteps, and without question, many of Crews's more damning and sensational claims are borrowed from this body of work, and from Swales's revelations in particular. It is a debt Crews acknowledges, though I'm not sure that he does so sufficiently.

Crews's account of Freud's life is essentially confined to the period between his enrollment at the University of Vienna in 1873 and the end of the nineteenth century—the period marked by the publication of *The Interpretation of Dreams* (1899), *The Psychopathology of Everyday Life* (1901), and his account of his failed analysis of "Dora," aka Ida Bauer (which was written in 1901 but not published until 1905). He thus omits most of the last four decades of Freud's life, though there is much in those years that could have served as grist for his mill. No matter: Crews does not find himself short of material.

Freud first pursued a career as a neurologist, but Crews demonstrates convincingly that in this he was an utter failure. Worse, he stumbled across cocaine, which he would use extensively for a decade and a half, publishing encomiums to its therapeutic properties, especially its utility to "cure" morphine addiction, and not desisting even in the face of devastating evidence to the contrary. Freud's puff piece "On Coca" proclaimed he had overseen the cure of a patient who had become addicted to morphine in the aftermath of a medical accident. This was, in fact, the distinguished neurophysiologist Ernst Fleischl, who had served Freud as a mentor and financial supporter. Fleischl's thumb, most of which had been amputated after he nicked it in the course of an autopsy, caused him immense pain, which led to his morphine addiction. Far from curing him, the cocaine produced a double addiction, a slow and disastrous physical decline, and an early and awful death. Freud, however, publicly proclaimed great success with "entirely harmless injections of cocaine" and blithely added, "I have taken the drug myself for several months"—he would go on to do so for many years—"without experiencing any condition similar to morphinism or any yearning for continued use of cocaine." He was, to use more neutral language than Crews chooses to employ, being rather economical with the truth, and in ways with damaging real-world consequences for those who believed him.

When a colleague, Carl Koller, discovered that cocaine could be used as a local anesthetic—an extraordinarily consequential discovery—Freud later sought to rearrange history to suggest that he had suggested this finding to Koller and ought to have been awarded the credit. As Freud put it in his *Autobiographical Study* of 1925, "It was the fault of my fiancée that I was not already famous at [a] youthful age." That falsehood, Crews argues, was all too typical of Freud. Who can accept his claim, later in the same passage, that "I bore my fiancée no grudge for the interruption [that prevented an announcement of the discovery]"? Grudge or not, the assertion was a lie. It was of a piece with the mendacity that Crews shows running all through Freud's work in the late nineteenth century, both before and after he sought fame for the treatment of hysteria and nervous disorders.

With his career foundering because of his failure to make any major progress as a neurologist, Freud secured a fellowship to study under the most eminent neurologist of the fin de siècle, Jean-Martin Charcot. What his sponsor thought would be neurophysiological work on brain tissue in the laboratory instead brought Freud into contact with Charcot's hysterical circus—his weekly exploitation of scantily dressed female patients who performed their rituals in front of tout Paris. Charcot, once the author of great neurological discoveries, was by this time a self-deceived charlatan; the performances of his pet patients, allegedly the product of hypnosis, were in reality the effects of suggestion and artifice on their part. In that sense, Crews suggests, he was an excellent role model for the ambitious and unscrupulous Freud, who cultivated what he took to be a powerful sponsor by promising to translate Charcot's lectures into German, Freud's execrable French notwithstanding. As a careerist move, Freud's sycophancy was largely a failure, since the major figures in Viennese medicine deplored Charcot's use of hypnosis. To make matters worse, when Charcot died suddenly in 1893, his disciples, freed from their fear of the notoriously spiteful and vengeful man, promptly abandoned his teachings. Classical Charcotian *grande hysterie* almost immediately vanished from the stage, never to be seen again.

But once Freud moved back to Vienna, hysteria soon came back in a different form, as the centerpiece of his otherwise faltering medical practice. Earlier, he had had trouble qualifying as a doctor. He was a clumsy and bungling practitioner who hated his patients, and, as he wrote to his fiancée in 1886, he found the whole business "a sad way of earning one's bread." For a decade after Freud's return to Austria, a senior colleague, Josef Breuer (who had an extraordinarily successful practice among the haut bourgeois Jews of Vienna), sent him patients and lent him money. Eventually, Freud persuaded his mentor that they should publish a joint paper and then a monograph, *Studies on Hysteria*. It was an endeavor that was the basis of Freud's more extended foray into psychotherapy, and it became the foundation of his later fame as the founder of psychoanalysis.

Freud's hagiographers have hailed these events, and the appearance of his books about dreams and slips of the tongue, as marking the decisive years in his career, a time of intellectual discoveries and breakthroughs that led to his emergence as the Copernicus of the unconscious, the man who transformed our understanding of the human mind. Crews devotes most of his attention to these same years, attending closely to what Freud was up to in his consulting rooms and at his writing desk, but also examining the most intimate features of his private life and his relations with his medical colleagues, Breuer among them. His mission is not to praise the conquistador who discovered psychoanalysis but to savage him and then bury him in mud (or worse). Ideas and therapeutic practices matter here, but only insofar as they serve to blacken Freud's name and to inflict what Crews hopes will be fatal damage on his reputation. If Jeffrey Masson titled his revisionist (and wildly speculative) treatment of Freud's abandonment of seduction theory *The Assault on Truth*,[7] Crews's weighty tome might more properly be called *The Assault on Freud*. A murderous assault it is too, one that does not scruple to use any scrap of evidence, however tenuous, as part of the effort to bury Freud.

Previously we were introduced to a Freud who spent a decade and a half abusing cocaine and who got one of his best friends addicted to the drug and eventually killed, all the while denying what he was up to, writing puff pieces for drug companies whose favor he sought, and proving himself an unscrupulous and incompetent laboratory scientist. Along the way, he is shown to have dabbled in the occult (an activity that scarcely disappeared in later years), sought credit for others' discoveries, and connived and schemed his way in devious and discreditable fashion toward a hoped-for fame and fortune. (Freud's obsessive love of and need for money and status are themes Crews returns to again and again.) But whatever dark deeds Freud committed in the first decade of his career, they pale beside those that Crews alleges he got up to in the second half of the 1890s.

Freud was a masturbator, and he shared his culture's neuroses about the practice. Crews suggests that as an adolescent he may have incestuously assaulted one or more of his sisters—though his evidence for this explosive allegation strikes me as remarkably thin and speculative, of precisely the ambiguous and dubious sort he repeatedly attacks Freud for relying on. But he is on surer ground when he turns to Freud's treatment of his wife, whom he seems to have humiliated and ignored, employing her to produce a string of offspring and cater to his domestic needs but stifling her personality, scorning her intellect, and crushing her originally vivacious nature. Finding her too tedious for his taste, he became enamored of her younger sister Minna, who lived under their roof, and with whom he elected to take his extended holidays and shared an intellectual bond. And more than an intellectual bond: drawing on some of Peter Swales's extraordinary detective work, as well as an astute reading of what turn out to be disguised autobiographical "dreams," Crews presents what I regard as an unanswerable case that Freud seduced his sister-in-law, took her as his mistress, and even procured an abortion for her when she became pregnant—an abortion that nearly killed her.

So, Freud stands accused (and likely convicted) of being an exploiter of women and the archetypical patriarchal chauvinist pig. That sits uneasily with the received portrait of him as a superhuman self-denying hero, the first human in recorded history to have the genius, the courage, and the capacity to psychoanalyze himself, and thus to pass from the conflicted neurotic state in which the rest of humanity wallows to a higher, more perfect state of being. Perhaps Freud's self-analysis was not so successful after all.

Crews is equally determined to undermine and then demolish the empirical foundations of the Freudian intellectual edifice. Here, discovering the identity of the patients who grace the pages of *Studies in Hysteria* in anonymous guise is a crucial first step—not just "Anna O." (Bertha Pappenheim), Breuer's sole contribution to the menagerie, but all the others, even the ones who made only the most fleeting of appearances on the stage. That work of excavation is something Crews owes mostly to others, but once these women (and they are virtually all women) have been identified, a ton of other evidence tumbles into view. With but a few exceptions—a young waitress at an Alpine lodge ("Katherina," in reality Aurelia Kronick) and an English governess ("Miss Lucy R.," never identified)— Freud's patients were rich, sometimes extremely rich. They included, for example, Anna von Lieben ("Frau Caecilie M."), a baroness, and reputedly one of the richest women in Europe; and another baroness, Fanny Moser

("Frau Emmy von N."). However difficult and demanding these ladies proved to be, there was generally some compensation in the form of the handsome fees they paid—at least for a time.

The harsh truth that emerges (and there is no disputing it, notwithstanding Crews's evident parti pris) is that all these cases, far from being the successes that heralded a new psychological approach to the treatment of hysteria and other nervous disordered, were unmitigated disasters. Bertha Pappenheim, for instance, terminated what she called "chimney-sweeping" with Breuer of her own volition. Allegedly, the meticulous retracing of her buried memories back to their traumatic source had induced a succession of catharses and brought about a complete recovery. Except that she wasn't cured at all. Within a matter of weeks, she had to be admitted to the expensive private Belleview Sanatorium in Kreuzlingen, Switzerland. Apparently, her symptoms had not been "permanently removed," as *Studies on Hysteria* would have it. True, she would later recover and embark on a highly successful career as a feminist, lecturer, and social reformer, but she was openly contemptuous of the claim that the "talking cure" had in any way contributed to her recovery.

Crews points out that Freud was a clumsy and ineffectual hypnotist, and later innovations in his therapeutic technique did not change the picture. He was a lousy clinician. His patients didn't improve, and in short order or long, they tired of his ministrations and abandoned him. Anna von Lieben, for example, on Crews's account (and there is ample reason to believe him), "was a spoiled, willful, histrionic tyrant whose self-absorption and self-pity were underwritten by her wealth." Freud attended to her once or twice a day, secretly administering morphine injections to the addict. But eventually she (or her husband) tired of him, and he was sent on his way. She had, he wrote to Minna Bernays, arrived at "a state in which she can't stand me, because it is a matter of suspecting that I don't treat her out of friendship, but only for money." It was almost certainly the correct (if obvious) conclusion.

A few years later, another of Freud's most famous patients, "Dora" (Ida Bauer), would also flounce out on him, decrying his ministrations. It is a case Crews is all too happy to rehearse, because it shows Freud behaving appallingly. The young woman was eighteen years of age when she entered analysis—involuntarily, at the insistence of her parents. Bauer's story is a shocking one: her syphilitic father had been carrying on an affair with another man's wife, who had previously served as his nurse. Herr K., the cuckolded husband, repeatedly attempted to kiss and subsequently to seduce Ida, and when she complained to her parents about his behavior, they dismissed her as delusionary. It was soon apparent that she had been offered as a prize to Herr K., the price of his tolerating relations between her father and his wife. Hence her depression. But Freud believed that her symptoms, which included a persistent cough that may well have had organic roots, and her reported disgust when the middle-aged man made advances disguised the fact that she really wanted to have sex with him. For Freud, this was further confirmed by her disposition to fiddle constantly with her purse—which was obviously, according to him, a stand-in for female genitals and demonstrated her habit of masturbation—and by a dream that involved a barn in flames—which he saw as a symbolic disguise for her flaming erotic desire for a middle-aged man. Freud repeatedly thrust this interpretation on her. Dora just as repeatedly rejected it, and after three months she had had enough. Even some analysts have acknowledged the truth. In Erik Erikson's words, "Dora had been traumatized, and Freud re-traumatized her."[8]

Crews attacks not just Freud's repeated therapeutic failures but also his deceptive accounts of what took place and his constant manipulation of evidence, a maneuver that required ever more ingenuity as his ideas about the source of hysterical symptoms evolved. By 1895, he was convinced (though Breuer was not) that the problem was always sexual. Committed to what is generally called the "seduction theory" (something Crews prefers to term the "molestation theory"), Freud alleged that his patients' symptoms derived from paternal assault. It was a theory he announced with great pride before the leading psychiatrists and neurologists of Vienna, but it "was given an icy reception by those asses," as Freud reported ruefully to his friend Wilhelm Fliess. The rejection was only made worse when the sexologist Richard Kraft-Ebbing, who was chairing the meeting, proclaimed that "it sound[ed] like a scientific fairy tale." Shortly thereafter, Freud had an epiphany: the molestations weren't real; they were the products of fantasy. It was a speculation, Crews shows, as ungrounded in any serious evidentiary basis as its predecessor.

Freud's mistreatment of his patients extended to submitting them to experimental nasal surgery at the hands of a man who for years was his best friend. Wilhelm Fliess (who, like Freud, embraced a mystical numerology) had convinced himself (and Freud) that there was an intimate reflex connection between certain regions of the nose, the sexual organs, and neuroses. Such problems were not confined to the female of the species, but surfaced particularly strongly among them. They could be treated by topical applications of the drug Freud had once hailed as magical, cocaine; by cauterizing the relevant spot; or in recalcitrant cases, by removing part of the bony structure of the nose. Freud's enthusiastic embrace of these ideas nearly cost the life of one of his patients, Emma Eckstein. Fliess botched her surgery, leaving a roll of gauze inside the wound. The resultant infection provoked a hemorrhage that nearly killed her. Freud was undeterred, seeing the bleeding (and subsequent further episodes of a less serious sort) as a sign of sexual longing.

Freud most certainly had homoerotic feelings for Fliess, a fact that Crews evidently sees as somehow discrediting and that he repeatedly emphasizes by using the word "congress" to describe their meetings. But eventually Freud grew jealous and tired of his friend and began to harbor murderous thoughts about him—thoughts that Fliess became aware of and that caused him to break off further ties. As always (because, as someone in his closest Viennese circle once remarked, Freud was a great hater: "Dass Freud allzeit ein grimmer Hasser war"), Freud responded by rejecting Fliess, a man who had once been one of his dearest friends. It was a pattern he had already put on display when he decided Breuer was of no further use to him, and one that would recur throughout his career, with particularly vicious score-settling with apostates such as Jung and Adler. The balance and maturity that a successful psychoanalysis supposedly produced is scarcely in evidence here.

Most of the serious charges Crews brings against Freud strike me as resting on a powerful array of evidence, much of it previously brought to light by others but here assembled in a damning and extended synthesis. The bulk of the book is an attack on the man and his character, and it succeeds, I think, in inflicting some grievous wounds on Freud's reputation. Some may be inclined to dismiss the whole exercise as nothing more than an ad hominem attack, and it most certainly is that. Crews weakens, not strengthens, his case when he resorts repeatedly to loaded and hyperbolic language, and when he routinely places the worst possible construction on the events he purports to describe. More troubling still are occasions when he simply can't resist a sensational charge—that Freud committed incest, for example—although the evidence for such propositions are as flimsy as some of the deductions Freud makes, about which Crews is appropriately scornful.

This is not a book that is centrally about Freud's ideas, and in that sense I suspect that psychoanalysts will be tempted to dismiss it and perhaps, as is often their wont, to allege that psychopathology lurks behind Crews's evident passion. But the evidence of Freud's duplicity and moral slipperiness, his carelessness, and his desperate search to be recognized as a genius inevitably creates a shadow that extends beyond his domestic failings and his often-disgraceful dealings with his colleagues, one that must raise doubts about the probity of his work. There is a serious case to answer here.

I'm left, though, with a question for Professor Crews: If psychoanalysis is nothing but an illusion, a giant confidence trick, how has it snared so many people, including (once upon a time) Crews himself, and held them in its thrall? Granting that Freud's legacy is now shriveling and apparently fading away, nowhere more evidently than among the ranks of psychiatrists, is that unambiguously a boon? Is there nothing left of value? It is a question (or series of questions) others may care to ponder as well. I suspect I know how Professor Crews would respond. For him, Freud seems to be the Devil, and his works must therefore be condemned as utterly diabolical.

Perhaps it is just a strange coincidence then (though the numerologically obsessed Freud might well think otherwise) that the text of this weighty polemic ends—and I am not making this up—on page 666.

7 Psychobiology, Psychiatry, and Psychoanalysis

THE INTERSECTING CAREERS OF ADOLF MEYER, PHYLLIS GREENACRE, AND CURT RICHTER

INTRODUCTION

By common consent, Adolf Meyer (1866–1950) was the most prominent and influential American psychiatrist of the first half of the twentieth century. Particularly after his appointment to Johns Hopkins, as its first professor of psychiatry, he dominated psychiatry in the United States until his retirement in 1941.[1] But his influence was almost equally strong in Britain, where his pragmatism and therapeutic eclecticism had a wide appeal.[2]

This chapter examines some central aspects of Meyer's life and work, focusing particularly on his role as a mentor and patron of the research and careers of two other major figures in twentieth-century psychiatry and psychobiology, broadly conceived. The first of these, Phyllis Greenacre (1894–1989), worked closely with Meyer from 1916, when she graduated from Chicago Rush medical school and joined his staff at Hopkins, until her abrupt departure from Baltimore in late 1927. For the next decade, Meyer continued to play an important role in her life and career, though to his dismay she was now progressively abandoning his distinctive type of psychiatry for psychoanalysis. Completing that process of intellectual transition just as Freud's followers were moving to a position of institutional and theoretical dominance in American psychiatry, Greenacre rose to remarkable prominence in those circles, one of the few nonrefugee analysts to become part of the psychoanalytic elite.

Curt Richter (1894–1988) was another promising young scientist attracted to Meyer's circle, initially through a decision to move from Harvard to Johns Hopkins to work with the founder of behaviorist psychology, John B. Watson. After Watson's resignation from the Hopkins faculty in the aftermath of a sex scandal, Meyer orchestrated Richter's succession to head the psychological laboratory, now renamed the psychobiology laboratory. Richter would remain at Hopkins for seven decades, a highly successful experimentalist whose early work did much to lend empirical substance to Meyer's programmatic calls to develop psychobiology.

Like Greenacre, to whom he was married for ten years, until their acrimonious divorce was finalized in 1930, Richter's career continued to flourish for decades after Meyer's forced retirement from his professorship in 1941, and like her, he emerged from Meyer's tutelage to become very much his own person. Still, in a variety of ways, the years the two younger figures spent as subordinates of Meyer exercised a decisive influence over their otherwise very disparate professional trajectories. And, among other things, we will see that the complex relationships between the three of them have a great deal to teach us about a topic to which much scholarly attention has been devoted in recent years: the role of gender in scientific careers.

ADOLF MEYER IN AMERICA

Adolf Meyer was born in Niederweningen, Switzerland, on September 13, 1866, the son of a Zwinglian minister. He trained as a neurologist under Auguste-Henri Forel at the University of Zurich. In the course of his studies, he spent a year abroad in Edinburgh, London, and Paris, where he worked under both John Hughlings Jackson and Jean-Martin Charcot, among others. Concluding that his career opportunities would be better in the United States, he emigrated immediately after receiving his MD in 1892, initially settling in Chicago, one of the major centers of neurology in the country. Despite his impressive European credentials, however, he was unable to find a full-time, salaried post at the new, Rockefeller-funded University of Chicago, and the following year, Meyer felt compelled to accept an appointment at the vast Illinois Eastern Hospital for the Insane at Kankakee, some ninety miles from the city.

It was not an auspicious beginning to his American career. Neurologists had been fiercely critical of institutional psychiatry in the preceding decade, and this criticism culminated in an excoriating address to the American Medico-Psychological Association in 1894 by the prominent Philadelphia neurologist Silas Weir Mitchell. Condemning psychiatrists for their scientific somnolence and ignorance, and for deliberately distancing themselves from the rest of the medical profession, Mitchell spoke scathingly of observing patients "who have lost even the memory of hope, sit in rows, too dull to know despair, watched by attendants: silent, grewsome [*sic*] machines which eat and sleep, sleep and eat."[3]

Mitchell could have been describing Meyer's own dispiriting encounter with the realities of institutional psychiatry. Indeed, just a few months later, Meyer wrote from Kankakee to G. Alder Blumer, superintendent of New York State's Utica State Hospital:

> [I have become] more and more convinced that the atmosphere of the place shows little sign of being improved to such a degree as to make life satisfactory enough to spare energy for the work I am longing for. Catering towards political effects, towards more show and granting insufficient liberty of action, the administration discourages progress along sound principles. The library facilities are poor and the whole mechanism of medical work little promising although much better than when I came here. My courses on neurology and mental disease have certainly roused the interest of the Staff, but the ground does not promise much fruit as long as the simplest means of clinical observation and examination are absent![4]

Meyer had begun his time at Kankakee by conducting large numbers of autopsies in an attempt to correlate brain lesions with psychiatric diagnoses. Soon, however, he realized that the disarray of the hospital's patient records and the absence of any systematic record of the patients' symptoms while they were alive made all such endeavors pointless.[5] Crucially, this led him toward a greater interest in studying the clinical course of psychiatric illness in living patients.[6] If he wanted to train the hospital staff in systematic history taking and record keeping, he had perforce to develop the necessary techniques himself. Assembling the hospital staff and employing a stenographer to take notes as he examined patients, Meyer thus pioneered a standardized case record. Soon, he was emphasizing the need to create a comprehensive record of all aspects of a patient's mental, physical, and developmental history, features that would become standard elements in Meyerian psychiatry and the central feature of his future teaching and mentoring of young psychiatrists.

Meyer's year at Chicago and two and a half years at Kankakee were decisive in bringing about his transition from neurology to psychiatry. Not only did these years see Meyer move from the morgue to the bedside and develop a key instrument for recording the shape of psychiatric disorder (and for keeping psychiatrists busy), but they also brought him into close contact with the ideas of John Dewey and Charles Peirce and with American pragmatism, a set of philosophic doctrines that henceforth exercised a considerable hold on him and helped to fuel his enthusiasm for collecting endless amounts of data. A later move to Massachusetts led him to create intellectual ties to the third major figure among American pragmatists, the Harvard psychologist William James. As one of Meyer's most prominent later students commented, before he became aware of these biographical linkages, "I had long been puzzled—since I first met Adolf Meyer and recognized the similarity of his teachings to those of James and Dewey—how it happened that a Swiss had embraced pragmatism, indeed had found in it his natural voice."[7]

Kankakee also provided ready access to a broad array of clinical material, allowing Meyer to make some of his few original contributions to the neurological literature while encouraging him to take a broader view of the problems of psychiatric illness. Meanwhile, the importance the pragmatists placed on naturalism and experimentalism as the keys to exploring the universe exercised a profound effect on Meyer. As he remarked many years later, "It was the work of American thinkers, especially of Charles S Peirce, of John Dewey and of William James, which justified in us a basic sense of pluralism, that is to say, a recognition that nature is not just one smooth continuity."[8] James would point out that "pragmatism is uncomfortable away from facts,"[9] and Meyer emphasized "the facts" like a mantra. His central conception of psychobiology can likewise be seen as echoing the pragmatists' focus on biological adaptation, the processes of problem solving, and whole-body activity.

In addition to suffering from the overcrowding, isolation, and lack of resources that were endemic features of most state hospitals in this period, the Illinois asylums were notoriously at the mercy of state politicians, who viewed them as patronage plums. Two years after Meyer had taken up his post, S. V. Clevenger, the superintendent at Kankakee, found himself under growing political pressure. He succumbed in a matter of months. Some observers concluded that his erratic behavior and "delirious delusions" were the product of his alcoholism. Meyer simply noted that he "broke down" under pressure "so that he was considered insane even by his friends." Meyer must by this point have begun to question his decision to leave Switzerland for the allegedly greener pastures of North America, and it was surely with great relief that he received an offer in 1895 to take over as director of research at Worcester State Hospital in Massachusetts.

Henceforth, Meyer's own career moved from strength to strength. Six years at Worcester led to an appointment as director of the Pathological Institute of the New York State Hospitals, and shortly thereafter he was offered a courtesy position as professor of clinical medicine at Cornell University Medical College. Then, in 1908, came the call to Johns Hopkins, where he occupied the first chair in psychiatry and headed the newly established and generously endowed Phipps Clinic.

At Worcester, modeling his approach on the best German clinics and mental hospitals, Meyer developed links to the local Clark University and developed a program to bring in four or five new assistants a year, recruited from the best mental hospitals in the country on the basis of their academic records and a competitive examination. Little or no formal instruction in psychiatry was provided at American medical schools in this period, a reflection of the specialty's marginality and low professional status. Meyer's new men (actually, the twenty-nine appointments he made included two women) were to be the shock troops of a new scientific psychiatry, employing serious and sustained clinical and pathological research to uncover the roots of mental disorder. With their aid, Meyer began to develop the eclectic approach he would soon dub "psychobiology," and in many instances, his young assistants went on to become the leaders of the

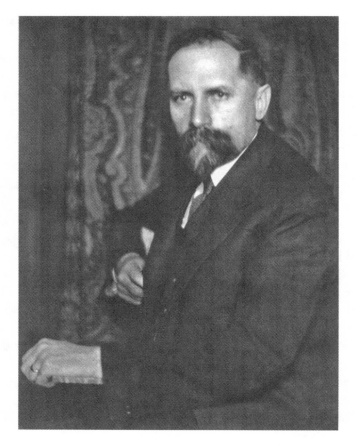

Figure 1. Adolf Meyer, c. 1900. (Reproduced by courtesy of the Alan Mason Chesney Medical Archives, Johns Hopkins Medical Institutions.)

next generation of American psychiatrists. Indeed, three of them subsequently served as presidents of the American Psychiatric Association.[10]

Meyer's move to New York was yet another step up the professional ladder. The New York State mental hospital system was by far the largest in the country, and its Pathological Institute, intended as a center of psychiatric research and training, was potentially a very influential bureaucratic niche. However, under its founding director, Ira Van Gieson, the institute had achieved little. A pathologist by training, Van Gieson was contemptuous of institutional psychiatry, viewing its practitioners as poorly trained and "ignorant" of medical science.[11] But the program of basic research he had sought to establish had little obvious therapeutic or intellectual payoff in its first half dozen years, leaving him politically vulnerable to the machinations of the superintendents and their political supporters, and by the autumn of 1901, he found himself out of a job.[12]

Meyer had been consulted privately about the deficiencies of the institute under Van Giesen, and after some hesitation, he agreed to take on the task of giving it a new direction. Far from being contemptuous of clinical psychiatry, Meyer embraced it, and this at once made for better relations with the superintendents. His work at Worcester had already begun to win him a national reputation, and he set about remaking the institute. He established an outpatient clinic, standardized record keeping and statistics statewide, and sought to provide research training for mental hospital staff throughout the system. His cooperative stance toward the hospitals, his expressed desire to "raise the standards of medical work in the State institutions," and his frequent visits to the various mental hospitals throughout the state helped to smooth ruffled feathers. But they did not, in the end, provoke a reciprocal engagement on the part of the heads of most institutions. And unfortunately, Meyer's insatiable appetite for collecting "facts" was not matched by any comparable creativity in organizing or making sense of this mass of material.[13]

Nonetheless, Meyer's intimidating Teutonic manner, the prestige of the institutions and individuals at which and under whom he had trained, his neurological background, and his extensive knowledge of the European, and particularly the German, literature on psychiatry all served to bolster his standing. Thus, the decision to appoint him as the first professor of psychiatry at Johns Hopkins was in some senses predictable. Not completely, however, for William Henry Welch, the dean of the medical school, had first approached Stewart "Felix" Paton, an immensely wealthy Princeton man who had studied in Europe, written one of the most widely used psychiatric texts of the time, and possessed more stellar social connections than Meyer. But Paton had no interest in being tied down by a full-time clinical appointment, and he urged Welch to appoint Meyer instead.

Hopkins had opened its doors in 1893, and it was the first American medical school to adopt the German model of combining medical education and research. By almost any measure, it was America's premier medical school in these years. Apart from its institutional innovations, the stature of its first four chairs—Welch, William Olser, William Halsted, and Howard Kelly—had done much to cement its dominance. In an era when most medical schools ignored psychiatry, Meyer's arrival in Baltimore represented a coup for the specialty, as well as for him personally.

Meyer's chair at Hopkins provided him with an extraordinarily powerful and prominent base on which to build his influence in the discipline, and he used it to great effect. The 1920s and 1930s saw the expansion of academic psychiatry across the United States, with much of the growth underwritten by the munificence of the Rockefeller Foundation, which had decided by the late 1920s to make the specialty its top priority in the field of medicine. The stream of students passing through Hopkins in these decades went on to prominent positions in these new departments, bearing with them the influence of Meyer's eclecticism and declaring their allegiance to Meyerian psychobiology. By one estimate, in 1937, as many as 10 percent of all academic psychiatrists in the United States had trained at Hopkins under him.[14] His influence extended abroad, particularly to Britain, where Aubrey Lewis in London and David Henderson in Edinburgh came to dominate the discipline, both having received extensive training at Hopkins under Meyer.[15] And his dominance was all the greater since so many of his pupils remained in his shadow. Smith Ely Jelliffe once commented waspishly that Meyer had put "partly castrated pupils in professional chairs" all across the country.[16]

Elected president of the American Psychiatric Association in 1928, Meyer also played a leading role in the establishment of the American Board of Psychiatry and Neurology in 1934, chairing its organizational meeting and serving on the committee that administered its first qualifying examination. Though he grew increasingly hostile toward Freud and psychoanalysis in the years before the outbreak of World War II[17]— a stance that helps explain the rapid eclipse of his supremacy following his retirement in 1941, for psychoanalysis was then about to cement its quarter-century long dominance of American psychiatry—his influence was all-pervasive. Yet his professional dominance rested more on the prestige of his European training, the power that flowed from his Hopkins position, and the number of academic psychiatrists who owed their careers to his sponsorship than on his intellectual contributions to the understanding and treatment of mental illness.

Meyer's original research in the fields of neurology and neuroanatomy virtually ceased once he arrived in Baltimore.[18] His psychiatric papers from his three decades at Hopkins were programmatic rather than substantive, and they were written in a notoriously dense and impenetrable prose. Meyer was faced with the bewildering complexities of an array of disorders whose etiology and treatment remained largely a matter of guesswork and improvisation. His talk of psychobiology provided an elastic overarching framework within which a whole array of hypotheses and interventions could be accommodated; and his stress on the meticulous collection of detailed case histories created a host of tasks with which his students could busy themselves.

BUILDING CAREERS AT JOHNS HOPKINS

Among those attracted to work under Meyer in his first decade at Hopkins were two young scientists with whom he would develop unusually close personal ties. The first of these, Phyllis Greenacre, was a talented and determined woman from Chicago who had overcome paternal disapproval (and her father's refusal to pay for her medical education) to secure both a BS and an MD from the University of Chicago. Her ambition led her to write to Meyer in 1916 asking for a position on his staff, and her intellectual talents (enthusiastically endorsed by Dean Dodson of the Chicago Rush Medical School), secured her the post. Two years later, Curt Richter, a Harvard graduate with a far more mixed academic record, arrived on the scene, initially to work with John B. Watson, the increasingly prominent behavioral psychologist.

Watson had recently moved his laboratory from the Psychology Department to Meyer's Phipps Clinic, so Richter found himself on the periphery of Meyer's academic empire. He had been attracted to Baltimore and to Watson by an interest in animal physiology,[19] and he quickly began work on the behavior of the ubiquitous laboratory rat. (By an odd coincidence, it was Meyer who had introduced the rat as an experimental subject to the American university.)[20] Largely left to his own devices, and

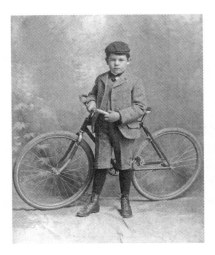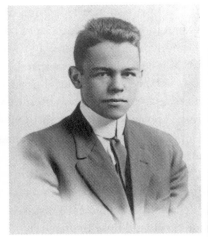

Figure 2. Curt Richter as a boy, 1905, and as a young man, 1912. (Reproduced by courtesy of the Alan Mason Chesney Archives, Johns Hopkins Medical Institutions.)

early on inclined to search for internally generated behavioral control mechanisms rather than focus on the external influences on behavior that fascinated Watson, Richter nonetheless quickly absorbed his mentor's emphasis on precise measurement and rigorous experimentation as the route to scientific legitimacy. Within three years, Richter had completed a PhD thesis on "The Behavior of the Rat: A Study of General and Specific Activities" (1921). By then, though, embroiled in a sex scandal that wrecked his first marriage, Watson had been forced to resign his Hopkins professorship, his unwilling departure fueled in part by some behind the scenes maneuvering by Meyer, with whom his relations had become increasingly acrimonious over the years.

Besides his fierce intellectual disagreements with Watson,[21] Meyer seems to have been motivated by his own sexual prudery[22] and concerns about the potential damage Watson's sexual dalliance threatened to impose on the university. He had engaged in an extensive private correspondence with Watson when rumors of the affair reached him from the psychologist Stanley Hall. In the course of what Watson must have thought was a private exchange of letters, he had revealed (foolishly as it would turn out) the depth of his unhappiness with his marriage and the crucial details of his affair.[23] In what many would regard as a serious violation of trust, Meyer subsequently passed this correspondence on to Hopkins's president, Frank Goodnow, and privately advised him that Watson must go: "Without clean cut and outspoken principles on these matters we could not run a coeducational institution, nor would we deserve a position of honor and respect before any kind of public, nor even before ourselves."[24] Six days later, under severe pressure from the university, Watson submitted his resignation. Disingenuously, when the New York cardiologist Robert Levy wrote to him about the matter eighteen months later, Meyer responded, "Personally, I did all in my power to smooth over the catastrophe, but there was nothing to be done in view of the fact that the authorities had evidently made up their minds to deal drastically with the matter."[25] One is tempted to conclude that a previous personal betrayal was here compounded by a lie.[26]

Meyer promptly appointed the inexperienced Richter to replace Watson as head of the psychological laboratory, a move that, over time, would pay large dividends to both men.[27] He also invited Richter to attend his staff rounds and to give some lectures, drawing the man away from Watson and into his own intimate circle.

Meanwhile, Phyllis Greenacre's first years at Hopkins had proved unexpectedly difficult. Her psychiatric training at Chicago Rush had been minimal, and the stress her relative inexperience created for her may have been one factor that led to a deep and for a time disabling depression, which eventually required temporary hospitalization. Meyer nonetheless kept her on staff, and during this period he developed a distinctly paternalistic interest in her future, one that almost amounted, as he himself confessed in a letter to her, to his assuming the role of a father figure, substituting for the estranged parent with whom Greenacre had little or no continuing contact. "Above all things," Meyer had urged her, "do not forget that hard as it may have been in the past to get help and a chance for free discussion with yr [sic] own family, you can count on an absolutely frank and thoughtful and yet not meddlesome hearing and discussion with your more neutral but none the less keenly interested 'chief' who has always felt himself to be, as far as this can be accepted, in *loco parentis* (and I hope without suggesting paternalism)."[28]

Greenacre had returned to work in the spring of 1918, and so when Richter was drawn into Meyer's orbit, it was inevitable that the two young

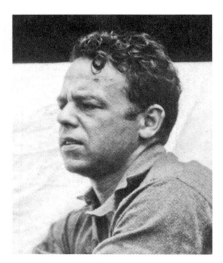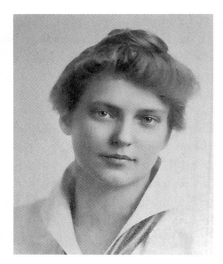

Figure 3. (*Left*) Curt Richter as a young scientist, 1930. (Reproduced by courtesy of the Alan Mason Chesney Archives, Johns Hopkins Medical Institutions.) (*Right*) Phyllis Greenacre while at medical school, c. 1916. (Photograph kindly provided by her grandson, Peter C. Richter.)

scientists would become acquainted. Within a matter of months, they developed a romantic relationship, and Greenacre was approaching her surrogate father for advice, just as he had urged her to do. Junior Hopkins staff in this era required the permission of the university's trustees before they could marry, and there were, besides, few precedents for married female staff members attempting to continue their professional careers.[29] Her "chief's" approval was thus of great importance to her on both a personal and a professional level.

Initially, however, it was not forthcoming. Instead, Meyer openly worried that her desire to marry might reflect the emotional turmoil she had gone through the year before. Greenacre hastened to assure him that this was not the case: "I have never looked upon marriage as an attempt at a therapeutic adjustment as promising of any success or stability. It has always seemed to me that the half-digested problems are bound to be augmented by the new complexities." As she hoped Meyer had observed, "I have been more at ease this past year. . . . Certainly less energy has gone into the vague states of tense depression which used to swamp me; and my thinking has, I believe, become more purposeful, with less of the depressive musing."[30]

But Meyer had misgivings that extended beyond a concern about Greenacre's emotional state. There were more practical objections to a marriage. Both Greenacre and Richter were in the early stages of building professional careers, an extremely demanding process from which marriage (and children) could prove a very significant distraction. "I have seen a few happy student marriages," Meyer conceded, "but also [know] how important it is to be free during the hard period during which one is tested out by the hard world for one's final career."

Her own career, he noted with evident satisfaction, was developing well, but Richter's had scarcely begun and seemed far less defined and secure. The uncertainties worried him. Richter's European training in engineering, his catholic intellectual tastes (which extended at this point in his career to an interest in psychoanalysis), his cleverness in the laboratory, and his biological bent all made for intriguing possibilities. But Meyer pointed out that his research agenda was still confused and inchoate: "He is a man whose potentialities I find it difficult to evaluate. . . . [He has] a certain difficulty in getting focused. I have had the feeling that whenever I thought Richter had focused on a point he was off on a tangent without having finished the starting point." He urged his protégée to try to weigh things rationally and carefully before she did anything irrevocable: "If the practical balance proves promising, there is no reason why your two careers could not blend to a reasonable extent. And the question in my mind is whether this balance cannot be gaged [*sic*] within a reasonable time and that without interfering with the frankness and sincerity of your relationship, but also without engaging *first* in the life-contract of marriage before the balance of *facts* is reasonably clear."

Seeking further arguments to dissuade her, Meyer spoke approvingly of how much Greenacre's work mattered to her. Marriage might jeopardize her career prospects, and how would she feel then? "I remember well your sensitiveness and reaction to the appearance of a slight in promotion a year ago when I had planned to lead you towards the laboratory and Dr. Fairbank [another young female associate] took a line for work for which she seemed better fitted, not than you, but better than for the other type of work." Greenacre had made her unhappiness vividly clear. He remarked that she should understand that "that type of preferences and deferments will be very [much] larger with a married couple, and I should feel it very wrong that you should be exposed to all of that instead of having a chance to become the vigorous and capable person you give every promise to become if at least you are not swamped by incidental difficulties and especially difficulties accruing to Mr. Richter."[31]

Meyer's prudential arguments, powerful as they may have been, failed to achieve their objective. Ignoring his strictures about the possible "complications which go with premature marriages," Greenacre seized on a passage in one of his letters that promised, "Whatever you may decide I shall try to be helpful."[32] She and Richter, she informed him, would marry on September 1, 1919, before the academic year got under way.[33] A clearly unhappy Meyer again urged caution but signaled, "If the course of things *must* be so, . . . I accept the situation."[34]

Perhaps disconcerted by her mentor's reaction, or perhaps because of a change of heart, Greenacre soon wrote to announce, "The plans of which I first wrote you have been entirely disrupted."[35] But the disruption proved only temporary. Meyer continued to counsel her not to proceed: "It is not your mutual affections, but the complications that go with premature marriage that I fear might be apt to create perplexities which may hinder the one or the other or both [of you], and especially also Mr. Richter and possibly in ways in which you may have to suffer without being able to help."[36] But he found himself ignored. In the spring of 1922, the two young scientists married, and within weeks Greenacre was pregnant.

Women pursuing careers in academic medicine were rare in the early twentieth century. Married women doing so were even scarcer. Married women with children attempting this were the rarest creatures of all. The expectation on all sides was that such women would gracefully retire from the fray, perhaps initially intending the break to be only temporary, though in reality the interruption generally proved fatal to any serious ambitions as a scientist. Marriage and a family were a normal part of most men's career trajectories. It was quite otherwise for women.

A few years earlier, for example, Dorothy Reed had been one of the most promising young medical scientists at Hopkins. After taking the necessary science courses at MIT in 1895–96, she entered the Hopkins medical school, where she finished fifth in her graduating class. Next she obtained posts under two of the leading figures at the school, serving first as an intern under William Osler in 1900 and then obtaining a fellowship in pathology with William Welch the following year. Two years later, she moved to take up a residency in pediatrics at Babies Hospital in New York.

During her time in the Hopkins laboratories, Reed definitively differentiated tuberculosis from Hodgkin's disease and discovered the blood cell disorder characteristic of the latter, the cells in question being eponymously dubbed "Reed cells." International recognition followed the publication of her results in 1902, and she seemed set for a major career in medicine—until her marriage in 1906 to a professor of physics at the University of Wisconsin, Charles Elwood Mendenhall. Immediately thereafter, she had four children in rapid succession (the first of whom died at one day old, and the second before he was two), and for eight years she stayed at home to care for the survivors. By that time, her once glittering professional prospects had all but vanished. When she returned to medicine, it was in the marginal and stigmatized field of public health—not, her male contemporaries sniffed, a serious branch of medicine.

Those who opposed allowing females into medicine saw her as a prime example of why it was foolish to "waste" precious medical space on the weaker sex. When Harvard debated the question of whether to open its medical school to women, Alice Hamilton (1869–1970), the first woman appointed to the Harvard faculty and an expert in industrial toxicology, informed Reed that the opponents of such a move specifically cited her case. Here, they proclaimed, "was an able woman who had married and failed to use her expensive medical education."[37] That it might be possible to balance a career in academic medicine with marriage and motherhood struck most contemporary observers as verging on the delusional, and Reed's career path confirmed it.

Greenacre, however, was determined to prove the conventional wisdom wrong. Her daughter Ann was born in February 1921, but even the birth of her son Peter in May 1922 did not shake her resolve. Not that Hopkins had made any attempt to ease her difficulties: for the first birth, she explained to Meyer, "the hospital was unwilling to grant me any extra time [off]," and she had to use her vacation allowance instead. In January 1922, she asked her mentor to try to secure her an extra "month or six weeks of vacation this summer. I shall have my second baby in May which will of necessity absorb three weeks of the usual allotment of four weeks." It is clear, however, that she did not expect the appeal for more time to spend with her infant son to succeed, and she announced in advance that she would not let that deter her: "If that is not possible next summer either, I shall accept the time in May as a good enough investment and let it go at that."[38] Greenacre hired a nanny to care for the children in her absence and just got on with her work.

But her work stagnated. In her early years at Hopkins, Greenacre had done extensive research on the pathophysiology of syphilis. Tertiary syphilis was responsible for between 10 and 20 percent of male mental hospital admissions in these years, and the work on the pathology of the central nervous system allowed Greenacre to draw more directly on her prior medical training in Chicago. Each time she sought to bring her research to closure, however, Meyer raised difficulties. The papers she wrote never seemed to satisfy him. Whenever she showed him a draft, he would raise a new objection or suggest a further extension of her research. In the end, the work never appeared in print, which damaged her efforts to begin to make a name for herself through publication.[39]

This wasn't the only difficulty she faced. Meyer had assured her during their exchange of letters about her impending marriage that he was "much less prejudiced than most organizers against favoring women and married couples."[40] Especially if the women remained single: Meyer had hired Ruth Fairbank and Esther Richards to work alongside Greenacre, and Richards served as Meyer's principal clinical associate and director of the outpatient service at the Phipps Clinic from 1920 until her retirement in 1951. But, as Greenacre found once she got married, "less prejudiced" still left much room for unequal treatment. Despite her obvious talents and her personal closeness to Meyer, she found her opportunities for professional advancement were sharply curtailed. Her salary remained static, and while the other women were given opportunities to expand their professional horizons, she remained stuck with the same rank and title, a source of growing embarrassment as well as frustration.

What made matters still worse was that she saw Richards and Fairbank as "second rate people" advancing "at the expense of first rate people" (among whom she clearly numbered herself). She considered Esther Richards, in particular, to be "much disliked, very cold, often cruel in front of patients, much disliked by the staff," someone afflicted with "scoliosis, a kind of hunchback," with a personality to match. To watch Meyer "lean over backwards" to help such people while she was left to struggle was immensely galling.[41]

Constantly pressed for funds, Greenacre took on other work on the side when she could in a frantic effort to make ends meet. This made for a punishing schedule. She organized and conducted a sex survey for the American Social Hygiene Association. She took a three-month rotation at a Maryland state hospital, which proved to be a dismal and daunting experience dealing with hopeless, chronic patients on badly overcrowded wards. Back at the Phipps, she supervised Meyer's laboratory for him and sought to find ways for "developing further work with students to include the relation of the laboratory examinations to the clinical material." Then there was the supervision of "the rotation of internes [sic] in the laboratory." This left her unable to do any original research of her own: "Follow-up work [with patients at the Phipps Clinic] is now absorbing all of the spare time I can manage during the day; usually 2 or 3 nights a week in interviews with patients who cannot come during the day; and 2 or 3 evenings a week spent in abstracting old histories at home. The unavoidable evening interviews [with patients] could be simplified if I were able to establish an office [nearby] . . . rather than making the extra night trips to the clinic. This, however, is quite out of the question on my present income which is limited strictly to the clinic salary."[42]

Meanwhile, the equally ambitious Curt Richter had thrown himself enthusiastically into an ever more elaborate research program of his own, working long hours in the laboratory on his animal experiments. Richter was proving to be something of a virtuoso at designing and constructing new pieces of equipment that allowed him to conduct his research, his hands-on skills allowing him to develop new ways of studying animal physiology and behavior. He developed numerous techniques to monitor the behavior of rats, constructing an "activity cage" filled with instruments that enabled him to observe and record patterns of activity and inactivity, and sleep and wakefulness, and to manipulate such things as light, temperature, and the availability of food and water.

On another front, Richter continued to work on the neurological basis of human behavior, a topic he had been introduced to by Watson. He studied the grasp reflex, conducting some experiments using human infants as

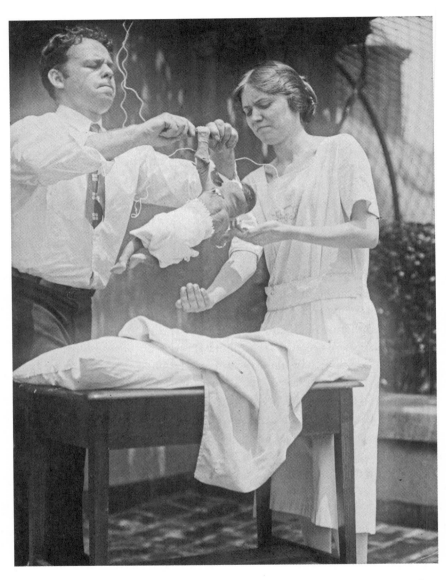

Figure 4. Curt Richter and Phyllis Greenacre conducting an experimental study of the grasp reflex in a human infant, c. 1923. (Reproduced by courtesy of the Alan Mason Chesney Archives, Johns Hopkins Medical Institutions.)

subjects. His wife initially assisted him with these studies in the laboratory, and they may have used their own children as experimental subjects.

Much of Richter's manual skill and dexterity, and his cleverness at inventing new instruments, derived from his childhood experiences. His parents had emigrated from Germany and set up an iron factory in Denver, a business his mother continued to run after his father was killed in a hunting accident when Richter was still a young boy. Hanging around the factory, assembling and disassembling clocks and other bits of machinery, Curt had honed his skills as an engineer and inventor.

Deeply committed to measurement and data, Richter quickly began to expand the work in his laboratory that sought to link biology and behavior, in the process giving substance to Meyer's programmatic commitment to psychobiology, particularly through an emphasis on self-regulation and behavioral adaptation to the environment. He had adopted Meyer's emphasis on the total organism and found Meyer's pragmatism equally congenial. Meyer visited the laboratory regularly, and the two men grew close. Meyer became a father figure for the fatherless Richter in much the same way as he had been something of a substitute parent for Greenacre, who was estranged from her parents. Meyer was someone whose advice and counsel Richter regularly sought, and on whom he depended for both material and emotional support. Meyer was generally viewed as an autocratic and intimidating figure, but the young couple enjoyed significant marks of his favor, including regular invitations to his home to dine with him and Mrs. Meyer.[43]

Richter interacted regularly with other Hopkins scientists outside Meyer's domain, and his experimental virtuosity and the meticulous care with which he conducted his investigations drew their admiration. Baffled as they might be by Professor Meyer's abstruse philosophical statements, they quickly recognized the worth and substance of Richter's work. Psychology, in Richter's hands, did seem to them to be developing into the science the infant discipline insistently proclaimed itself to be. During the 1920s, Richter's work was of growing importance scientifically and also played a very substantial role in legitimizing Meyer's whole enterprise.[44] Richter's first series of publications, appearing between 1921 and 1925, adumbrates themes that would resonate through all his later work, extending even into the 1980s: the determinants of spontaneous activity; the importance of biological clocks; endocrine control of behavior; the origin

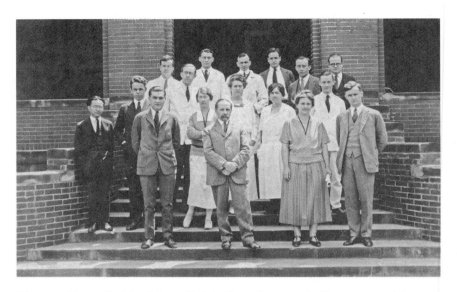

Figure 5. The staff of the Phipps Clinic in the mid-1920s. Phyllis Greenacre (*first row, second from the right*) is positioned next to Adolf Meyer (*first row, second from the left*). Curt Richter (*second row, second from the left*) is standing about as far from her as possible. (Reproduced by courtesy of the Alan Mason Chesney Archives, Johns Hopkins Medical Institutions.)

of the electrical resistance of the skin; brain control of the motor system; and the measurement of salivation.[45] Particularly striking was his discovery of circadian biological rhythms, an instance where his childhood fascination with clocks led indirectly to a quite profound set of insights into the role of internal clocks in animal and human activity and inactivity.

For all Phyllis Greenacre's frustrations, to most outside observers during the early 1920s, she and Curt Richter seemed to be a remarkable couple, both launched on careers of exceptional scientific promise. Among the handful of women on the Hopkins staff, only Greenacre had managed to combine work, marriage, and motherhood, and her determination to succeed professionally seemed undaunted by the obstacles she faced. In reality, however, Meyer's worries about the stresses the pair would face were proving prescient, though his own actions were helping to make his prophecy a self-fulfilling one.

The severe financial constraints the two young academics faced were exacerbated as their children grew beyond infancy. Adding to the strains on their relationship, their workaholic schedules gave them little time together. The marriage began to fall apart, and, as part of a vicious cycle, Greenacre experienced new episodes of depression and began to overeat. She gained some forty or fifty pounds in the months after the birth of her son Peter, which led to a dramatic change in her appearance, though no one around her seemed to grasp the significance of this development. Divorce seemed out of the question. Its stigma remained great, and in any event, it would have compounded the couple's financial problems. The path of least resistance was to immerse themselves more deeply in their work, which kept them apart and in the short term reduced the opportunity to fight. But inevitably, this course of action only further weakened the ties between them.

Generally shy and reserved, and diffident about promoting herself, Greenacre nonetheless made several efforts to alleviate the financial difficulties her family faced and confront the frustrations she was experiencing in her professional life. On the first such occasion, she complained to Meyer: "I find myself right now in a situation where I am neither consulted nor usually even informed of those few clinic arrangements which do concern me and my work." He had chosen to restrict her opportunities mostly to the laboratory, but even there, her position as head of the laboratory needed clarification, and she informed him that she would like to expand her role working with students in this setting. Making matters worse, she told him, "I think I am alone in the clinic in maintaining in the sixth year the same official rank that I achieved automatically when I was accepted as an interne." Since her official title was "the only available index [of her standing available] to strangers and students," the situation was, to understate the matter, "occasionally embarrassing." Meanwhile, she was forced to endure the spectacle of others around her "advancing by flattery, glittering talk, obsequiousness, and insincerity, too often with deliberate falsifications and distortions of the facts"—experiences to which she reacted with "discomfort and revulsion [and] disillusionment."[46]

It is perhaps a measure of the strength of the ties between Greenacre and her superior that she was bold enough to send this letter to him. She insisted: "I do not wish to present these matters as grievances or demands"—although, of course, this is exactly what they were—"but as more or less imperative factors in my work and interests." By way of justifying her actions, she invoked Meyer's own teachings: "My years at the clinic have taught me the necessity of getting dissatisfactions cleared up and talked out rather than storing up for a cumulative explosion. . . . Such an accumulation is taking place." One possible solution to her financial difficulties, she proposed, might be an increase in her clinical responsibilities. Here, perhaps, she undermined her own case by conceding that she made this proposal "as a means to increase my income rather than [from] any deeply rooted ambition. But as a practical means of easing urgent financial needs, I should welcome it." Listing her income since arriving at Hopkins in 1916, she stressed that "the apparent increase in salary during the last 2–3 years has not been a real one, amounting to no gain in actual cash at all over the year 1919–1920." It was an impossible state of affairs. She went on to explain that an increased salary "is an urgent need for me, and one which must have just now a governing influence on my plans. The present struggle is one which I cannot keep up and must find some way of relieving."[47] But nothing changed except for the proffer of a new title.

Seven months later, she was worrying that the new title Associate in Clinical Psychiatry was one reserved "for people who were not full time." Once more she expressed eagerness "if possible to have the privilege of practicing this year both because it would give me certain active contacts with patients which I am now missing, and because of the possible financial help."[48] Again, she was left unsatisfied.

Two years later, her situation had still not improved. Once more she appealed to Meyer, asking him to intervene with the Hopkins trustees to obtain an increased salary for her. After several weeks of ominous silence, he wrote back just as he left for Santa Barbara for a lucrative consultation on the mental state of Stanley McCormick, heir to the International Harvester fortune.[49] "I certainly owe you an apology," he began, "for this long delay in answering your letter. If I had anything pleasant or favorable to report to you, I should feel better about it." But the word from the treasurer's office was "to the effect, that the University owed you nothing. . . . I hardly know what the next step should be."[50]

Greenacre's response to this ostentatious wringing of hands was swift and fierce. She began with what, if one reads between the lines, appears to be an implied threat to leave, informing Meyer that she had recently turned down a "position offered me by the National Committee for Mental

Hygiene." For the present, she continued, "There are certain concrete problems which I have started [at Hopkins] which I feel I *must finish.*" But her commitment was not open-ended: "I *should not wish to continue,* however, *unless* I can foresee *greater development* and more *contacts through publication and* especially through *teaching,* than have yet seemed to come to me." And once more she returned to the issue of her inadequate salary: "I have just received the annual appointment notice from the President's office, and find myself officially reappointed as an associate in psychiatry with a salary of *$2,500* [$700 more than she had made in 1921–22]. I did not know whether in the event of my return to the clinic, this was intended to constitute the whole of the salary. I should find that *extremely difficult,* as I think you will understand."[51]

Meyer does seem to have understood at last that he was in grave danger of losing one of his closest and most valued associates. In San Francisco, he drafted a lengthy response to her memorandum, one that contained what was a remarkable set of concessions to his junior if one recalls his strong sense of hierarchy and his usual role as the bully rather than the bullied. First, he promised to address her complaints about teaching and publication. He would set in motion a plan for her to take "every other Thursday for a topic of clinical discussion, or a series of Thursdays if you prefer." He would also "arrange with Dr Richards a certain amount of group teaching." These alterations would form part of a general "readjustment . . . in which the aims of research and teaching of both yourself and the clinic come to best fruition." And he acknowledged the need to ensure that "the problem of publication is adjusted (which is my first concern)." That would remove "a cause of grievance . . . which I regret very much."[52]

There remained the crucial issue of her financial compensation. He announced that he could do little about the Hopkins salary. Somewhat feebly, he assured her that "concerning the sex studies, the same amount of money will be available as last year."[53] But, as if conscious that he had to offer more on this front, he made a fateful proposal, one that would have important consequences for himself, for Greenacre, and for Richter. He proposed that she undertake a special research project for him in return for an augmented salary.

Another of Meyer's protégés, from all the way back to his days at Worcester, Henry Cotton, had been appointed as the superintendent of the New Jersey

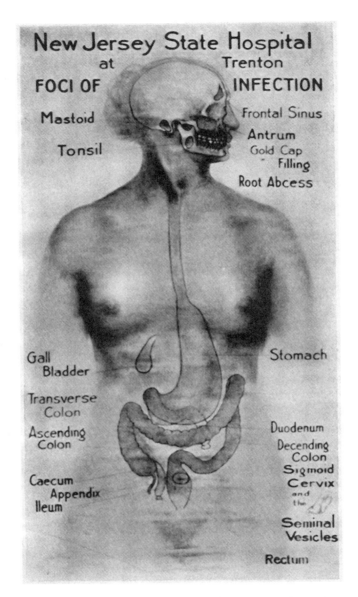

Figure 6. The sites of focal infection. Henry Cotton used a version of this diagram on multiple occasions to illustrate the often obscure nooks and crannies where focal sepsis could lurk undetected, spreading its poisons into the system and prompting a descent into madness as those toxins reached the brain. According to him, any of these infections might require surgical excision. (Reproduced by courtesy of the Trenton State Hospital Archives.)

State Hospital at Trenton in 1907, in large part because of Meyer's firm recommendation. In 1916, Cotton had put forth the bold hypothesis that mental symptoms were epiphenomenal and that the singular source of mental illness was the impact of chronic, undiagnosed, and untreated infections in the body, infections that produced toxins that poisoned the brain. His preferred solution was surgical extirpation of the offending organs: teeth, tonsils, spleens, stomachs, colons, uteri, and so forth—operations that, so he claimed, led to cure rates exceeding 80 percent. He was invited to give the prestigious Vanuxem lecture series at Princeton University in 1921, and he secured a typically ambiguous but largely favorable foreword from Meyer for the published version of the lectures.[54]

But Meyer's apparent endorsement did not prove sufficient to head off a bitter professional controversy over Cotton's claims. Though the Trenton superintendent had attracted powerful support among some American and British psychiatrists, others, particularly in North America, had sharply questioned his results, with major debates breaking out over his focal sepsis theory at both the 1922 and the 1923 meetings of the American Medico-Psychological Association (now the American Psychiatric Association). Fearing a hostile outside inquiry into Cotton's work, the Trenton asylum board of governors had decided to institute an assessment of its own and had approached Meyer about undertaking the task—a curious choice given that Meyer was Cotton's mentor and the godfather of his second son, Adolph.

It was this assessment that Meyer now offered to Greenacre. The plan was for her to work, under Meyer's supervision, two or three days each week to conduct an independent review of Cotton's methods and results. For Greenacre, the attractions were obvious: she would gain a generous supplement to her income (one that almost doubled her salary), to be paid by the New Jersey authorities, and the opportunity to publish the results of her researches into a topic that was attracting enormous professional and public attention. Meyer reminded her that the study would require her to spend considerable time away from her husband and children, for the amount of information to be gathered was substantial—but then so was the potential importance of her findings for the profession.[55] For Greenacre, the decision was easy.

The work, however, turned out to be hard, taking almost eighteen months to complete. Meticulously documented, and reflecting many hours in the field, Greenacre's findings delivered an apparently fatal blow to Cotton's claims. She found that Cotton's treatments, far from helping cure patients, were actively harmful, and often fatal. Supported by four volumes of case notes, her report concluded that *"the lowest recovery rate and the highest death rate occurs among the functional cases who have been thoroughly treated. . . . The least treatment was found in the recovered cases and the most thorough treatment in the unimproved and dead groups. . . . Thorough treatment, including abdominal operation, is not only dangerous to life, but ineffective in the cases of those who survive."*[56] Thousands of patients, it would transpire, had been maimed by Cotton's operations, and hundreds had died.

Cotton's reaction, when he, Meyer, and Greenacre met in Baltimore in January 1926 to discuss the findings, was to reject them out of hand. Furious, Cotton accused Greenacre of bias against him and refused to accept any hint of criticism. Meyer sat passively by for the most part as Cotton attempted to bully Greenacre, and when the meeting ended abruptly, with Cotton leaving for Trenton, Meyer forbade Greenacre to disseminate her findings until the two sides could reach common ground. Meanwhile, the hospital board at Trenton sided with its superintendent.

At first, Meyer's reluctance to take action appeared to be a temporizing move, but as the months went by, Greenacre came to the realization that nothing would be done to stop Cotton's experiments and that she stood little or no chance of publishing her findings—unless she was willing to commit professional suicide by disobeying her superior. As he had done with her earlier research on syphilis, Meyer had blocked Greenacre's work from going into print, but in this case she bore the additional burden of knowing of the deaths and damage that inaction was producing. For the next year and a half, she periodically pressed Meyer for a change of heart, but with no success. Meanwhile, she learned that Cotton was continuing to operate on his patients and had journeyed to Britain, where he had been lionized by leading members of the medical profession as psychiatry's Lister.

Adding to the personal pressure, the prolonged absences Greenacre's work had necessarily entailed had put further strains on a marriage that was already in deep trouble. It cannot have helped that Richter, too, had found ways to disappear from Baltimore, sometimes for extended periods. In 1924 and 1925, for example, with Meyer's support and encouragement, he spent several months at a field station in Panama, where he extended his work with sloths and other mammals.[57] Mutually alienated, Greenacre and Richter were by this point essentially living separate lives. And yet when she finally discovered that her husband was having an affair with a young woman she had considered a family friend, Greenacre was devastated. It was a crushing blow to her self-esteem, leaving her unable to sleep and in "vivid pain."[58]

She approached Meyer with the news, and he promptly shared what he had learned with his brother Hermann: "I was absolutely bowled over when Dr. Greenacre came to tell me the tale of disaster." For years, "everyone had thought she was one of the few who had succeeded in combining scientific and professional work with homemaking."[59] Beneath the surface, however, as Greenacre would learn in the months to come, as their impending divorce turned bitter, her husband had long resented her decision to continue her academic career. Richter wrote to his mother, "I will fight her to the end,"[60] and in a series of wounding letters, he began to do just that. He bitterly accused her of "a lack of affection for the children as shown by her continuing in medicine" and complained of "her inability to create a home that would have attracted him."[61]

In the meantime, the parallel with the Watson case was uppermost in Meyer's mind, and he confided to Hermann that Richter would have to go. He hoped that he would not lose Richter's wife as well, but, he wrote, "I do not know whether Dr. Greenacre can or will stay."[62] A month later, she told him she simply could not remain on staff,[63] leaving him to lament the discomfiture her departure would cause him: "Dr. Greenacre leaves at a time when I should have had all her help." He also openly worried that she would experience another mental collapse: "I am afraid she is not going to have an easy road. She may get into the depressive condition again which she had in 1917 and 1918."[64]

A BITTER SEPARATION AND ITS AFTERMATH

Between Christmas and the New Year, Greenacre abruptly left Baltimore for New York, leaving the children briefly with Mrs. Meyer while she located a place to live. Within weeks, with Meyer's assistance, she had obtained a new job in suburban White Plains, but it was "a far cry from the intensive work at the Phipps."[65] She served as a staff psychiatrist at the juvenile court and department of child welfare, a dreary, low-level routine job that left her ever more dissatisfied. Making matters worse, Richter was refusing to provide any financial support for their children, informing her that since she had chosen to take them to New York and had her own professional career and income, he regarded them as her responsibility. Betrayed by Meyer over the Cotton affair; forced to leave behind the Phipps Clinic, which "stands more in the place of [a] familial roof to me than any other place can";[66] embroiled in a poisonous break-up with her husband; and facing a grim professional future, her depression deepened, and she sought psychotherapeutic help.

Repeatedly, Greenacre confided her troubles to Meyer, sharing with him the grievously hurtful and obdurate letters she was receiving from Richter and seeking advice and intervention from her "chief." Sympathy was forthcoming, but not action. Years earlier, Meyer had intervened decisively with the Hopkins administration to ensure Watson's departure. With Richter, he did no such thing. Though his first reaction had been that his younger colleague would have to resign, he made no move to secure that result. On the contrary, he allowed the younger man to become even more indispensable to his enterprise, and rather bizarrely, he chose to inform Greenacre of this development: "Dr. R. has evidently changed his attitude towards my courses and instead of a cold blanket, the students with whom he deals seem to fall in line with a more favorable spirit—both the 1st and the 2nd year classes. I do not think it is mere policy [i.e., calculation on his part]. I really feel it is the first time he has approached the teaching with a fairer spirit, and I myself seem to feel the relief in the rather heavy load I have taken on."[67]

By June, Meyer was confessing to Greenacre to some hesitancy and indecision about his own course of action: "Whether Dr. R. had best go . . . is a question. I wish he wd go to Russia where he wd like to see the Pavlov lab—and stay there to prepare for another place in this country. I shd find it terribly hard to find anyone in his place just yet."[68] And he never had to do so. The acrimony over the impending divorce between Richter and Greenacre dragged on and on, with Meyer in the middle trying feebly to broker peace between the two fiercely contending sides.[69] Even when Richter submitted a formal resignation in 1929, Meyer allowed him to withdraw it, and the two men then reached an understanding, one that would allow them to put the whole "unfortunate" episode behind them.

On August 26, Richter wrote:

> I am writing to tell you what I would like to do next year and to offer a concrete Plan which I hope will serve the purpose of helping us to arrive at a constructive working agreement and thereby bring to a close what has been for me a very unhappy period. I am glad to state at once that I should like to withdraw my resignation and assume all my old responsibilities along with others concerned with working out the course in psychobiology. The latter responsibility I assume willingly and gladly since during the summer my resistance to giving a course of this kind has largely disappeared. I feel that now I can undertake this work with confidence as well as with enthusiasm. I may also state at once that I will give you my word that I will take care of the settlement of marital difficulties and the associated complications in a way that is in harmony with your own personal wishes and the interests of the Phipps clinic.[70]

Almost certainly, it was not just Richter's willingness to play a vital role in Meyer's teaching program that persuaded Meyer to keep him on. Richter's friendship with many of the leading Hopkins scientists, and the respect with which they viewed his work, with its clever instrumentation and meticulous data collection, would undoubtedly have complicated any decision to seek his dismissal. Meyer was much further up in the institutional hierarchy, but he had been unable to improve his discipline's lowly rank in the intellectual pecking order, and his wordy pronouncements were rightly seen as programmatic rather than scientific. There were signs that his colleagues were seeing an emperor bereft of clothes. On one notorious occasion, the medical students put on a play with the bearded "Meyer" as a central character, giving a lecture in "Chinese," interspersed with favorite bits of Meyerian jargon: integration concept, family formation, experiment of nature, the ergasias, and so forth. Unlike his colleagues, the great man was not amused, and he induced the medical board to ban all future performances of that kind.[71] In this context, Richter's work provided vital evidence for the scientific fruitfulness of Meyer's concept of psychobiology. Meyer's puritanical instincts notwithstanding, Richter may have been simply too valuable to dismiss.

We do know that Meyer felt guilty about his treatment of Phyllis Greenacre. Both Greenacre and her son, Peter Richter, commented separately that Meyer's efforts on her behalf in the 1930s reflected a sense of guilt and obligation.[72] Such sentiments are also evident in his private notes to himself. Some time in the summer of 1928, he wrote self-reproachfully about his behavior toward her. For all her ability and experience, and the invaluable work she had done for him, he had neglected to advance her over the years, so that both her title and her income had lagged far behind her responsibilities: "Dr. Greenacre should have been . . . instructor and director of the lab. . . . Justly or unjustly, I considered her as a potential rather than a fully active member of the staff, on account of the family responsibilities."[73]

He tried to make amends, sometimes ham-handedly. Only two months after Greenacre's abrupt departure for New York, he invited her back for a reunion of the Phipps Clinic staff.[74] Still traumatized, she responded: "I want if possible to attend, for the Phipps will always have my loyalty and interest, . . . [but] I do not know whether I shall find it possible to face again, in the setting of a family reunion, the whole physical situation which swamps me with such painful conflicts and memories. . . . The thought of this past year and a half gives me a comprehensive shudder."[75] Six weeks later, she had made up her mind: "There is much that draws me and I should like to come. But I have about decided not to attempt it, because it still stirs me up too much,—and in addition I do not know that I should really be able to live up to the conventional surface demanded. . . . I do not want to take the risk of exposing my personal feelings in a general gathering of that kind."[76]

In mid-June, Meyer had an even more audacious proposal. He was setting up a new research project on schizophrenia. Would she return to direct it? He knew she had expressed an interest in "practice with patients whom you can treat according to emergency, outside of hospital . . . [and] were inclined to make any special research and teaching incidental to practice. The research position I can offer naturally assumes a somewhat different orientation," but he was convinced it could be "an ideal position for you. . . . Now it is just a question whether such leadership in handling the material appeals to you and whether it would help you overcome preoccupations of memories of the past."[77]

The proposal was, from Greenacre's perspective, impossible to accept, even though Meyer had assured her that he had arranged for the departure of Richter's mistress before she would need to arrive in Baltimore and had emphasized, "I am terribly anxious to make possible a harmonious active working group during the rest of my working years at Hopkins."[78] Though her New York situation was an unhappy one, she wrote, "I find that going back there [to Baltimore] even for a short time, precipitates a depression that takes several weeks to deal with. I know that ultimately I will come to a better immunization, but it seems to be a bewilderingly slow process. . . . In addition, I would hesitate before taking the children back now into an atmosphere in which there would be the possibility of stirring up further conflict for them. They accept Curt's not living with us now,—as we are on new ground, but they think that if we went back to Baltimore, it would mean a re-establishment of joint family life."[79]

In her New York exile, Greenacre set about rebuilding her life and career. To deal with her depression, she began psychoanalytic treatment, first with the Jungian analyst Beatrice Hinkle; then with Freud's first biographer, Fritz Wittels;[80] and lastly with Edith Jacobson.[81] Beyond whatever therapeutic value these encounters may have had in troubled times, they gave her insight into a new intellectual universe and ultimately launched her on a radically different career path. As she began to recover some semblance of stability in her life, the endless round of mundane activities that her job at the juvenile court entailed left her feeling increasingly trapped. It had been "something I could carry . . . adequately even through a period of intense personal preoccupation." Three years on, however, she lamented, "[The position] furnishes relatively little opportunity for developement [sic] and I do not feel that I can stick by it indefinitely without danger of atrophy."[82]

Hence came a renewed appeal to Meyer: "Since you know my capacities and limitations better than anyone else, I would appreciate very much your advice and help if you know of any opening which I might satisfactorily fill."[83] For months, little help was forthcoming. Meyer did suggest that she approach some prominent New York psychiatrists—William L. Russell, Frederick Wells, and George Stevenson—to see if they knew of a position for her. More than a year later, he at last intervened more forcefully and secured her a post as director of outpatient psychiatric treatment at the Cornell Medical Center in New York. "I am ever so grateful,"[84] Greenacre informed him. She had at last obtained a new academic appointment, almost four years after her abrupt departure from Hopkins.

Greenacre's new role overseeing the treatment of patients not confined in a mental hospital now provided the material basis on which she rebuilt her career along novel lines. Her second analyst, Fritz Wittels, was a powerful figure in the oldest and most important Freudian center in the United States, the New York Psychoanalytic Society and Institute. Within a few months of the society deciding to set up a formal program of psychoanalytic education, Greenacre joined the institute as a candidate, and by 1937, to Meyer's considerable dismay, she had begun to practice as an analyst.[85]

Thereafter, her rise was rapid and remarkable, if somewhat surprising. The society and its companion institute were dominated, by the late 1930s, by an oligarchy of European refugees who had fled the Nazis. These exiles, for the most part, exhibited a barely concealed contempt for American analysts and tended to keep power firmly in their own hands.[86] Greenacre succeeded in penetrating this inner circle of Viennese exiles (many of them Freud's intimates), virtually the only one of her native-born contemporaries to do so. As early as 1942, she was granted the coveted status of training analyst and became a member of the society's Education Committee. These were critical steps in her new career. "Being a training analyst conferred great prestige within the organization, as well as referrals, economic security, and the mystique of authority."[87]

By the 1950s, Greenacre was training more analysts than anyone else at the institute. Her status had been recognized by her election first as president of the institute, a position she held from 1948 to 1950, and then as president of the society itself half a dozen years later. And she became "the analyst of analysts, particularly those who were troubled."[88] Leaving her Meyerian training far behind, she became an expert on the psychoanalytic study of childhood and adolescence[89] and wrote psychohistorical studies of such figures as Jonathan Swift, Lewis Carroll, and Charles Darwin.[90]

Between the end of World War II and the late 1960s, psychoanalysis temporarily dominated American psychiatry. During this quarter-century of Freudian hegemony, the New York Psychoanalytic Society and Institute was without question one of the most prestigious centers of Freudian ideas and training in the country—one writer termed it "the Harvard of American analysis."[91] Greenacre's leading position in its councils thus made her arguably one of the most influential psychiatrists and analysts in the country. Such, indeed, was the conclusion reached by the American

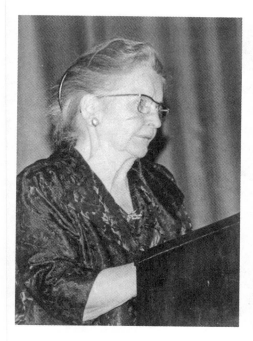

Figure 7. Phyllis Greenacre lecturing during her New York years, most probably in the 1960s. (Reproduced by courtesy of the New York Psychoanalytic Institute and Society Archive.)

political scientist Arnold Rogow in 1970. After conducting a survey of psychiatrists, he found that Greenacre was considered the fourth most influential living analyst, ranking behind only Anna Freud, Heinz Hartmann, and Erik Erikson.[92] It was a remarkable rise from the emotional turmoil and professional marginality that had confronted her in the late 1920s.

Her ex-husband had an equally stellar career, and Meyer's faith in Richter would be amply repaid over the ensuing years. His protégé's accumulating body of scientific work would lead to Richter being elected to such august institutions as the National Academy of Sciences and the American Philosophical Society, and it earned him a serious nomination for a Nobel Prize. Out of a lifetime of laboratory labors, his elaboration of the significance of the biological clock and his work on homeostasis and the behavioral regulation of the internal milieu within the context of nutritional choice were of particular importance, stimulating a host of later researches.[93]

From the late 1920s until the 1950s, Richter was at the forefront of those creating a psychology that eschewed the introspective and marginalized

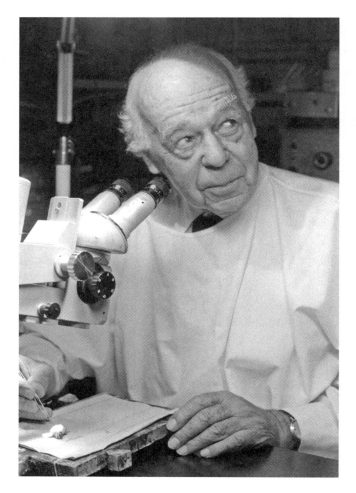

Figure 8. Curt Richter at his microscope, 1976. (Reproduced by courtesy of the Alan Mason Chesney Archives, Johns Hopkins Medical Institutions.)

the human in favor of experimental studies of the psychobiology of laboratory animals—the very antithesis of the intellectual approach his ex-wife was embracing and advancing. Over and over again, he sought ways to take the body apart and put it together again, honing his surgical skills, creating new instruments, and constructing novel experiments to examine behavioral and biological adaptation. Even his formal retirement in the late 1950s brought no letup in his work. To the very end of his life—and to the evident dismay of the university, which found itself unable to eject so distinguished a scientist from his laboratory (even turning off the heat did not dissuade him from remaining in situ)—Richter continued to occupy his space in the Phipps Clinic, turning out papers on growth hormone and cortisol secretion in rats, guinea pigs, and monkeys in his seventh decade on the staff, even as the rest of the building was torn apart and renovated around him.

CONCLUSION

This chapter has examined some aspects of the development of American psychiatry, psychoanalysis, and psychobiology through the prism of three overlapping and interlocking lives and scientific careers. Adolf Meyer, the most senior of the three, played a vital but ambiguous role in the development of his two protégés. It was his recognition of their talents and the environment that he created at the Phipps that allowed Phyllis Greenacre and Curt Richter to manage the crucial transition from promising student to established professional. A notoriously controlling figure, Meyer for more than a decade played a large role in even the personal lives of his two associates, a role that was all the more expansive, perhaps, because Greenacre was thoroughly estranged from her parents and, at more than one time in her Hopkins career, emotionally vulnerable; and because Richter had lost his father as a young child.

Yet although Meyer advanced Greenacre's career, he also held it back. He encouraged her early researches into the neurobiology of syphilis, but he then stood in the way of her publishing her results. He constrained her opportunities for clinical work and failed to advance her in rank or salary, even as her experience grew and her value to his enterprise soared. (Latterly, he would concede that this might have reflected an unconscious prejudice against a female associate who remained ambitious to develop her career alongside marriage and motherhood.) He prevailed on her to invest eighteen months of her career investigating the experimental treatments of another of his protégés, Henry Cotton, but then suppressed her findings, placing her in an almost impossible ethical dilemma.[94] (The bigger price in this instance, of course, was paid by yet more mental patients

who found themselves subjected to maiming and even fatal rounds of surgery while Meyer remained silent and complicit in Baltimore.) Finally, he
allowed, and perhaps indirectly forced, her departure from Hopkins and
Baltimore when, having been informed of Richter's sexual indiscretions,
he kept her husband on the staff, creating an intolerable environment for
Greenacre.

Unintentionally, of course, Greenacre's forced flight to New York, and
the emotional turmoil associated with it, paved the way for her intellectual
transformation from a Meyerian to a Freudian psychiatrist. Her success in
the latter coincided with the emergence of psychoanalysis as the dominant
strand in American psychiatry and helped to catapult her to the highest
reaches of her chosen profession. Obviously, the very qualities that had
marked her during her time at Hopkins—her intellectual acumen, her
capacity for hard work, her discretion, her curiosity—did much to foster
her advancement even in the peculiar environment that was New York psychoanalysis, where she became one of the few figures to advance into the
inner circle of analysts who was not a Jewish Middle European refugee.

Greenacre professed a continuing gratitude to Meyer for the training
he had provided, but it was a gratitude increasingly tempered by a sense
of the limitations of his worldview. As she acknowledged in the 1970s, late
on in her career, "The training to observe," which she had received under
Meyer's tutelage, "has been of incalculable benefit to me and I owe a debt
of gratitude for it." But by then, she had distanced herself from "an obsessional and probably futile search for accuracy" and had long reached the
conclusion that "the emphasis on recording all possible phenomenological
details" about a patient's life history had "sometimes reached fantastic
proportions." Not the least part of what she had taken from her experience
at Hopkins was thus a negative lesson, "The warning not to drive recording observation to a stage of the infinite and the absurd in the effort to
cover everything."[95]

For Meyer, indeed, nothing had been too trivial or inconsequential to
record and enter on a patient's life chart.[96] "A fact," he proclaimed, "is anything which makes a difference."[97] But his system advanced no clear criteria for determining what *did* make a difference. By contrast, in becoming
an orthodox Freudian (and one suspects that this transition was no accident), Greenacre had moved from this sort of catholic eclecticism, where

interpretation was loose, unstructured, and lacking any way of discovering what was etiologically significant, to a highly deterministic intellectual system that was in many ways its polar opposite.

If Greenacre's success after she left Hopkins is the more remarkable because it was achieved in the face of such obstacles—her gender, her national origin, the sharp shift in intellectual focus and identity that it required—her former husband's progress is in some ways less remarkable, even if he achieved a comparable level of distinction in his chosen field. Curt Richter had no gender handicaps to overcome. He remained in the environment that had first nurtured his scientific career and could thus build cumulatively on the foundations he had created during the 1920s. His extraordinary usefulness to Meyer ensured his initial survival beyond the crisis that had emerged with the exposure of his affair, and his creativity and ingenuity as an experimentalist, his drive, and his compulsion to work make the accomplishments of his later years somewhat unsurprising, if nonetheless notable. His and Meyer's relationship was, in part, a marriage of convenience, with the older man benefiting indirectly from the prestige that Richter's laboratory brought to the field of psychobiology but contributing very little of a concrete sort to the enterprise.

Not surprisingly, Richter's career continued to flourish in the decades after Meyer's retirement. Indeed, Richter and Greenacre were professionally active almost to the end of their remarkably long lives. Born in the same year, 1894, both died within less than ten months of one another, Richter in December 1988 and Greenacre in October the following year.

Having both lived for almost a century, Richter and Greenacre had grown up in a world that was unfriendly, even hostile, to the idea of women having active careers in science and academic medicine, most especially if they further tempted fate by presuming to marry and have children. Their own marriage had foundered under the attendant strains. After their partnership broke apart, Richter remarried and had another child by a wife content to play the supportive female role then prescribed by the culture. Greenacre, by contrast, eschewed further matrimonial entanglements, refused to rein in her ambitions, and overcame the powerful obstacles presented by her status as a woman and a single parent to build a life of remarkable professional accomplishment. In the process, she helped to create a world of very different norms and structural possibilities for the generation coming to maturity at her death—albeit one not immune, of course, to its own inequalities and prejudices.

Meyer's position at the forefront of American psychiatry was in substantial part the product of his strategically important post as a professor at Hopkins at a time when it was almost certainly the premier medical school in the United States. His resistance to the schemes promoted by the Rockefeller Foundation to have medical school faculty appointed to full-time salaried positions (rather than subsisting on clinical income)[98] left him bereft of the generous funding more compliant departments received from Rockefeller's General Education Board, and though he trained a whole generation of leading American psychiatrists (and developed techniques like the life chart, which provided some structure to the practice of psychiatry), it was his institutional location, rather than the power of his ideas, that made him so central to what remained at his death a marginal and stigmatized specialty. Hence, perhaps, his depressed musings, in characteristically unidiomatic prose, just three years before his death: "What was it that failed to go across? Did I pussyfoot too much? *Wherein did I fail?*"[99] And hence as well the evanescence of his influence, once he had passed from the scene.

Curt Richter's career might well have been set back by his extramarital affair. After all, something very similar had cost his patron, John Watson, both his Hopkins post and any future in academia; and one of Watson's predecessors as a professor of psychology, James Mark Baldwin, had likewise been forced to resign his Hopkins post in 1908 when he was caught in a black brothel during a police raid.[100] Meyer had supported both earlier dismissals,[101] but, as shown above, in Richter's case he prevaricated and then let his subordinate remain. Deviance that in two cases spelled professional ruin was ignored for someone of such central importance to the Meyerian project.

It was Richter's talents, though, that let him escape from Meyer's shadow and go on to develop a distinguished and independent scientific career. But that career extended into the era of big science and a bureaucratic, peer-reviewed grant process, an environment for which the independent and idiosyncratic Richter was ill-suited, and of which he was increasingly critical.[102] By the end of his long and illustrious scientific career, Richter was something of an intellectual oddity, someone who left few students of his own and whose influence was largely indirect and often unacknowledged.

Finally, this chapter has emphasized the gendered discrimination that marked Phyllis Greenacre's career and made her accomplishments the more striking. But it was precisely because psychiatry was so little valued by the medical profession that it provided a niche in the professional division of labor that was in general more receptive than most to women. And that was even more true of psychoanalysis, where a number of female analysts besides Greenacre came to occupy positions of considerable prominence: Helene Deutsch, Karen Horney, Frieda Fromm-Reichmann, and Melanie Klein and her bitter antagonist Anna Freud, to name but a handful of obvious examples. Within American psychoanalysis, Greenacre long occupied a position of great prestige and influence at what was the very center of Freudian orthodoxy, the New York Psychoanalytic Society and Institute. And in the 1950s and 1960s, while psychoanalysis occupied the commanding heights of American psychiatry, that meant she was a figure of some moment in the psychiatric profession broadly construed. But the very possibility of such a career and set of accomplishments arose out of her willingness during the 1920s to be silenced; to acknowledge her subordinate state; to abide by the norms that enjoined junior researchers to acknowledge the absolute authority of their superiors; and her decision to eschew the lonely (and usually fatal) role of the whistle-blower.[103] Finally, she lived long enough to see her form of science become an anachronism. The resurgence of biological psychiatry in the 1980s meant that the branch of the enterprise in which she had achieved prominence lost its luster, intellectual prominence, and appeal. Greenacre had had her analysands, but, by the late twentieth century, that scarcely seemed to matter.

8 Mangling Memories

On November 19, 1948, the two most enthusiastic and prolific lobotomists in the Western world faced off against each other in the operating theater at the Institute of Living in Hartford, Connecticut. They performed before an audience of more than two dozen neurosurgeons, neurologists, and psychiatrists. Each had developed a different technique for mutilating the brains of the patients they operated on, and each had his turn on the stage.

William Beecher Scoville, professor of neurosurgery at Yale, went first. His patient was conscious. The administration of a local anesthetic allowed the surgeon to slice through the scalp and peel down the skin from the patient's forehead, exposing her skull. Quick work with a drill opened two holes, one over each eye. Now Scoville could see her frontal lobes. He levered each side up with a flat blade so that he could perform what he called "orbital undercutting." Although what followed was not quite cutting: instead, Scoville inserted a suction catheter—a small electrical vacuum cleaner—and sucked out a portion of the patient's frontal lobes.

The patient was then wheeled out and a replacement was secured to the operating table. Walter Freeman, a professor of neurology at George Washington University, was next. He had no surgical training and no Connecticut medical license, so he was operating illegally—not that such

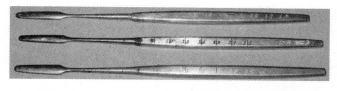

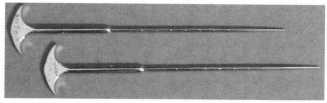

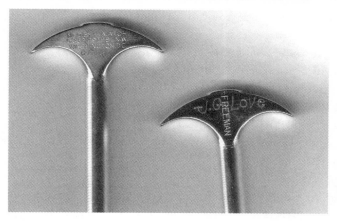

Figure 9. (Top) Conventional lobotomy knives, with centimeters engraved on them to provide a guide to "precision" cutting. *(Middle)* A pair of orbitoclasts, the modified icepick developed by Walter Freeman to perform transorbital lobotomies (note the centimeter markings, which were used as a guide to how far to drive the instrument into the frontal lobes of the brain). *(Bottom)* The heads of two orbitoclasts, engraved with the name of the instrument maker in Washington, DC (H. A. Ator), and stamped "Freeman," since this was Walter Freeman's proprietary design. These instruments were owned by Dr. J. O. Love and used at the Rochester State Hospital in Minnesota. They were later thrown into the trash. Dr. Robert Coffey rescued them from oblivion and kindly shared these photographs with me.

a minor matter seemed to bother anyone present. Freeman was working on developing an assembly-line approach so that lobotomies could be performed quickly and easily. His technique allowed him to perform twenty or more operations in a single day. He proceeded to use shocks from an electroconvulsive therapy machine to render his female patient unconscious and then inserted an ice pick beneath one of her eyelids until the point rested on the thin bony structure in the orbit. A few quick taps with a hammer broke through the bone and allowed him to sever portions of the frontal lobes using a sweeping motion with the ice pick. The instrument was withdrawn and inserted into the other orbit, and within minutes, the process was over. It was, Freeman boasted, so simple an operation that he could teach any damned fool, even a psychiatrist, to perform it in twenty minutes or so.

Tens of thousands of lobotomies were performed in the United States from 1936 onward, and both these men would continue operating for decades. Lobotomy's inventor, the Portuguese neurologist Egas Moniz, received the Nobel Prize in Medicine for his pains in 1949. Major medical centers in the United States—Harvard, Yale, Columbia, the University of Pennsylvania—regularly performed variations on the basic operation well into the 1950s.

It has become fashionable in recent years among some medical historians to argue that the operation was not the medical horror story that popular culture portrays it as being. These scholars suggest that, when considered within the context of the times, lobotomy was perhaps a defensible response to massively overcrowded mental hospitals and the therapeutic impotence of the psychiatry of the time. That is not my view, and Luke Dittrich's book *Patient H.M.: A Story of Memory, Madness and Family Secrets* (2017) adds to evidence from elsewhere that Scoville (like Freeman) was a moral monster—ambitious, driven, self-centered, and willing to inflict grave and irreversible damage on his patients in his search for fame. He certainly had no time for the Hippocratic injunction: "First, do no harm."

Ironically, Scoville was quick to denounce the crudity of Freeman's procedure, a position the neurosurgeons in the audience were happy to endorse. Freeman, in turn, was scornful of the notion that his rival's suctioning away of portions of the brain was "precise," as Scoville and his supporters contended. On these points, at least, both men were for once correct.

Dittrich devotes considerable space to this remarkable surgical contest in Hartford, which he views with a suitably skeptical eye. But he opens his narrative much earlier, with the story of an accident that befell Henry Molaison, a young boy of six or seven, one summer evening. En route home for dinner, Henry stepped into the street and was struck from behind by a bicycle. The impact threw him through the air, and he landed on his head, sustaining a concussion that temporarily rendered him unconscious. Henry eventually recovered from his injuries, but only partially. He began to suffer from epileptic seizures that increased in frequency and severity as the years went by and made his life a misery. Drugs didn't help. Finally, in 1953, Henry's parents brought him to see Dr. Scoville. Unlike most of the other patients subjected to psychosurgery, Henry was sane. Scoville informed the family that the epilepsy might be tamed by the brain surgery he was pioneering, and within a matter of months, Henry was wheeled into the operating theater. What occurred next made him one of the most famous patients of the twentieth century.

Following his usual procedure, Scoville cut into Henry's skull, exposing portions of his brain to view. His target on this occasion, however, lay further back, behind the frontal lobes that he usually targeted for his lobotomies. The electroencephalograph had failed to reveal any epileptic focus. Now, using a flat brain spatula, Scoville pushed aside the frontal lobes to expose deeper structures in the temporal lobe—the amygdala, the uncus, the entorhinal cortex—searching for any obvious defects or atrophied tissue. Nothing. At this point, a cautious surgeon would have cut the surgery short, since there was no obvious lesion to justify further intervention. Scoville was not such a person. In his own words, "I prefer action to thought, which is why I am a surgeon. I like to see results."[1] Results he obtained, although not the ones his patient was hoping for. Using a suction catheter, Scoville proceeded to destroy all three regions of the temporal lobe bilaterally.

Patient H. M., as Henry became known in the trade, suffered absolutely devastating losses. Though his intellect remained intact, he had in those few minutes lost all but the very shortest of short-term memory. Henceforth, as Scoville noted, he was left essentially helpless and hopeless, with *"very grave"* memory loss, *"so severe as to prevent the patient from remembering the location of the rooms in which he lives, the names of*

his close associates, or even the way to the toilet or the urinal." And, of
course, much else besides. Those words constituted, as Dittrich puts it,
"the birth announcement of Patient H. M. It was also the obituary of
Henry Molaison."[2]

The first of many surprises Dittrich springs on the reader is the news
that William Beecher Scoville was his grandfather, someone he came to
know well over many years. Those family ties gave Dittrich access to all
manner of materials that no outsider could have obtained, and he is clearly
both a talented and persistent journalist and an excellent storyteller. I
found it all the more disappointing, then, that he and his publisher elected
to provide neither footnotes nor any systematic documentation of his
sources. What we are left with is a gripping story, but one whose provenance is at times unfortunately quite murky. A second surprise concerns
Dittrich's grandmother, Emily Barrett Learned, whom he affectionately
refers to as Bam Bam. Emily had been a high-spirited young woman
before she married the handsome Bill Scoville in June 1934. By 1944, they
had three children, and Bill was serving in the Army medical corps, leaving her alone much of the time in the small town of Walla Walla in eastern
Washington State. Then she found out that her husband was having an
affair. She began to hallucinate and tried to hang herself. She was placed
in a secure ward of a local hospital until, a few weeks later, the entire family left for Hartford, Connecticut. There, she was rushed to the Institute of
Living, one of America's oldest mental hospitals, and where her husband
would perform most of his lobotomies (though not the operation on
H. M.). Scoville had been on staff there since 1941.

The Institute of Living (previously the Hartford Retreat for the Insane)
was a ritzy private establishment catering to the wealthy in surroundings
that superficially resembled a country club. Its grounds had been laid out by
Frederick Olmstead, the architect of Central Park in New York. Its inmates
were referred to as "guests," though these were guests deprived of any voice
in their fate. The superintendent, Dr. Burlingame, aggressively employed all
the latest weapons of 1940s psychiatry: insulin comas, metrazol seizures,
hydrotherapy, pyrotherapy (insertion into a coffin-like device that allowed
the patient to be heated until the body's homeostatic mechanism failed and
an artificial fever of 105 or 106 degrees Fahrenheit was achieved), and electroshock therapy (ECT) in its unmodified form (which produced violent

seizures). Emily received many of these so-called treatments, to little effect. Her unsympathetic psychiatrist commented that her husband's infidelity "has upset her to an unusual degree,"[3] and her case notes reveal someone frightened of the ECT and still in the grip of psychotic ideation. Her subsequent release seems a bit mysterious. She was henceforth withdrawn and rather lacking initiative, a pattern that makes more sense when we learn, in the book's closing pages, that Dr. Scoville had personally lobotomized her. One of the many poignant scenes in Dittrich's book is his recital of a Thanksgiving dinner at his grandparents' house, during which Emily sat silently amid her family while her ex-husband and his new wife (a younger, more attractive model) presided over the proceedings.

His book's title notwithstanding, Dittrich spends many pages exposing these kinds of family secrets. But he eventually returns to the case of the memory-less H.M. Here was a scientific prize. Unlike the legions of lobotomized patients Scoville left in his wake (he continued to perform his orbital undercutting procedure into the 1970s, claiming it was "safe and almost harmless"), H.M. was not mentally ill, and his intellectual abilities remained intact after the surgery. That made him an ideal subject for research on human memory, and the findings of that research were what made Henry so famous (not that he was capable of appreciating that). Early on, an eminent neuroscientist from McGill University in Montreal, Dr. Brenda Milner, was the primary psychologist studying H.M., and she made a number of pathbreaking discoveries about memory through her work with him, including the finding that humans possess two distinct and independent memory systems. One of these had survived in H.M., the one that allowed him to acquire and improve on learned skills. The other, memory for events, was utterly extinguished.

Dr. Milner soon moved her research in a different direction and lost touch with H.M. In her place, one of her graduate students, Suzanne Corkin, took over. Subsequently, Corkin obtained a faculty position at MIT. H.M. became, in effect, her possession. For as long as he lived, Corkin controlled access to him, forcing other researchers who wanted to examine him to dance to her tune, and building a good deal of her career as one of the first women scientists at MIT on her privileged access to this fascinating subject. From 1953 until his death in 2008, H.M. was regularly whisked away to MIT from the Hartford family he had been placed with, and later from the board-and-care home where he resided, to be poked and prodded, examined and re-examined, each time encountering the site and Dr. Corkin as though for the first time.

Corkin, it turns out, also had a connection to Dittrich. She had lived directly across the street from the Scoville family and had been Dittrich's mother's best friend when the two girls were young—not that it seems to have helped Dittrich much when he sought to interview her for his book. She first evaded meeting him and then sought to put crippling limitations on his ability to use whatever he learned from talking to her. How much this affected Dittrich's attitude toward her is difficult to say, but it seems inarguable that he developed an extremely negative view of her behavior.

As Dittrich points out, Corkin and MIT obtained millions of dollars in research grants due to her control over H. M. Not a penny of it reached poor Henry's pockets. He subsisted on small disability payments from the government, and not once did he receive any compensation for his time and sometimes suffering. He once returned to Hartford, for example, with a series of small second-degree burns on his chest—the result of an experiment to determine his pain threshold. After all, he couldn't remember the experiment, so why not subject him to it? Belatedly, it seems to have occurred to Corkin that she should get some legal authorization for her experiments, since H. M. was manifestly incapable of giving informed consent. Making no effort to locate a living blood relative (a first cousin lived only a few miles away), she instead secured the court-ordered appointment of a conservator who never visited H. M. but who routinely signed off on any proposal she put in front of him.

Henry Molaison does not seem to have had much luck at the hands of those who experimented on him. Scoville cavalierly made use of him to see what would happen when large sections of his brain were suctioned out, and Corkin seems to have taken virtual ownership of him and then exploited her good fortune for all it was worth. According to Dittrich, H. M.'s travails did not end with his death. Quickly preserved, his remains were transported to the West Coast, where Jacopo Annese, a neuroanatomist and radiologist at the University of California at San Diego, carefully harvested his brain and began to reveal its secrets. The Italian-born physician Annese comes across as a superb scientist, eager to share what he was finding with the world, but also a naïf in shark-infested waters.

As his work proceeded, he discovered an old lesion in H. M.'s frontal lobes, presumably brought about when Scoville maneuvered them out of the way to reach the deeper structures in the brain he sought to remove. All the memory research on H. M., including Corkin's work, rested on the assumption that only temporal lobe structures had been damaged, so this was a potentially important finding. Coincidentally or not, after being alerted to this discovery, Corkin called on MIT's lawyers to reclaim H. M.'s brain and all the photographs and slides Annese had meticulously prepared. Annese had neglected to secure any sort of paper trail documenting his right to these materials, and UCSD's lawyers hung him out to dry. Waiving a document she had secured from the court-appointed guardian she had personally nominated, Corkin, aided by MIT's attorneys, successfully reclaimed the lot. Annese promptly resigned his faculty appointment, his research career in tatters and his slides and photographs now lost. According to Dittrich, Corkin then made one final twist of the knife. In an interview with him before she died of liver cancer in May 2016, she announced that she planned to shred all her raw materials and the laboratory records relating to her work with Henry Molaison and that she had already shredded many of them. For the last fifty years of H. M.'s life, Corkin had essentially owned him. And she planned to carry with her to her grave whatever secrets lay hidden in her files.

9 Creating a New Psychiatry

ON THE ROCKEFELLER FOUNDATION AND
THE RISE OF ACADEMIC PSYCHIATRY

Like its counterparts elsewhere, American psychiatry was born of the asylum, the massive institutional solution to the problem of serious mental illness that was adopted all across Western Europe and North America in the first half of the nineteenth century.[1] These days, of course, the geography of madness has changed beyond all recognition, and the center of gravity of the psychiatric profession has moved decisively out of the mental hospital and into clinics, general hospitals, and outpatient forms of practice. The end of World War II seems to have marked the crucial moment in this transformation. Certainly, the census of mental hospitals in the United States continued to increase for another decade after 1945, but long before inpatient numbers started to decline at the national level, mental hospitals began to lose favor. New recruits to the profession of psychiatry were abandoning institutional practice in droves, and these deserters rapidly outnumbered their colleagues working in mental hospitals.[2] Yet if the move beyond the institution was decisively and irrevocably made in the years after 1945, its origins can be traced back to developments that took place in the last decades of the nineteenth century and the first decades of the twentieth.

Freud famously visited the United States in 1909 to speak at the anniversary celebrations at Clark University and to receive the only honorary degree of his lifetime. Because of the quarter-century long psychoanalytic domination of American psychiatry that began in the mid-1940s, it is tempting to assume that the wave of earlier experiments with a psychiatry outside the walls of the asylum were closely bound up with the advent of Freudian psychodynamic psychiatry. Tempting, but wrong.

Long before Freud set sail on his lone visit to America, there existed a segment of the profession that had begun to gather under the label "psychiatry" that had commenced practicing in extrainstitutional settings. While most psychiatrists still practiced in mental hospitals and dealt with those legally certified as insane, in the aftermath of the Civil War, practitioners of the newly emerging specialty of neurology had found that many of the patients crowding into their waiting rooms complained of a variety of nervous disorders. Some were veterans of combat who carried no signs of overt physical pathology but complained of a variety of ills. Others were society matrons (or their daughters). Even bankers and captains of industry were showing up. Suffering from the ancient disease of hysteria or the newly fashionable disorder of neurasthenia, all these patients turned to nerve doctors after general practitioners had failed them.[3] Victims of train accidents soon joined them, and "railway spine" became part of an expanding lexicon of functional disorders—complaints that often manifested themselves via physical symptoms but often seemed at odds with what anatomy and physiology taught about the makeup of the body. Nervous patients not disturbed enough to require seclusion in an asylum or even in a sanitarium created a demand for a new kind of nerve doctor, and neurologists willing to accept the challenge (and the lucre) soon found their ranks augmented by refugees from the asylum sector, alienists who had tired of the asylum routine and its atmosphere of hopelessness.[4] A somewhat heterogeneous and disorganized group, these practitioners existed alongside, though at a considerable intellectual and experiential remove from, traditional alienists.

Within a decade or so, the Great War and its aftermath saw a slow but distinct increase in the numbers of such practitioners. The late entrance of the United States into World War I had curtailed, but not prevented, the emergence of shell shock among the troops. Army medics, perforce, found themselves treating both traumatic injuries to the brain and the central nervous system and war neuroses of a far more mysterious sort. Though some continued to proclaim that the shell shocked were malingerers or just

degenerates whose underlying defects had surfaced under combat conditions, there was growing acceptance among other medical men of the view
that the horrors of combat were to blame. Madness was not just a condition found among the biologically inferior who thronged the wards of the
asylum but rather existed along a continuum, from psychoneurosis to psychosis, and the belief was that early intervention in a noninstitutional setting might perhaps head off more serious forms of disturbance.

In the first three decades of the twentieth century, when these psychiatrists working outside institutions looked for an intellectual justification
of their daily practice, it was the murky writings of Adolf Meyer, rather
than the doctrines of Sigmund Freud, that most of them embraced. From
his prominent positions first at the New York Pathological Institute and
then at Johns Hopkins, Meyer advanced the proposition that mental illnesses formed a continuum and represented, however slight or serious
their manifestations, a failure of adjustment. Acute psychosis, mania or
depression, obsessions and chronic unease, even "the trivial fears . . . and
petty foibles of everyday life" were but variants on a theme, the product of
an individual's psychobiological makeup and the environmental challenges she or he confronted. Those at less disturbed points on the continuum might more readily be coaxed and induced to abandon their pathological habits, or so these psychiatrists argued and their patients hoped.

Faced with the bewildering complexities of an array of disorders whose
etiology and treatment remained largely a matter of guesswork and
improvisation, Meyer's notion of psychobiology provided an elastic overarching framework within which a whole array of hypotheses and interventions could be accommodated. His related stress on the meticulous
collection of detailed case histories created a host of tasks with which his
students and the profession at large could occupy their time, consoled by
the illusion that piling up facts would somehow inductively lead to a solution to the problems posed by mental disturbances, both slight and serious. Meyer's prose was notoriously dense and impenetrable, but the word
"psychobiology" seemed comfortably to gesture toward a scientific basis
for psychiatry that brought together all the myriad features of human
existence: psyche and soma, social context, consciousness, and the complexities of human biology. In the more straightforward words of one of
his disciples, Franklin Ebaugh, "Mental disorders are considered to result

from the gradual accumulation of unhealthy reaction tendencies, . . . [and their treatment requires] the study of all previous experiences of the patient, the total biography of the individual and the forces he may be reacting to, whether physical, organic, psychogenic or constitutional."[5]

Meyer's emphasis on the possible relevance of the patient's prior life experiences, as well as on documenting his or her presenting symptoms led him to invent and pass along to his many students something he called "the life chart,"[6] a structured array of techniques to reduce a life history to a standardized record. For Meyer, nothing was too trivial or inconsequential to record and to enter on a patient's life chart. Even the color of the wallpaper in a childhood nursery might have some bearing on the distress of the adult patient in front of him. "A fact," he proclaimed, "is anything which makes a difference."[7] But his system advanced no clear criteria for how to determine what made a difference. In later years, Phyllis Greenacre, who had served as one of his assistants from 1916 to 1927, recalled that this approach rested on "an obsessional and probably futile search for accuracy," one in which "the emphasis on recording all possible phenomenological details" about a patient's life history "sometimes reached fantastic proportions." Meyer's intimidating effect on his students had led most of them "to drive recording observation to a stage of the infinite and the absurd in the effort to cover everything."[8] Constructing such charts, however, did add some structure to psychiatrists' practice and reinforced their sense of active engagement, even though it contributed little to the cure of their patients.

Meyer claimed that his was a "common-sense psychiatry." If mental illness was a problem of ingrained bad habits, psychotherapy should seek to modify them. "Habit-training," Meyer pronounced, "is the backbone of psychotherapy; suggestion is merely a step to the end and only of use to one who knows what that end can and must be attained. Action with flesh and bone is the only safe criterion of efficient mental activity; and actions and attitude and their adaptation is the issue in psychotherapy."[9] Meyer had been heavily influenced by American pragmatism—first by Pierce and Dewey, and later by William James. The problem, of course, was that James had proclaimed that the character and habits of most people, even those who had not succumbed to mental illness, had "set like plaster" by the age of thirty "and will never soften again."[10]

Perhaps that explained the Meyerians' poor therapeutic results with the seriously mentally ill, whose defective habits were simply too deeply engraved on their systems. But the logic of this position also suggested that early intervention might have better results. "Every kind of training," as James had pointed out, quoting from the English physiologist William Carpenter, "is both far more effective, and leaves a more permanent impress, on the growing organism, than when brought to bear on an adult."[11]

The years immediately before the Great War had seen the birth of the National Committee for Mental Hygiene (NCMH), the outgrowth of a campaign by a former mental patient, Clifford Beers, whose own mistreatment in a series of institutions, public and private, had led him to launch a campaign to reform the treatment of the mentally ill. Beers's bestselling autobiography, *A Mind That Found Itself*,[12] written in part while he was a patient at the Hartford Retreat and published in 1908, had made him a national celebrity and had brought him into contact with Adolf Meyer. Meyer sought, without much success, to rein in Beers's grandiosity, ultimately prompting a break between the two men. Meyer suggested Beers should work as an attendant at the mental hospital run by his protégé Henry Cotton; then, when Beers rejected that idea and sought to launch a national campaign of mental health reform, Meyer tried gently to persuade him to limit his ambitions to his native state of Connecticut. He succeeded in arousing Beers's suspicion of his motives, but not before he had planted the idea that, instead of trying to reform mental hospitals, Beers should focus on "mental hygiene," the attempt to promote mental health and head off outbreaks of insanity.

The mutual estrangement between the two men deepened when Beers successfully sought funds from Henry Phipps, the industrial magnate who had funded Meyer's clinic at Johns Hopkins. For three years after the NCMH was founded in 1909, financial difficulties had made it little more than a cipher, but with the help of the Phipps money, it was eventually able to secure further funds from the Rockefeller Foundation. In 1912, an office was established in New York, and a new director, the psychiatrist Thomas Salmon, was recruited to run the organization. Two years later, the Rockefeller Foundation began to pay Salmon's salary and provide funds for national surveys of mental health issues—a forerunner of the foundation's far more extensive involvement in psychiatry during the 1930s and 1940s. Salmon's brief period as an army psychiatrist in the closing months of World War I had brought him into direct contact with victims of shell shock and cemented his commitment to a psychiatry practicing outside the traditional asylums and to a program of mental hygiene that would help to prevent mental illness.

To Salmon and his organization, the most promising way to prevent insanity was to treat the young, an idea Salmon soon sold to another of the great foundations created by America's robber barons, the Commonwealth Fund.[13] Preventing juvenile delinquency became a major goal, and child guidance clinics and marriage guidance clinics were the new institutions to serve as the weapons in that fight. With foundation money, demonstration clinics were established, allowing some psychiatrists to find work outside the walls of traditional institutions.[14] A handful of others found employment in industry, and a handful more worked in the outpatient clinics that progressive states like New York, Pennsylvania, Michigan, and Massachusetts had begun to establish in the second decade of the twentieth century. The plan was to treat incipient cases of insanity among children and adults to slow or reverse the remorseless increase in the number of mental patients confined in state mental hospitals. In that regard, these programs were an abysmal failure, but they did mark a tentative effort by a small minority of psychiatrists to escape from the drudgery of institutional practice.[15] Meanwhile, efforts to establish outpatient clinics in general hospitals were met with resistance or, more often, simply ignored. Hospitals had little interest in treating those exhibiting even mild symptoms of mental disorders and little confidence that psychiatrists possessed the capacity to do so. A 1930 survey by the NCMH found that a mere 3 percent of the general hospitals responding made provision for psychiatric patients, and even that number was likely an overestimate given the tendency to conflate psychiatric and neurological conditions.[16]

Psychiatry remained the most poorly paid and despised of medical specialties, and the efforts it made to break out of its institutional straitjacket enjoyed only limited success. Thomas Salmon left the NCMH in 1922 for a post at Columbia University and the following year became the first psychiatrist without a background in institutional psychiatry to assume the presidency of the American Psychiatric Association. But his death in a boating accident on Long Island Sound in 1927 silenced one of the main advocates for noninstitutional psychiatry.

After Salmon's departure from the NCMH, the Rockefeller Foundation began to distance itself from the organization. The foundation stood aloof from the initiatives sponsored by the Commonwealth Fund, and Rockefeller staff privately voiced increasing mistrust and disdain for the whole mental hygiene enterprise. Alan Gregg, for example, who had become director of the foundation's Division of Medical Sciences in 1930, spoke repeatedly in his official diary of his sense that "mental hygiene has been much oversold and expectations excited beyond likelihood of gratification," a feeling that he found was "widespread" as he traveled around the country.[17]

In the preceding two decades, the General Education Board, and then its successor, the Rockefeller Foundation, had sought to transform American medical education, bribing and cajoling medical schools to reform their practices and investing vast sums in universities that embraced its vision.[18] Just as important, the two organizations had sought to drive out of business the proprietary and substandard medical schools that had been so notable a feature of the American scene in the nineteenth century—those whose admissions standards, laboratory facilities, and clinical instruction were so poor as to be beyond rescue. Ultimately, as many as a third of the existing schools closed their doors. In other respects, though, the Rockefeller Foundation had considerable, though mixed, success in creating medical schools in the mold it sought—schools that emphasized biomedicine, the laboratory, and the production of new medical knowledge, to the detriment, some have argued, of the clinical care of patients.[19]

Be that as it may, there can be little question that the financial resources the foundation mobilized had a transformational influence on American medical education, a result that reflected the fact that in important respects, medicine was otherwise an orphan.[20] Since Big Pharma had yet to enter the picture in any major way (the transformative effect of antibiotics still lay in the future), alternative nongovernmental sources of funding were few and far between. Likewise, government funding of universities, science, and medicine was essentially nonexistent—as it would remain until World War II turned the world upside down and ushered in the era of the imperial state. One of the unintended consequences of that growth of federal power and influence was to give birth to Big Science and Big Medicine, transforming universities from finishing schools for the elite into knowledge factories. In the absence of the federal largesse that,

some decades later, would underwrite research on the etiology and therapeutics of disease (and reconfigure work in the basic sciences), it was
funding from the great private foundations that provided universities with
research equipment and support, and even underwrote the establishment
of new specialized academic departments. And in the medical arena, the
Rockefeller Foundation was the preeminent actor.

It was thus of great consequence when, in the late 1920s, the Rockefeller
Foundation shifted its focus away from the reform of American medical
schools and toward a much greater emphasis on research and the generation of new knowledge. Two divisions were soon established to implement
this new policy: the Division of Natural Sciences, headed by Warren
Weaver from 1932 to 1955; and the Division of Medical Sciences, run by
Richard Pearce from 1927 to 1930. When Pearce died unexpectedly, he
was replaced by his deputy, Alan Gregg. In the early thirties, Weaver and
Gregg faced the task of setting the agenda for their respective divisions,
subject to the approval of the Rockefeller trustees, and both rapidly set
their priorities. For Weaver, a mathematician impressed by the advances
in physics and chemistry that quantitative work had brought in its train,
these priorities quickly became genetics and molecular biology. Gregg's
surprising choice was the highly unfashionable field of psychiatry.

The parlous state of psychiatry had not gone unnoticed by the foundation even before the 1932 decision to focus on the field. The foundation
had debated the matter internally during the late 1920s, and in 1930 its
leadership solicited a memorandum from David Edsall, one of its trustees
and the dean of the Harvard Medical School, to assist their deliberations.
Edsall was hardly encouraging, noting that "traditionally, psychiatry has
been distinctly separated from general medical interests and thought to
such a degree that, to very many medical men it seems a wholly distinct
thing with which they have no relation." Nor was this state of affairs surprising: "In most places psychiatry now is dominated by elusive and inex-
act methods of study and by speculative thought. Any efforts to employ
the more precise methods that are available have been slight and spo-
radic." He dismissed psychoanalysis as "speculative" and argued that any
assistance to the field "would seem to have an element of real danger. . . .
It has a strong emotional appeal to many able young men, and I have
known a number of men highly trained in science who began activities in

psychiatry but, through the fascination of psychoanalysis, gave up their scientific training practically entirely for the more immediate returns of psycho-analysis." And Edsall was equally dubious about the value of "the psychological or sociological aspects of psychiatry, . . . romantic and appealing" as they might appear to be.[21]

On taking up his position as head of the Division of Medical Sciences, Alan Gregg had spent several months in conversation with a wide variety of psychiatrists: Adolf Meyer of Hopkins; his own brother, Donald Gregg, who ran an exclusive private sanitarium in the Boston suburbs; W. G. Hoskins of the Worcester State Hospital in Massachusetts (whose work on dementia praecox was already supported by a sizeable grant from Mrs. Stanley McCormick); and Franklin McLean of the University of Chicago, among many others.[22] Edsall's memorandum had accurately reflected the widespread skepticism, if not contempt, most mainstream physicians had for psychiatry, but Gregg seems to have become increasingly convinced that this status as medicine's stepchild provided precisely the opportunity he was looking for. Psychiatry was, he granted, "one of the most backward fields of science. In some particulars, it was an island rather than an integral part of the mainland of scientific medicine. . . . Teaching was poor, research was fragmentary and application was feeble and incomplete." Ironically, these defects were precisely what attracted him.

Prudence might have argued for directing the foundation's resources into other fields of medicine, where the prospects for advances were better and the bets safer. But Gregg decided to roll the dice and urge the trustees to make psychiatry the foundation's top priority in medicine. It was a bold decision by the newly appointed director, but his chances of persuading his superiors of the virtues of this approach were greatly heightened by the fact that at least two leading figures at the foundation had personal experience of the problems posed by serious mental illness. Max Mason, who nominally served as president of the foundation from 1929 to 1936 (in fact, his unsuitability for the job led to him being largely sidelined for his last two years at the helm), had had to institutionalize his wife for schizophrenia in the 1920s, and she had recently died.[23] Raymond Fosdick, who succeeded him (and had previously been John D. Rockefeller Jr.'s personal attorney and close advisor), had had to cope with an even more tragic set of circumstances: on April 4, 1932, his mentally ill wife had shot and killed their two children and then taken her own life—an outcome that haunted him for the rest of his days.[24] By late 1932, the trustees had endorsed Gregg's recommendation, and the new policy went into effect the following year.[25]

Within the Division of Medical Sciences, it was broadly accepted that because the field of medicine was so wide, it was necessary to proceed on a highly selective basis in order to do effective work. The strategic decision to focus on psychiatry reflected this consensus. When Gregg spoke to the Rockefeller Foundation trustees in April 1933, he outlined the rationale for the priority he proposed establishing: the major reason he gave for why the foundation should throw support behind the development of psychiatry and neurological science was "because it is the most backward, the most needed, and probably the most fruitful field in medicine." Implicit in according psychiatry this priority was Gregg's recognition that the population of America's mental hospitals was rapidly approaching four hundred thousand souls on any given day and that the mental health sector was the largest single element in many states' budgets.[26]

A decade later, in a confidential memorandum to the trustees designed to justify the fact that "approximately three fourths of the Foundation's allotment for work in the medical [field] is devoted to projects in psychiatry and related or contributory fields," Gregg returned to these themes: the costs associated with mental illness were "tremendous and oppressive. In New York, for example, more than a third of the state budget (apart from debt service) is being spent for the care of the mentally defective and diseased." In tackling this issue, "because teaching was poor, research was fragmentary and application was feeble and incomplete, . . . the first problem was to strengthen the teaching of psychiatry."[27]

Gregg was relatively clear-eyed about the difficulties associated with his choice of priorities, and he sought as well to advance research in the discipline. Though intrigued by psychoanalysis, he was not at first disposed to provide support to it.[28] The fields he initially proposed to concentrate the foundation's resources on were the "sciences underlying psychiatry," which he enumerated as including "the functions of the nervous system, the role of internal secretions, the factors of heredity, the diseases affecting the mental and psychic phenomena of the entity we have been accustomed erroneously to divide into mind and body." The way forward was complicated, however, by the fact that these were not medical specialties "in which the finest minds are now at work, nor in the field[s] intrinsically easiest for the application of the scientific method."

Some historians have suggested that Gregg simply sought to draw on Adolf Meyer's work at Johns Hopkins and have it serve as the basis for his new program.[29] Certainly, Hopkins had by far the largest academic department of psychiatry in the country—indeed, some might argue that it was the only department in the country that came close to matching the intellectual range and numbers of personnel that would be found in other areas of medicine at first-rate medical schools. And it is also true that the term "psychobiology" was frequently bandied about when the Rockefeller officers discussed their support for psychiatry. But a useful turn of phrase by itself has little significance, and there are ample grounds for skepticism about the claims that Meyer's work represented the core element of the foundation's support of psychiatry. This becomes apparent, for example, when one moves beyond the employment of bits and pieces of jargon and looks at the substance of what the foundation funded.

Early on, the foundation acknowledged that "in point of equipment and staff [Johns Hopkins] is the leading laboratory in psychiatry in the United States."[30] But such apparent praise for Meyer's operations has to be read alongside the thoroughly negative assessment of the state of psychiatry in 1933 that Gregg made to the Rockefeller Foundation trustees—a report that in some ways echoed the earlier opinions of David Edsall (though where Edsall saw the backwardness as irremediable, Gregg saw it as an opportunity). What really reinforces this sense that (while having respect for two or three individuals working at the Phipps) Gregg and his colleagues did not see Meyer's empire as one they wanted to model their program on, or make central to the foundation's dispensation of funds, is the record of Rockefeller philanthropy, and the patterns of funding stand out starkly in the archival records.[31]

If one can glean from the financial records an implicit index of what the officers and trustees saw as their intellectual and institutional priorities, it would seem that Meyer's domain was not one they saw as crucial to psychiatry's development. Individual researchers at Hopkins were supported: Horsley Gantt for work on Pavlovian ideas in relation to mental disturbances, most notably attempts over a four-year period to create neurotic dogs; Curt Richter for his laboratory research on such topics as the existence of an internal clock in humans and other organisms;[32] and subsequently, in 1934, Leo Kanner for his work on child psychiatry (although Kanner was awarded a smaller sum than the other two). But Meyer himself was not given much support, nor was his department the recipient of major funding. That remained the case even though Gregg recognized that Meyer was constantly short of funds and was paying for much of his operation from his clinical income and some rather odd donors. In 1932, for example, Gregg reported that Meyer had supported his laboratories with $12,000 of a $15,000 gift from a grateful patient: "This patient is a spiritualist and cannot endure the mention of the word death and . . . his other main support comes from a Christian Scientist."[33]

Instead, the lion's share of the Rockefeller money went toward underwriting a massive expansion of the small and inadequate academic programs in psychiatry at other major medical schools and to creating entire new departments from scratch. The total support for Hopkins was dwarfed by the resources directed to Stanley Cobb's work at Harvard (Cobb received five times as much as the Hopkins researchers put together). Yale's department of psychiatry was funded even more munificently; Gregg noted: "The RF [Rockefeller Foundation] has maintained the department since 1929 to the tune of $1,600,000."[34]

Hopkins also received much less than the amounts directed to McGill, Rochester, the Illinois Medical Center in Chicago, Duke, Tulane, Washington University in St. Louis, and the University of Chicago, where entire departments of psychiatry were founded with Rockefeller money. Though some funds continued to be provided to individual researchers at Hopkins after Meyer's much postponed retirement in 1941, and though Alan Gregg voiced initial support for the appointment of John C. Whitehorn as Meyer's successor,[35] the expectation the foundation had that Whitehorn's background in biochemistry and physiology would foster a closer engagement between psychiatry and the basic sciences proved misplaced. In the words of a department colleague, Jerome Frank, Whitehorn was "taciturn and retiring and often seemed depressed" and devoted "his clinical, reaching, and research efforts to psychotherapy." Even in that discipline, one of his residents commented, "he took only tiny steps forward."[36] When the Rockefeller Foundation provided funds in 1948 for Fritz Redlich to tour a number of departments of psychiatry prior to taking up his post as the new chair of psychiatry at Yale, Robert A. Lambert reported that Redlich was "somewhat disappointed in the psychiatry setup at Johns Hopkins. This is epitomized in his remark that it seemed like autumn there instead of spring."[37]

A 1943 memorandum to the trustees of the Rockefeller Foundation titled "The Emphasis on Psychiatry" noted that "approximately three-fourths of the Foundation's allotment for work in medical sickness is devoted to projects in psychiatry and related or contributory fields,"[38] and that pattern continued into the years immediately following the end of World War II.[39] Where did it all go? Much of it, of course, went to underwriting the creation or expansion of departments of psychiatry, where, it was hoped, a new generation of psychiatrists with academic training—instead of the previous catch-as-catch-can apprenticeships on the back wards of state hospitals—would foster a closer relationship with mainstream medicine and advance the prospects of the specialty. But a good deal of money went to underwrite research that the foundation officers, led by Gregg, hoped would lead to therapeutic breakthroughs.

In this latter endeavor, the major obstacle, given the backward state of the field, was that setting research priorities was extremely difficult. The foundation's solution was to fund an extraordinarily heterogeneous array of projects. Throw enough money at the problem, and one or more lines of inquiry would surely yield results. As early as the late 1920s, Rockefeller money had flowed to Germany, to Kraepelin's Munich institute and elsewhere, to fund research on genetics and mental illness. The accession of Hitler to power and the growing racial dimension of this line of research brought about no change of heart from the foundation, and its money continued to go to German researchers with a commitment to Nazi racial policies until the outbreak of war.[40] At McGill in Montreal, Gregg put large amounts of money behind the young neurologist and neurosurgeon Wilder Penfield and sought to bring together neurology, neurophysiology, and neurosurgery, a project whose scientific value was easy to present to the trustees. At Harvard, large sums were mobilized to create a psychiatric service within a general hospital, while at Yale, originally under the aegis of the interdisciplinary Institute of Human Relations, funds were found for everything from psychoanalysis to primate neurophysiology. Neurotic disorders, seen as a less extreme form of mental disturbance than psychoses, were treated as a function of the autonomic nervous system on the one hand and as an example of psychosocial maladjustment on the other. Horsley Gannt's research on neurotic dogs at Hopkins was matched by Cornell's program to study neurotic pigs and work on conditioned reflexes in sheep. The latter proved particularly problematic because sheep "are so markedly gregarious that they cannot endure the loneliness of the labora- tory alone and only perform satisfactorily when another sheep is tethered in the corner."[41] Elsewhere in the Ivy League, George Draper of Columbia University was given money to examine the relationship between person- ality and body types. In other words, a thoroughgoing eclecticism charac- terized the way money was allocated, and the term "psychobiology" simply provided a convenient umbrella that lent some sort of spurious coherence to the whole.

Although the teenaged Alan Gregg had met Freud after his visit to Clark University and Donald Gregg, Alan's older brother, dabbled in psychoana- lytic techniques at his elite New England sanitarium, the Rockefeller Foundation at first shied away from Freud's creation. A staff conference held on October 7, 1930, concluded that "psychoanalysis is in a stage of development where it cannot be attacked philosophically and can be left to its own devices—does not need money but needs maturity and needs defeat in places where it does not stand up. . . . Psychoanalysts are fighting enough among themselves to winnow out a great deal of chaff—nothing for us to do; but may not be dismissed as non-existent."[42]

At just that moment, one of Freud's closest disciples, Franz Alexander, had arrived from Berlin to lecture on psychoanalysis at the invitation of Robert Hutchings, the president of the University of Chicago. The lectures went very badly, and at the end of the year, Alexander retreated to Boston to lick his wounds.[43] By chance, however, during his time in Chicago, he had analyzed Alfred K. Stern, who claimed the sessions cured him of a stomach ulcer. Stern had inherited a banking fortune and had also had the good fortune to marry Marion Rosenwald, the daughter of Julius Rosenwald, one of the richest of Chicago plutocrats and the driving force behind the emergence of Sears Roebuck. Stern became the sort of Dollar Onkel for Alexander that Freud had long fantasized finding. By 1932, Alexander was back in Chicago as head of the newly established Chicago Psychoanalytic Institute, a position he would occupy until 1956. Stern was installed as chair of its lay board of trustees, and with his assistance, Alexander was soon raising funds from other wealthy Chicagoans, including Julius Rosenwald and the Macys, and adding other former patients to his board. The presence of Alexander's analysands in this role ensured that he exercised almost autocratic power over the institute, which became a central focus for psychoanalytic training in America.[44] It was there, for example, that both Karl Menninger and, more briefly, his younger brother Will became acquainted with psychoanalysis.

Alexander thought he deserved the income and standing of a German Herr Doktor Professor, and he paid himself accordingly. When he attracted Karen Horney, another prominent refugee analyst from Berlin, to his staff in 1934, she too was paid very well, earning $15,000 a year as his deputy before the two of them fell out and she removed to Boston. But before then, Alexander and Stern had succeeded in gaining an audience with Alan Gregg to seek Rockefeller money. Gregg initially demurred, indicating that he thought "it unwise to back a non-university Institut of Psychoanalysis at Chicago, where there is as yet not even a department of psychiatry."[45] Alexander and Stern were persistent, and finally, in early 1934, Gregg relented and agreed to recommend Rockefeller Foundation assistance to the institute. In the end, the foundation awarded a total of $220,000 to the institute over an eight-year period, from 1935 to 1943. Some of the money was earmarked for psychoanalytic training, but the bulk of it was intended to support a program of work on psychosomatic disorders.[46] Alexander had been shrewd enough to grasp that the latter emphasis was key to obtaining Rockefeller funds.[47]

Here was still another example of research that could fit under the elastic umbrella provided by the term "psychobiology." The idea that the study of psychosomatic illnesses could help to create close linkages between psychoanalysis and mainstream medicine, and the fact that this approach seemed to inject a concern with the patient as a person into a laboratory medicine that Gregg and his associates feared was unduly reductionist, seem to have convinced Gregg to overcome his initial misgivings about supporting Alexander.[48] Troubled by the fact that the Chicago institute was a freestanding organization with no formal links to a university, Gregg early on nudged Alexander to develop such ties. Since it was obviously impossible to form such a relationship with the University of Chicago, where the influential

Pearce Bailey and others would have no truck with psychoanalysis, the University of Illinois for a time seemed promising.[49] In the end, though, Alexander preferred to keep tight control over his personal fiefdom—quickly quarreling with his main internal rival, Karen Horney, and ensuring her departure—and so Gregg's hopes of a university tie-in proved vain.

As early as 1937, there were signs that Gregg's confidence in Alexander was beginning to fray. He acknowledged that the training program seemed to be functioning but complained that "the physiological correlations they are attempting are not in competent hands" and that the place seemed to be "a one-man show or at least rather too much dominated by Alexander." With some hesitation, he recommended renewing funding for three to five years but insisted that any further support "should be based on a clear understanding of termination at the end of the period."[50] Gregg's junior associates were even blunter when they exchanged their assessment of the institute a year later. Robert Lambert noted: "I still don't think much of the Chicago Institute crowd. Maybe Alexander has contributed a little something towards making psychoanalysis respectable but he certainly has not brought it into the scientific fold. I shall feel relief when the RF [Rockefeller Foundation] award terminates—and is not renewed." His colleague Daniel O'Brien concurred: "I have the same general hesitation as you about Alexander and some of the other people at Chicago. . . . Frankly, I would like to see the directorship of any institute of psychoanalysis turned over to, say, a sound physiologist or a good internist in medicine."[51]

There were further signs of disenchantment over the next four years, with Alexander's lavish salary the source of repeated negative commentary. Finally, at a tense meeting held on October 31, 1941, Gregg rejected Alexander's overtures. Marion Rosenwald, who had divorced Stern in the aftermath of his affair with Martha Dodd, the daughter of the American ambassador to Berlin,[52] was still a reliable source of funds, but Gregg had had enough. The psychosomatic researches seemed to have led nowhere, and the salaries paid at the institute, partly financed by Rockefeller money, were "too large." There was, he informed Alexander, "no chance" that he would recommend further support from the foundation. It was "up to the Institute to find its own essential funds for continuance," and he "did not see any likelihood that the RF [Rockefeller Foundation] would contribute to this."[53]

The only significant involvement of the Rockefeller Foundation with psychoanalysis in North America thus came to an abrupt end. It had never amounted to much. There were a few crumbs thrown to psychoanalytic psychiatry in the form of grants to universities like Harvard, Yale, the University of Chicago, and Washington University in St. Louis, but not much more than that. Even the flirtation with Alexander's institute had cost less than 2 percent of the money the foundation used to underwrite American psychiatry. When Gregg received a proposal to provide support for an international institute of psychoanalysis in Vienna headed by Freud, he wanted nothing to do with it. The amount requested was small—$30,000 to $60,000—but the project struck him as worthless "in view of the present status of psychoanalysis," in particular its "Cinderella position in point of academic status" and the fact that "Vienna as a locus has not optimum prospects from the standpoint of racial liberties."[54]

And yet, inadvertently and without intending to do so, another branch of the Rockefeller Foundation had much to do with creating some of the pre-conditions for the flourishing state of psychoanalysis in the United States in the aftermath of World War II. Beginning in 1933, and subject to much internal debate and handwringing, the foundation had started a program of "Special Aid to Displaced Scholars," designed to help persecuted European scholars escape fascist Europe. It was this program, among others, that allowed almost two hundred psychoanalysts and psychiatrists sympathetic to analysis to relocate to the United States. In the period following the war, such refugee analysts would dominate psychoanalysis along the East Coast, and most especially in New York, and at the time they constituted more than half the psychoanalytic community in the New World.

Inevitably, during World War II, new initiatives on the part of the foundation were few and far between, and after the war, the landscape of aca-demic medicine, and perforce of psychiatry, was irrevocably changed by the enormous expansion of the federal government and its growing involvement in funding scientific and medical research. No one was ini-tially sure what the impact of agencies like the National Science Foundation, the National Institutes of Health, and the National Institute of Mental Health would be, but by the early 1950s, it was clear that America had entered the era of Big Science and Big Medicine and that the previously enormous influence of organizations like the Rockefeller

Foundation was inevitably waning. Even the enormous endowment of the largest private foundations was dwarfed by the resources that could be mobilized by the modern state.

It was in part these structural changes that prompted soul-searching at the Rockefeller Foundation, not least because the model its officers had long leaned on—picking out prominent scholars and relying on the judgments of its officers and personal inspections Gregg and his associates conducted to determine the allocation of funds—was increasingly being challenged and supplanted by something approximating the peer review system. But it was also brought about by the advent of a new president of the foundation, the management theorist Chester Barnard, who took over from Raymond Fosdick in 1948 after serving on the foundation's board of trustees. Barnard raised questions about what the foundation's massive investments in medicine and the sciences over the preceding two decades had produced.

In the case of the Division of Natural Sciences led by Warren Weaver, the answer was quite reassuring. Weaver had coined the term "molecular biology," and the grants he had administered had largely created the field.[55] The technologies, laboratories, and scientists Weaver had funded had proved their worth in the just-concluded war, and his own activities in organizing the Applied Mathematics Panel when seconded to the United States Office of Scientific Research and Development in wartime further cemented his reputation. Of the eighteen molecular biologists who received a Nobel Prize between 1954 and 1965, fifteen had received funds from the Rockefeller Foundation, and on average, they had received their first support "more than nineteen years before the Nobel Prize was awarded." Even in the late 1940s, Barnard could feel assured that the Division of Natural Sciences grants had been money well spent.[56]

What about Gregg's program in support of psychiatry? Here, matters were more complicated. The various somatic therapies—malaria therapy, insulin comas, metrazol, ECT, lobotomy, and the like, which were still mostly seen as having some therapeutic value—had all originated in Europe and owed nothing to Rockefeller funding. Nor could Gregg and his team point to any other breakthrough that owed anything to their investments over nearly two decades. In 1944, Gregg had acquired an able deputy, the neurophysiologist Robert Morison, and four years later, as

Barnard settled into the presidency of the foundation, Morison attempted a survey of the state of psychiatry. What he confronted and had to explain was the inescapable reality that "a generation of funding [had] yielded painfully little in tangible results."[57]

Morison's conclusions did not make for very encouraging reading. Of the approximately $16 million in grants the foundation gave to psychiatry between 1931 and 1946, only about a quarter went to departments that already existed, and little of that money went to research. About half had been spent on "establishing entirely new or to expanding negligibly small university departments of psychology or psychiatry." What had all this wrought? According to Morison, not much: "One cannot point to any definitive advances in our knowledge of the causes or treatment of any major mental disease." He could identify some progress in the treatment of epilepsy and some "slow but steady progress . . . in the understanding of the elementary functions of nervous tissue. But the total is not distinguished or dramatic." What should be done? "The relative lack of specific results in the form of contributions to knowledge only serves to emphasize the continuing need for providing the basic tools to do the job. . . . A sound beginning has been made."[58]

Having spent so much money, it must have been difficult for the foundation to confront the meager progress that had been made, and Barnard was not slow in communicating his unease. In August 1948, he sent a sharp memorandum to both Gregg and Morison after reading the latter's report. The portrait of the state of psychiatry Morison presented was something he found "terribly disturbing, [though] somehow it wasn't terribly surprising to me. Isn't there a way," he asked, "to blast this situation?"[59]

In private, Morison, who was not afraid to differ from Gregg, had complained on multiple occasions that the profession's heightened emphasis on psychotherapy had not been accompanied by any effort to test the efficacy of such forms of treatment. Indeed, psychiatry's leadership, instead of looking for ways to address the issue, seemed to throw up its collective hands, declare the problem beyond solution, and content itself with relying on anecdotal evidence. After being made aware of these concerns, Barnard was obviously unimpressed. Rather bluntly, he confronted his officers: "Doesn't a continued and general refusal to permit or attempt validation of psychotherapeutic methods put everyone concerned, including ourselves, in a position of promoting or carrying on a social racket? How can the charlatans be dealt with if the good men will give no validation but their own individual say-sos?"[60]

A month and a half later, after consulting with Gregg, Morison attempted to answer these pointed questions. His report, he noted, was "to be regarded as a collection of data relevant to the present situation but not necessarily a complete or conclusive description of it." But what followed cannot have made for very reassuring reading. Medicine, Morison claimed, had long displayed "an almost complete neglect of the less easily analyzed psychological factors." Combined with "the very rapid increase in scientific knowledge about the organic elements in disease," the upshot was that "the prestige of psychiatry, which had never been very high, declined almost to a disappearing point during the Twenties and Thirties." There had, Morison hastened to add, "been an extraordinary change [since then], due in part to the interest of the RF [Rockefeller Foundation]." Faced with the problem of their professional marginality, "the younger generation of psychiatrists have naturally devoted a large proportion of their energies to gaining acceptance on the part of the rest of the medical profession."

How had they done so? "Since their art was too primitive to be defended on the basis of scientific evidence," Morison wrote, "psychiatrists have relied largely on rhetorical persuasion in their campaign for recognition. A large part of this persuasiveness has rested upon the revelatory nature of Freudian concepts." That accords with my own reading of what had been happening in the 1940s. But it scarcely advanced Morison's defense of the profession very far, because, as he was immediately forced to concede, "It is certainly very difficult to give in any clear and simple way one's reasons for believing that the basic Freudian hypotheses are correct." The best he could offer was, "There is no question in my mind . . . that the concept of unconscious motivation has enabled us to understand the meaning of psychiatric symptoms which have hitherto been incomprehensible"—a proposition whose force was immediately undercut by his acknowledgment that, "as Whitehorn has recently pointed out, there is probably a great difference in understanding the meaning of a symptom and understanding its 'cause.'"

It was on this (rather slender) reed that "modern psychiatry has convinced the liberal members of the medical profession that psychiatry deserves a hearing. . . . [However,] since this improvement in status has been won with little reference to scientific evidence, it is natural that psychiatrists under-rate the necessity of providing such evidence in the future. It is here," Morison concluded, "that they are making their greatest mistake for I believe they under-rate the tentativeness with which acceptance has been extended. [The rest of medicine is] still waiting, however, for evidence of the sort which has validated, for instance, the use of antibiotics. If this is not forthcoming within the next ten to fifteen years, [physicians] may react rather violently, partly out of embarrassment for having extended a welcoming hand to a group which finally failed to produce."[61]

One doubts whether Chester Barnard's skepticism was allayed by reading these statements, even without what followed. But toward the end of his lengthy assessment of the state of contemporary psychiatry, Morison provided some direct evidence of some of the problems he had identified. He indicated that he was enclosing a recent report prepared by "the Committee on Research of the Group for the Advancement of Psychiatry" and proceeded to itemize its troubling features.

GAP, as it liked to call itself, was an organization of Young Turks who saw themselves as being at the forefront of psychiatric progress. GAP was a product in many ways of the changes in the psychiatric profession that World War II had brought about, most notably the doubling and tripling of the size of the profession, the shift in its center of gravity away from the traditional mental hospital and toward office-based practice, and the concomitant move among a younger generation away from biological theories of mental illness and toward "psychodynamic psychiatry," or an Americanized version of Freud. GAP had successfully installed its de facto leader, William Menninger, as president of the American Psychiatric Association in 1948, defeating the candidate of the Old Guard, Francis Braceland. Its propensity for overreach and the diffuseness of its aims would eventually marginalize the organization, but when Morison assessed the terrain, it could plausibly be seen as living up to its own claims of being the psychiatric vanguard.

GAP's report on psychotherapy did not make for reassuring reading so far as Morison was concerned. It spent a lot of time talking about "the intrinsic difficulty of doing research in psychotherapy . . . [and] seems more concerned with explaining why it is impossible to do a good job of validation than to find ways of circumventing the difficulties. It would be so much more comfortable"—a note of sarcasm creeps into Morison's bureaucratic prose at this point—"if one could only maintain the status quo of acceptance on rhetorical grounds rather than risking the whole reputation of the art by submitting it to scientific study." There was, however, something even more worrisome, to which he drew Barnard's attention: "The ease with which the Group for the Advancement of Psychiatry has adopted the committee approach to situations of this sort. There have been several times recently when I have felt that the leaders of American psychiatry are trying to establish the truth on the basis of majority vote. This is, of course, quite contrary to the usual scientific procedure of submitting evidence which can stand on its own merits in a candid world."[62]

It would remain a device, however, that organized psychiatry would repeatedly resort to all the way to the present. It would be the basis, for example, on which the profession would decide that homosexuality was no longer a mental illness,[63] and it has underpinned, indeed been the defining feature, of each successive version of the American Psychiatric Association's *Diagnostic and Statistical Manual,* from the third edition, published in 1980, all the way to the fifth edition, released in 2013.

Had the decision to focus the Rockefeller Foundation's efforts on remaking psychiatry been a terrible error? Morison realized that such a conclusion would be easy to draw, and he immediately sought some way to avoid such a devastating judgment: "I very much hope that this frank statement of my misgivings about current trends in psychiatry will not give the impression that I feel we have made a mistake in helping these trends to develop." Why not? "There is absolutely no doubt that something had to be done fifteen years ago to increase the medical interest in psychiatry and to recruit and train personnel," he argued. "One had to begin somewhere, and it was impossible to start on the basis of tested scientific knowledge." Perhaps conscious that statements like this risked damning the whole program with faint praise, Morison changed tack. Contrary to the impression his previous remarks surely would have given, he insisted that, looking at the program as a whole, "the gains so far have really been surprisingly large. For example, it is really of immense importance that the oncoming generation of medical students is being shown that the emotions play an important role in almost all their patients. It is equally significant that there is now a large group of able young men who have been attracted to the field of psychiatry and who may, if properly handled, be able to take the necessary next step. I therefore do not feel that we are supporting a racket when we continue to aid psychiatry in its present, admittedly imperfect state." It was, in any event, no time for "blasting" but rather for "some less drastic handling," perhaps a shift away from psychiatric teaching toward a greater emphasis on psychiatric research.

Other documents suggest how worried Morison was becoming about the directions psychiatry was taking. On August 28, 1948, for example, he made a record of a lunch with Douglas Bond, chair of the Department of Psychiatry at Case Western Reserve, and a man Morison seems to have held in high regard: "One of my objectives in this trip was to find evidence against my increasing skepticism of the leaders of American psychiatry and GAP in particular. Unfortunately, the reverse occurred. B[ond] has just finished a brief monograph on his experience in military psychiatry which will have a good deal of documentation of the uselessness of psychological selection procedures and psychiatric therapy as practiced during the last war. . . . He also more than shares my feeling that the current leaders of dynamic psychiatry are throwing their weight around in a way quite unjustified by the minute amount of really tested knowledge on which their procedures are based."[64] He found similar doubts being expressed by Bernard Wortis at New York University: "He feels that there is far too much acceptance of untried views, especially on the psychoanalytic side and seems to be as disturbed as RSM [Robert S. Morison] at the tendency of the leaders in the Group for the Advancement of Psychiatry to set themselves up as high priests."[65]

Four years later, Morison's patience was wearing even thinner. He lamented that "most [psychiatrists] refuse to recognize that the brain may have something to do with the mind." And his hopes that the internal opposition to research on the efficacy of psychotherapy would diminish with time had dimmed. In an interoffice memorandum, he complained that "the development of research has lagged badly so that psychiatric practice is still without a scientific foundation." Rather than continue to throw more money in that direction, Morison suggested a different route: "For some time to come it seems likely that university departments of psychology will offer better research possibilities than most departments of medical psychiatry."[66] And with that, with a whimper more than a bang, the Rockefeller Foundation essentially exited from its support of psychiatry.

In March 1951, aware that his authority was at an end and that the foundation was moving on, Alan Gregg wrote to Chester Barnard and asked to be relieved of his position as director of the Division of Medical Sciences. Barnard proceeded to merge the Division of International Public Health and the Division of Medical Sciences into a single entity, and he put Gregg's former deputy, Robert Morison, in charge of it. A fig leaf was found for public relations purposes and to salve Gregg's pride: he was appointed as vice president of the foundation and charged with writing and speaking about medicine and its broader role in society. He joined various boards and traveled the country, and then in 1956, at the age of sixty-five, he had to retire (the Rockefeller Foundation had a strict rule on the matter). A year later, Gregg was dead.

In the end, for all its disappointments, the Rockefeller Foundation's extended involvement in and support of American psychiatry did have two major consequences for the profession, both of which were largely unintended. The support the foundation offered to émigré psychoanalysts can be weighed in the balance against its support for Nazi research centers in the 1930s. More importantly, it helped to create a critical mass of highly educated, committed Freudians in the United States, which was an important factor in the postwar domination of American psychiatry by psychoanalytic perspectives on mental illness—a hegemony that would last for a quarter-century.

Of at least equal importance, while Rockefeller money had not fueled any intellectual breakthroughs of significance in the years before it largely abandoned the field (and would have no role in the transformative impact of the psychopharmacological revolution, which began quite independently in Europe), it did have a massive impact on the demographic composition of the profession—an impact that began in the 1930s, but that was more fully realized after the war. All the money spent on building up departments of psychiatry had succeeded in creating a whole generation of psychiatrists schooled in academic psychiatry rather than in the practical institutional forms of knowledge and practice that had dominated the field in the United States until the 1930s. These men—and they were overwhelmingly, though not exclusively, men—saw themselves as very different from ill-educated asylum hacks and had little interest in entering the world of the state hospital. The pay in these institutions was dismal, the work was dominated by bureaucratic routine, mental hospitals were underfunded and on the point of collapse, and the patients were mostly beyond hope, or at least were seen as beyond hope. Here was one of the sources of the massive shift away from institutional psychiatry that was so central to the evolution of postwar psychiatry. As the late Gerald Grob rightly remarked, "In seeking to integrate their specialty with scientific medicine, psychiatrists were unaware that their efforts would lead them to modify"—"abandon" is perhaps a better descriptor—"their commitment to institutional care."[67] With that development, a deep rift opened up between the professional elite and institutional psychiatry, and over time, much of psychiatry's commitment to treatment of the most severely disturbed, most desperate mental patients was sharply diminished.

PART III Transformations and Interpretations

10 Shrinks

DOCTOR PANGLOSS

Over the past half-century, the history of psychiatry has flourished as never before. In the 1970s and 1980s, much of the most innovative scholarship came from social historians. By 1990, the profession had acquired a flagship journal (*History of Psychiatry*), and the social historians had been joined by a number of clinician-historians such as Joel Braslow, German Berrios, David Healy, and George Makari,[1] who combined psychiatric expertise and serious historical scholarship in ways that greatly enriched the sophistication and the range of questions that have come to characterize work in the field. Dozens and dozens of monographs on a variety of topics appear annually, along with hundreds of academic papers from researchers across the globe.

In *Shrinks,* Jeffrey Lieberman, who is currently chair of the Department of Psychiatry at Columbia University and served as president of the American Psychiatric Association (APA) from 2013 to 2014, sets out to tell readers what he assures us is "the untold story" of his discipline's history, concluding with a paean to its glorious present. He writes with the assistance of a ghostwriter (more on this anon) and is apparently blissfully ignorant of the work of the serious scholars who have preceded him. His is history as morality tale, a story of heroes and villains (mostly the latter), of charlatans and hucksters who inflicted extraordinary harm on those they purported to treat and understand, and of a handful of visionaries who anticipated or helped usher in the golden age that now awaits the mentally ill—if they could only be made aware of psychiatry's emergence from its "long sojourn in the scientific wilderness." At last we have emerged from centuries of superstition and barbaric treatments doled out by earlier generations of alienists. Since 1980, science has been in the saddle, and there have been "dazzling" advances in the treatment and understanding of mental illness. We stand on the cusp of many more. "The modern psychiatrist," Lieberman assures us, "now possesses the tools to lead any person out of a maze of mental chaos into a place of clarity, care, and recovery."[2] Would that this were so.

Lieberman's portrait of the first two centuries of psychiatry's existence occupies almost two-thirds of his book. Time after time, we are shown a profession that is "the black sheep of the medical family." It is a history full of "rogues" and "red herrings," "false leads and dead ends," "ideology and dubious science," "mumbo jumbo" and "worthless treatments"—therapies that often maimed and killed, or that extracted large sums of money from desperate patients without producing any noticeable improvements, save in the psychiatrists' bank accounts. From Mesmer's animal magnetism and Reich's orgone therapy to near-drowning devices and frontal lobotomies, nothing was too extreme for psychiatrists to peddle and to try. And then there is Sigmund Freud, who looses psychoanalysis on the world. Freud is a little less of a cardboard cutout than the other heroes and villains who populate Lieberman's pages. Or rather, Freud is recorded as "a tragic visionary far ahead of his time, . . . simultaneously psychiatry's greatest hero and its most calamitous rogue."[3] If that seems an incongruous combination of qualities, it is Lieberman's apparently considered judgment.

Nevertheless, when Lieberman entered the practice of psychiatry in the 1970s, Freud's followers dominated American psychiatry. They were the shrinks of his title. On his account, they were nothing more than an unscientific (indeed antiscientific) cult, engaged mostly in treating the "worried well," relentlessly expanding the boundaries of pathology by assuring all their patients that they were a little bit mad. The analysts used their entrenched position atop the departments of most medical schools to enforce their dogmatic orthodoxy. They were "omen-divining wizards," "*consiglieri* for the wealthy, educated, and influential."[4] Everyone who aspired to a professional career as a psychiatrist had "to demonstrate fealty to psychoanalytic theory" and undergo a training analysis "with someone who would use this deeply intimate material to determine how devoted you were to Freudian principles."[5] Meanwhile, diagnosis was scorned (madness was "infinitely variable and could not be neatly packaged into diagnostic boxes"[6]), and the brain and biology were ignored, for they were irrelevant to a condition the analysts were convinced had its origins in unconscious conflicts and murdered memories.

Lieberman's strategy in presenting what he claims is an unvarnished history of his profession is clear: the blacker the hues in which he presents the past, the more glorious the present can be seen to be by contrast as we move from the horrors of lobotomies and insulin comas and "from a psychoanalytic cult of shrinks into a scientific medicine of the brain."[7] It is a history quite deliberately bereft of nuance or context, full of anachronistic and moralistic judgments, unreliable in its details, and presented in a prose riddled with clichés and breathless proclamations that reminds me of nothing so much as *Time* magazine at its nadir. One must presume this is the contribution of Dr. Lieberman's ghostwriter, Ogi Ogas, who was recruited for his expertise in writing about pop psychology and for eighteen months became Lieberman's "Siamese twin."

As befits a ghost, Ogas remains barely visible. Though his name appears on the dust jacket and he is thanked in the acknowledgments, we learn only that he is a game show winner and computational neuroscientist. Ogas did indeed win $500,000 on the game show *Who Wants to Be a Millionaire?* and has a PhD from Boston University. His other claim to fame is having coauthored a pop psychology book on Internet pornography that has attracted criticism for its shoddy research design, wholly speculative biological reductionism, and circumvention of the basic forms of ethical oversight that are standard for research in this field. An odd choice of Siamese twin, one might think.

If heroes are in short supply for much of Lieberman's book, they surface more noticeably once he turns his attention to the revolution that he claims has swept over psychiatry in the past thirty-five years. Prominent among the revolutionaries is Robert Spitzer, one of Lieberman's predecessors at Columbia's Department of Psychiatry. This is why: Psychiatry's inability to agree on questions of diagnosis became an ever more serious source of scandal and public embarrassment in the 1970s, in no case more so than when the Stanford psychologist David Rosenhan published a study in the august pages of *Science*, one of the two most prominent general-circulation science journals in the world, describing how a series of pseudopatients had succeeded in repeatedly duping psychiatrists, who failed to recognize that they were sham patients, into institutionalizing them, usually with a diagnosis of schizophrenia.[8] Faced with a crisis of legitimacy, psychiatry's leaders sought to revamp the profession's diagnostic processes to ensure its members could agree on what labels to assign to the patients who came their way. Spitzer took charge of this task force and swiftly staffed it with biologically inclined psychiatrists who had no truck with what they called Freudian dogma.

Lieberman is right to see the document Spitzer produced as marking a defining moment in the history of his profession. The third edition of the *Diagnostic and Statistical Manual of Mental Disorders* (routinely referred to as *DSM III*) was officially adopted by the still psychoanalytically dominated APA through Spitzer's skillful political maneuvering. Its content, too, reflected his organizational skills and dedication. As Lieberman gleefully notes, in approving this document, the Freudians dug their own grave. Their seemingly impregnable position atop the profession's commanding heights, such as they were, vanished abruptly, like Lewis Carroll's Cheshire Cat—though instead of a smile, what was left behind was a collection of squabbling sectarians. Lieberman's account of these developments is tendentious but often revealing. He dismisses the analysts as antiscientific ideologues and lionizes Spitzer and his task force as tough-minded scientists. But his own account shows that, for all their claims that their changes to the previous edition of the *DSM* rested on hard data, Spitzer and his colleagues were forced at many turns to make use of unpublished research that had not undergone the test of peer review and to rely on the "clinical experience" of those working in the field—precisely the sorts of shaky evidence he condemns the Freudians for using. Spitzer's task force was a political animal, and its aim was to simplify the diagnostic process by reducing it to a tick-the-boxes approach. The presence of a certain number of symptoms (the number was arrived at by a vote because it "seemed right," on Spitzer's account) was sufficient to warrant the assignment of a particular diagnosis.

What this approach succeeded in doing was in increasing the chances that psychiatrists would agree with one another about what was wrong with a patient—that is, it increased the reliability of psychiatric diagnoses. What it did not do, and could not do, was increase their validity, to give us diagnoses that correspond to "real" diseases. It paid no attention to whether the entities it identified existed in nature, independent of psychiatric judgment, being satisfied with concocting labels that were consistently applied. Spitzer's fundamental approach has continued to underpin successive editions of the diagnostic manual, right up to the most recent edition, *DSM 5*, which appeared in 2013, the same year that Lieberman assumed the presidency of the APA. The fundamental difficulty is that we simply do not understand the etiology of most major mental disorders, and we have no blood tests, MRIs, or other tests that can distinguish the mentally ill from the rest of us and assign mental disturbances to one category of illness or another. Instead, like eighteenth-century physicians, psychiatrists use symptoms as their touchstone. So serious are the problems that flow from this situation that two past directors of the National Institute of Mental Health, Steven Hyman (now at Harvard) and Thomas Insel (now at a startup, Mindstrong Health, after a brief period at Google Health Sciences) have denounced the new manual as a scientific nightmare that stood in the way of making progress and have objected that even its most important diagnostic categories, depression and schizophrenia, were artificial constructs, not real diseases.[9]

So much for the first part of Lieberman's vaunted revolution. To be sure, in the crisis atmosphere that ensued when Insel published his comments, he and Lieberman got together to issue a public relations statement that papered over the cracks.[10] But the fault lines remained, and the damage was done.

The other side of the *DSM* revolution was the way it portended a switch away from psychodynamic and social perspectives on mental illness, and back to biology. Increasingly, psychiatrists embraced psychopharmacology as the major treatment modality for the most serious disorders they encountered, and for many of the minor ones as well, with a more or less ritual genuflection in the direction of another form of psychotherapy: laboratory-tested cognitive behavioral therapy. Those links between psychiatry and psychoactive drugs have become increasingly close and controversial as the years have gone by. Lieberman's triumphant account of these developments is, like the rest of his recital of psychiatry's "unknown" history, partial (in more than one sense of the term) and unreliable.

On Lieberman's account, the last sixty years, since the advent of Miltown and Thorazine, has been a story of uninterrupted progress as hard medical science has replaced foolish Freudian dogma, psychiatry has assumed its rightful place as a legitimate part of the medical enterprise, and patients have benefited from a stream of discoveries that have liberated them from the scourge of mental illness. The only thing presently holding us back from entering this Panglossian universe has been a public (and perhaps even a medical profession) that has remained unaware of these remarkable breakthroughs and thus continues to regard "shrinks" with suspicion, and to spurn and stigmatize the mentally ill. Just take your pills, and keep taking them after you feel better, and all will be well. Schizophrenia, for example, is "highly treatable." Clinical triumphs have ensured that psychiatrists can often provide, "not merely the relief of a patient's symptoms, but the utter transformation of a patient's life."[11]

Throughout Lieberman's discussion of these issues, the benefits of psychopharmacology are vastly oversold. Antipsychotic medications, for example, damp down the florid manifestations of schizophrenia but have little or no impact on the negative symptoms that are a central part of patients' suffering—the flattened affect, the lack of initiative, social withdrawal, and cognitive deterioration that mark the disease. For some, they provide a measure of symptomatic relief, and that is welcome, but they are far from being some sort of psychiatric penicillin. Moreover, and this is something Lieberman essentially skates over in silence, the major psychiatric drugs are associated with very severe side effects, some of them life-threatening (such as serious metabolic disorders), and others stigmatizing, profoundly distressing, and often irreversible (like tardive dyskinesia, unbearable restlessness or akathisia, and Parkinson's-like syndromes).[12]

Psychiatry is in thrall to the drug companies, which underwrite much of the research that the profession and public rely on (and suppress the scientific data they don't like, transforming evidence-based medicine into evidence-biased medicine).[13] This is a topic Lieberman entirely ignores, which is perhaps not surprising when one learns how much his own career has been bolstered by his ties to the drug industry.[14] Furthermore, all the money that has been poured into research on new pharmaceutical treatments hasn't proved to be of much value to patients, though the patenting of new and supposedly improved pills have had extraordinary effects on Big Pharma's profits.

Lieberman knows all this very well. After all, he was the lead author on a major government-financed study known as CATIE (Clinical Antipsychotic Trials of Intervention Effectiveness), which compared four second-generation drugs, so-called atypical antipsychotics (whose annual sales amount to $10 billion), with a much older first-generation antipsychotic. Published in the *New England Journal of Medicine* in 2005, the study had two notable results, neither of which finds its way into *Shrinks*. The new drugs offered few, if any, benefits over the older drugs, and they not only carried the same risk of neurological symptoms such as stiffness or tremors[15] but also were often associated with massive weight gain and heightened risk of contracting diabetes. The side effects and lack of efficacy of all of the drugs tested were so marked that 64 percent of patients put on the second-generation drug Zyprexa and at least 74 percent of the patients put on the other four drugs had refused to keep taking their medications.[16] For years, drug companies had claimed that "the introduction of second-generation or 'atypical' antipsychotic drugs promised enhanced efficacy and safety." On that basis, they had acquired "a 90 percent market share in the United States, resulting in burgeoning costs."[17] The CATIE study suggests that these claims are simply false. Its authors acknowledge that "antipsychotic drugs . . . have substantial limitations in their effectiveness in patients with chronic schizophrenia" and concede that "there were no significant differences in effectiveness between the conventional drug perphenazine [the first-generation antipsychotic] and the other second-generation drugs." As for side effects, "There were no significant differences among the groups in the incidence of extrapyramidal side effects, akathisia, or movement disorders." Finally, depending on which of the drugs they were receiving, between 11 and 20 percent of the study participants had to be "hospitalized for an exacerbation of schizophrenia."[18] No magic bullets in evidence here.

The results of the CATIE study were subsequently confirmed in a wide-ranging meta-analysis of 150 randomized trials comparing first- and second-generation antipsychotics published in *The Lancet*. In an editorial summarizing the results, two British psychiatrists, Peter Tyrer and Tim Kendall, spoke of "the spurious advance of antipsychotic drug therapy." Contrary to the claims of Big Pharma, "The second-generation drugs have no special atypical characteristics that separate them from the typical, or first-generation, antipsychotics. As a group, they are no more efficacious, do not improve specific symptoms, have no clearly different side-effect profiles than first-generation antipsychotics, and are less cost effective." Far from marking an advance in the treatment of schizophrenia, "the atypicals can now be regarded as an invention only, cleverly manipulated by the drug industry for marketing purposes." This disturbing reality had emerged despite sustained efforts by the drug industry to manipulate the data. For example, the trials mostly compared new drugs to "a high-potency first-generation antipsychotic [haloperidol] likely to be associated with a high rate of extrapyramidal side-effects." And doses of the first-generation drug were often higher than normal, which was intended to increase the side effects these patients would experience and thus bias the trial in favor of the newer drugs.[19]

Lieberman sings a song of progress. His Harvard colleague Steven Hyman sings from a very different hymn sheet. Asked to provide an assessment of the landscape of the psychiatric profession over the course of his career, Hyman notes the excitement that swept the field following the discovery of the first antipsychotic and antidepressant drugs in the early 1950s, a development that, he contends, "promised both therapeutic progress and significant probes of brain function. Looking back, the picture is painfully different. The efficacy of psychotherapeutic drugs plateaued by 1955. Subsequent progress has been limited largely to tolerability [and as the CATIE study shows, has not even occurred on that front]. Strikingly, we still do not know how psychotherapeutics exert their desired effects."

Nor, Hyman continues, has research on the genetic basis of mental illness made much headway. He recalls the confidence once expressed that "we might soon identify causal mutations." No such luck. Twin and adoption studies seemed to point to the existence of a certain role for genetic factors, and "the field focused on families in which schizophrenia or bipolar disorder seemed to be transmitted with tragic certainty. Only later were the striking phenotype differences even within such 'high density' families recognized as significant harbingers of genetic complexity, along with a plethora of other disconcerting observations." It turns out that "the genetic, epigenetic, and other environmental risks of psychopathology are etiologically complex and heterogeneous. For example, the many risk genes that might contribute to schizophrenia are not transmitted together across generations."[20] Time, it would seem, for a major rethink rather than a celebration of a largely mythical "progress."

One last statistic that nowhere graces the pages of Lieberman's Panglossian account of the enormous strides his profession has made in treating serious mental illness: British and American studies have found that the life expectancy of people with serious mental illness is between one and two decades less than for the rest of us.[21] Despite the dazzling advances that Dr. Lieberman claims psychiatry has made in recent decades, we obviously still have a long way to go.

11 The Hunting of the Snark

THE SEARCH FOR A HISTORY OF NEUROPSYCHIATRY

"Psychiatry" as the preferred term of art for those specializing in the treatment of mental disorders was invented in early nineteenth-century Germany. Its adoption was long resisted in Anglo-American circles— Henry Maudsley, for example, arguably the leading English alienist of the late nineteenth century and founder of London's Maudsley Hospital, detested the word. But by the early twentieth century, it had been broadly embraced by the profession, a shift signaled in the United States by a change in the title of the specialism's flagship journal in 1921, from the *American Journal of Insanity* to the *American Journal of Psychiatry*. The term "neuropsychiatry" has enjoyed an even briefer time on the stage, and it has had a somewhat checkered history. It began to be used in World War I, during the epidemic of shell shock that marked that appalling period of mass slaughter, perhaps prompted by the fact that many of the medical men who found themselves compelled to treat its casualties came from a neurological background.[1] It may also have been part of an effort to persuade skeptical army brass that those suffering from the ravages of shell shock were genuinely ill, not malingerers or cowards. In the interwar years, the term fell into disuse as the traditional fissures between neurology and psychiatry re-emerged. Attempts by a small minority of medical men to revive the label in the aftermath of World War II were largely ineffectual, and it was not until the 1980s that there was a renewed effort to revive the concept.

This time, its advocates enjoyed a measure of success. The British Neuropsychiatric Association was formed in 1987, the American Neuropsychiatric Association was created in 1988, and the International Neuropsychiatric Association was established in 1996. Quite what "neuropsychiatry" means, however, has remained a somewhat controversial question. Some adopt a relatively circumscribed definition of the field, one that sees its practitioners focusing their research and clinical care on psychiatric conditions with a demonstrable neurological basis and on the psychiatric disturbances that frequently accompany neurological disease, such as the depressive symptoms that surface among those with Parkinson's disease. Others have adopted a much more expansive definition of the field, in keeping with the more general shift among psychiatrists in the past half-century toward a biologically reductionist view of mental illness. If (and of course it is a very big *if* indeed) mental illness is actually no more than brain disease, the psychiatric symptomatology being the epiphenomenal manifestation of neural pathology, then the "mental" part of the label is a misnomer. It would follow that schizophrenia, bipolar disorder, and the like are in reality brain diseases, and neuroscience and neuropsychiatry are the appropriate disciplines to which to entrust the future.

The subtitle of Michael Trimble's 2016 book, *The Intentional Brain: Motion, Emotion, and the Development of Modern Neuropsychiatry,* indicates that he seeks to provide a history of the development of modern neuropsychiatry. Accordingly, one might expect him to focus heavily on the past century or so, the period when some specialists began to self-consciously refer to themselves as neuropsychiatrists. In reality, however, that relatively recent history occupies no more than the final third of the book. The bulk of the text has a much broader remit, starting in ancient Greece and then taking us through the Dark Ages, the Renaissance, the era of Romanticism, and the nineteenth century. Only in the closing chapters do we move from a discussion of antecedents and anticipations of contemporary understandings toward a focus on present realities.

Attempting to survey two and a half millennia in the space of less than two hundred pages is, of course, a Herculean task. It is all the more difficult when one's quarry is singularly elusive, not to mention not really there. If one is looking for neuropsychiatry in the many centuries when such an animal simply didn't exist, the search will inevitably be an unproductive one. Trimble is thus forced to hunt for a rather different target, speculations about brain and behavior and about the neural origins of madness.

Trimble's chapters on the ancient world and the transition from the Dark Ages to medieval civilization focus much of their attention on conditions that involve seizures. He narrates the well-known story of Hippocrates and the "sacred disease," or epilepsy, and the physician's insistence that its roots lay in the brain, not in the realm of the metaphysical; and he discusses hysteria, another syndrome closely associated with convulsions. It is a theme that persists prominently in his chapter on the Renaissance, where he notes the coexistence of a uterine theory of hysteria's origins alongside the growth of a more careful attention to human anatomy and even some early speculations about the localization of brain function. Already, he argues, "things were on the move."[2]

Especially in these opening chapters, Trimble displays a tendency to wander all over the place. A paragraph on the Reformation is swiftly followed by two on Vesalius and the teaching of anatomy, then a couple on Paracelsus and Robert Burton on melancholy. Abruptly, the text then veers off into the realm of art (Dürer) and literature (Shakespeare) before lurching off into the realms of theology and philosophy, where Descartes and Spinoza make all-too-brief appearances. It is all rather dizzying. It is also a jumble, a hodgepodge of fleeting references and simplistic observations that make little overall sense and have only the most tenuous of relationships to the book's purported theme, the development of neuropsychiatry.

We appear to be in the presence of someone who has combed through a variety of texts in search of anything that might possibly have some relevance to the linkages of body and mind, and of brain and behavior, and that image of an intellectual magpie seeking shiny objects is only amplified in the chapters that follow. Trimble is a self-confessed sufferer from bibliomania,[3] and one can imagine him in his personal library, scanning one famous text after another and piecing together one or two paragraphs—perhaps on occasion five or six—to somehow fit them into the story he wants to tell. The range of items consulted is considerable, reflecting Trimble's own wide-ranging intellect and his collector's mania, but it scarcely conduces to the construction of a coherent narrative or thesis. At times, his disjointed prose comes close to mere list-making, so void of serious content or attention to context that it appears to be mere name-dropping, a jumbled amalgam put together simply for the purposes of display. In a single twenty-eight-line paragraph in chapter 11, for example, we move from William James to James Joyce, thence to Virginia Woolf and William Faulkner (with a tangential allusion to Proust), before diverting off to Verdi, Puccini, Wagner, Ravel, Schoenberg, and Stravinsky.[4] Somehow, this parade of luminaries and the varying characteristics of their work are adduced as helping us to understand why "neuroscience too lost track of the self and interest in studying consciousness." And then, just to pile another series of observations on top of these, we are invited to contemplate what is apparently the related rupture of psychiatry from neurology—that is, psychiatrists' embrace of Freud—and psychiatry's simultaneous distancing of itself from a psychology dominated by Pavlov's dogs and Skinner's pigeons.

Conventional history—even conventional storytelling—Trimble's book most certainly is not. Trimble's introductory chapter sees him nail his colors to the mast: "I am not a professional historian. . . . This book is not intended to be a historical exegesis."[5] As for the attention to music, literature and the arts, he writes: "I make no apology for linking neuroscience perspectives to poetry, literature, or developments of musical style. Literature is an essential pathway to feeling the human situation and examining an individual's responses to the environment."[6] Fair enough, but if one wants to range across this exceptionally broad terrain, there needs to be some sustained effort to connect neuroscience to these other realms of human endeavor, not just to gesture feebly in that direction. And one can eschew the discipline and aims of the professional historian, but any attempt to substitute the researcher and practitioner's "interest and curiosity to understand from whence [his] discipline came and how we got to where we are today"[7] must extend beyond potted histories of great men and what they had to say and contribute. Trimble does try to avoid one set of errors to which retired scientists often fall prey when they write the history of their subject, adopting a linear narrative of progress and a teleological account of the past. It is unclear, however, what he intends to put in their place: History as just one damned thing after another?

According to Trimble, the heroic age of neuropsychiatry (before there supervened a tragic break between neurology and psychiatry that he dates to the early twentieth century) was the late nineteenth century. Two major neurologists, Jean-Marie Charcot in Paris and John Hughlings Jackson in London, are seen as major figures in this development, and their ideas are given more extended and coherent analysis than most others in the book. Both trafficked across the boundaries that normally existed between psychiatry and neurology, showing interest in mental illness as well as paying more sustained attention to syndromes then and now regarded as classically neurological. Disorders involving seizures were a focus of sustained work by the two of them, though for Jackson that meant epilepsy, while for Charcot it was hysteria, a disorder he was convinced, for most of his career, was as deeply rooted in organic changes in the brain as the scleroses he had initially made his reputation studying. Trimble is interested in comparing and contrasting these contemporary figures and in attending to the very different fate of their reputations after their deaths—Jackson's status as a major contributor to neurology endured, while Charcot's experimental circus in Paris and his use of hypnosis to display his favorite female patients brought opprobrium and neglect once he departed from the scene and colleagues no longer feared his vengeful nature. In many ways, this chapter is the strongest in the book.

Neuropsychiatry tended to lose its way for much of the twentieth century. Trimble is inclined to blame the situation on Freud, and secondarily on Pavlov and the founder of behaviorism, John Watson. If the psychoanalytic revolution brought into being a brainless psychiatry, Watson's theories were worse yet: brainless *and* mindless. To be sure, a handful of figures sought to keep the neuropsychiatric flag flying, but they were marginalized (particularly in America) by a profession that focused almost exclusively on the psychological. Trimble argues that it was this psychoanalytical revolution that ruptured the links between neurology and psychiatry, and sabotaged for a time any hope of integrating the two.

The historical picture is actually far more complex than this account allows. Charcot and Jackson notwithstanding, psychiatry and neurology developed along almost completely separate paths in the nineteenth century. Psychiatrists were creatures of the vast museums of madness that the Victorians built, places that continued to house legions of the seriously mentally ill into the second half of the twentieth century. Neurologists had a more impressive pedigree, more closely connected to the laboratory and the growing links between science and medicine. Their therapeutic impotence notwithstanding, neurologists were well served by their increasing knowledge about the nervous system and their increasing diagnostic and prognostic skills. Neurologists had high status; psychiatrists were practically professional pariahs. And even the patients who crowded neurological waiting rooms with conditions that might arguably have fit better in the psychiatric ambit—sufferers of hysteria, neurasthenia, and other conversion disorders—were generally a far more affluent and attractive crowd than the psychotics with whom institutional psychiatrists dwelt. With their claims to jurisdiction over the whole range of disorders rooted in the brain and the nervous system, neurologists were in principle disposed to lay claim to expertise in diagnosing and treating the mad. But in practice, they recoiled from the stigmatizing and unpleasant work such patients brought in their train, contenting themselves with fiercely attacking the credentials and competence of those who actually ran the asylums. The divisions and tensions between neurology and psychiatry thus ran deep and had a much longer history than Trimble seems aware of.

Certainly, the collapse of the psychoanalytic enterprise in the last quarter of the twentieth century, and the associated shift of psychiatry (particularly American psychiatry) in a biologically reductionist direction, has reduced some of the distance between the neurologists and academic psychiatrists. Neuroscientists now rule the roost in many university departments of psychiatry, and psychiatric practice has moved out of the old barracks-asylums and into general hospitals and clinics. Trimble recognizes that these developments contributed to the reshaping of the psychiatric enterprise and helped to lay the groundwork for the re-emergence of his subspecialty. But he also stresses that the consolidation of neuropsychiatry can be traced in part to certain technological advances, first the advent of electroencephalography and then the growth of ever more sophisticated imaging techniques. These were among the developments that spurred advances in our understanding of neuroanatomy and neurochemistry. Finally, perhaps reflecting his own expertise, he sees the increased interest in "the links between epilepsy and psychopathology"[8] as helping bring about the consolidation of his chosen branch of the profession.

Trimble closes with a qualified optimism about the future of neuropsychiatry. He discounts the idea that the field is simply the "'bridge' between neurology and psychiatry" or "the derivative idea that it forms an indiscrete narrow space shaded in between neurology and psychiatry in a Venn diagram. The current status of an independent neuropsychiatry seems secure, and its importance as a recognized discipline within the clinical neurosciences is increasingly accepted."[9] But he sees a cloud on the horizon. The overwhelming embrace of psychoanalysis as both theory and practice during the first two-thirds of the past century "wiped out the psychopathologists' contributions of the previous 100 years."[10] In short order, "the introduction of *DSM 3* and its successors . . . toppled the house that Freud built."[11] It was a revolution, however, that depended on the imposition of a new ruling ideology that was "politically driven and committee-based"[12]—atheoretical and with no secure foundation in science. "There is every reason to believe," he concludes, "that this house of cards will tumble in the future, and where the residence of neuropsychiatry will be then, no one can tell."[13]

12 Contending Professions

SCIENCES OF THE BRAIN AND MIND IN
THE UNITED STATES, 1900–2013

The history of American psychiatry as a profession in the twentieth century is marked by three major shifts in its intellectual orientation—dramatic breaks with past ideologies that have been associated with equally profound changes in the nature of psychiatric practice. These resonate in important ways with changes in the mind and brain sciences in general—psychiatry, neurology, and physiology—and at least some of the changes in psychiatry reflect clashes between its practitioners and those in neighboring disciplines, most especially psychology. In turn, these three eras have been marked by broader alterations in the meanings ascribed by the larger culture and in social practices to mental illnesses and to what appear to be unambiguously nerve diseases rooted in physiology. I speak here of the dominant tendencies that can be observed, because there have always been undercurrents of dissent—vocal or otherwise—against the hegemonic ideas of a particular era, but the existence of radically different organizing ideologies and the rapidity with which change has overtaken the profession are remarkable features of the psychiatric universe. There is every sign, moreover, as we move into a new millennium, that these wrenching changes may not be at an end. Despite frantic efforts to shore up the epistemological framework that has dominated psychiatry since

1980, a new sense of crisis is enveloping the field, and only the absence of a new organizing paradigm seems to stand in the way of the collapse of the current ruling ideology.

What, then, are the defining characteristics of the three eras I have spoken of? When did their respective periods of dominance manifest themselves? What are some of the fundamental forces that seem to underlie the shift from one era to another? And why does a profession that proclaims its practices are founded on "science" (implicitly portrayed as a progressive and cumulative process) instead seem to lurch periodically toward radically incompatible ends. What I have to offer here, after all, is a narrative that is fundamentally at odds with any such "march of progress" rhetoric.

Ordinarily, one has difficulty attaching precise dates to major transformations like the ones we are discussing here, and to be sure, social phenomena like these have no neat and precise chronological boundaries—they exist in embryonic form before briefly achieving hegemonic status and then enjoy a half-life that extends into the succeeding era. But bearing that caveat in mind, I think one can indeed treat each of these successive historical moments as having an identifiable beginning and (in all but the last case) end that are remarkably definite, to which one can attach a chronology that is anything but arbitrary or purely conventional. First, there is the period where institutional psychiatry predominates and a veritable mania for experimenting on the bodies of the mentally ill sweeps through the profession, which lasts from the turn of the century through 1945. The second period, running from 1945 to 1980, is when psychoanalysis rules the roost, madness is declared to be rooted in meaning, and the profession begins to desert the old institutions in droves; it is an era marked, in its later stages, by sharp declines in the in-patient census and the relocation of most of the seriously mentally ill into the "community," whatever that term came to mean. Finally, there is the third period, the so-called neo-Kraeplinian era, when psychiatry is rebiologized, shifts drastically away from psychodynamic accounts of mental illness and psychotherapeutic approaches to treatment, and embraces the twin gods of psychopharmacology and an ever-expanding universe of psychiatric disorders defined purely conventionally and descriptively.

The asylum era in the United States was largely the product of the last two-thirds of the nineteenth century.[1] To be sure, a handful of corporate asylums predate the 1830s, having served as a conduit for the transmission of the contemporary European infatuation with the virtues of the well-ordered institution conceived as an engine of reformation, a means of reclaiming the mad.[2] But it was the opening in 1833 of the first state asylum run along moral treatment lines, the Worcester State Asylum in Massachusetts, that truly marks the decisive moment in the American "discovery of the asylum."[3] From then on, and particularly once that remarkable moral entrepreneur Dorothea Dix launched her crusade to "rescue" the insane from the barbarities and neglect that she claimed were their lot in the community,[4] the asylum was transformed into the ideal weapon in the battle against the ravages of mental disturbance. "Ideal" is the appropriate word in this context, for the earliest reform asylums were born in an atmosphere of utopian optimism about the opportunities they offered for cure[5] and a veritable "cult of curability" operated in the 1830s and 1840s, with claims to cure upward of 70 to 80 percent of recent cases, which did much to loosen the purse strings of otherwise parsimonious state legislatures. Enlightenment convictions that human beings were the product of their experiences and environments helped to foster such optimism and underpin the claims that the controlled environment of the asylum could provide the tools for reworking the human raw materials, thus promoting recovery.

By the end of the Civil War in 1865, however, such optimism had faded. As the first generation of alienists disappeared from the scene, they were replaced by a generation that accommodated without evident strain to an essentially custodial role for themselves.[6] The nineteenth-century asylum, it seems, was both the means and the end of psychiatry. Psychiatry thus reconstituted itself as a managerial specialism, content to minister to the hordes of the hopeless who thronged the increasingly overcrowded wards of ever-larger institutions, asylums that grew to contain thousands of patients apiece. They became places that resembled miniature towns (and sometimes not so miniature: Milledgeville in Georgia contained some 14,000 inhabitants early in the twentieth century). Branded by their captors as degenerates, the patients they housed were seen as biologically defective creatures largely beyond the reach of medical remedies or relief,[7] a heterogeneous mass of jetsam and flotsam that crowded asylum hallways. They included the senile; the alcoholic; those suffering from want and malnutrition; women in the throes of postpartum depression; the victims of heavy metal poisoning or of the ravages of tertiary syphilis (then called general paralysis of the insane, after the progressive physical decay that accompanied its lurid psychiatric symptomatology); not to mention a host of other raving and melancholic inmates whose mental troubles were as mysterious then as they remain now.

States sought to pare the costs of these warehouses of the unwanted, though few in the community expressed much enthusiasm for lunatics to be left at large. Madness of all sorts was profoundly unsettling to the social order, both symbolically and practically. Those familiar with the internal life of the asylums knew that they were littered with mostly chronic patients, many of them reduced, as the Philadelphia neurologist Silas Weir Mitchell remarked, to little more than "silent, grewsome machines that eat and sleep, sleep and eat."[8] But the remote locations and physical barriers to the outside world that typified asylums of this era ensured that few outside the ranks of the alienists who ran them had much direct knowledge of their human contents. Why, the public might ask, were such mad folk locked up unless they were a menace to society? This sentiment was doubtless reinforced by occasional dramatic crimes of violence adjudged to be the product of insanity, not to mention the growing sense that the mentally ill were a biologically defective lot, shorn of the usual restraints that reined in the passions of the sane, and hence liable to propagate their kind uncontrollably were they to remain free.

But the profession paid a steep price for embracing the role of being glorified boarding house keepers. Increasingly, beginning with the creation of the State Board of Charities in Massachusetts in 1867, psychiatrists found themselves subjected to tighter state control, and along with this loss of autonomy came decreased budgets and political interference.[9] In states like Illinois, positions in asylums became political patronage plums, with superintendents' tenure at the mercy of the political winds. In New York State, grumblings about political interference grew markedly in the 1890s and led to the departure of G. Alden Blumer, superintendent of the state's foremost asylum at Utica. (To prevent the profession's flagship journal, the *American Journal of Insanity*—now sadly renamed the *American Journal of Psychiatry*—from falling into state hands, for it had been owned and published by the Utica superintendent since its first issue in 1844, ownership was abruptly transferred to the American Medico-Psychological

Association just before Blumer's resignation.)[10] And worse still, a specialty that had felt secure enough to rebuff the entreaties of a nascent American Medical Association to join with it in the late 1840s, when its members were more economically secure and professionally respected than most physicians, now found itself the target of contemptuous criticism from both the public and its professional brethren. Sharp censure from lay quarters, particularly the National Association for the Protection of the Insane and the Prevention of Insanity had been amplified in the 1870s and 1880s by scathing complaints from the emerging specialism of neurology that alienists knew more about sewage pipes, heating systems, and animal husbandry on asylum farms than they did about mental illness. The brash Edward Spitka condemned asylum superintendents as "experts at everything except the diagnosis, pathology and treatment of insanity." "Psychiatry," he declared, "is but a subsidiary branch of neurology. . . . The study of insanity should be considered a sub-division of neurology."[11] His New York colleague William Hammond, who had served as surgeon general of the Union army in the Civil War, insisted that "there is nothing surprisingly difficult, obscure, or mysterious about diseases of the brain which can only be learned within the walls of the asylum." Not trapped in the isolated world of the mental hospital, general practitioners with a modicum of training in "cerebral pathology and physiology [were] more capable of treating successfully a case of insanity than the average asylum physician."[12] Conflicting claims about the relevance and role of pathophysiology would play a scarcely concealed part in creating ongoing tensions between psychiatry, psychology, and neurology in decades to come.

It hardly mattered that the neurologists' claims to superior scientific standing and more effective techniques with which to intervene were dubious if not delusional. They resonated with a public that saw asylums as expensive mausoleums of the mad that little could be expected of beyond safekeeping. Psychiatrists maintained control over the institutions from which they derived their authority, but their marginality was manifest, and the need to escape from the nihilistic position they occupied was ever more pressing, something felt with particular force among psychiatrists who retained some semblance of ambition.

In 1894, at the fiftieth anniversary of the American Medico-Psychological Association, the assembled psychiatrists listened sullenly as the keynote speaker their own leadership had invited, Silas Weir Mitchell, America's most prominent neurologist, excoriated their performance and called into question their claims to be competent medical scientists. In his opening blast, he noted that while medicine and surgery had made extraordinary progress over the past half-century, psychiatry had been stagnant: "Your hospitals are not our hospitals; your ways are not our ways." He stated that psychiatrists lived in isolation, had cut themselves off from healthy criticism and scientific progress, and had become "almost a sect apart," and he warned that the consequences for profession and patient alike were "evil." The very title to which the more senior members of his audience clung, "medical superintendent," was "absurd." Many listening to him had won their jobs through political patronage, still another "grave evil."

The invective rained down on his audience for over an hour. Mitchell denounced the "senile characteristics" of asylum boards, the repetition of "old stupidities in brick and stone," and the "neat little comedy" of outside inspections that were known about in advance and thus incapable of getting at the truth. But these were the least of the profession's issues. The medical superintendent was the "monarch" of all he surveyed, but, Mitchell asserted, he was an emperor with no scientific clothes: "Where, we ask, are your annual reports of scientific study, of the psychology and pathology of your patients? . . . We commonly get as your contributions to science, odd little statements, reports of a case or two, a few useless pages of isolated post-mortem records, and these are sandwiched among incomprehensible statistics and farm balance sheets." Asylum case records put on display an appalling state of affairs, an "amazing lack of complete physical study of the insane, . . . the failure to see obvious lesions," and a complete ignorance of the diagnostic technologies indispensable to the practice of modern medicine—problems as visible in the most prominent and best-endowed asylums for the rich as in the meanest, most overcrowded state hospitals.

According to Mitchell, psychiatrists had spent a half-century attempting to persuade the public of the "superstition . . . that an asylum is in itself curative. You hear the regret in every report that patients are not sent soon enough, as if you had ways of curing which we have not. Upon my word, I think asylum life is deadly to the insane." Far from being therapeutic environments, he insisted, mental hospitals (as they were ironically beginning to be called) had the air of prisons, with "grated windows and locked doors. . . . I presume that you have, by habit, lost the sense of jail and jailor which troubles me when I walk behind one of you and he unlocks door after door. Do you think it is not felt by some of your patients?"

The upshot of such conditions was what he himself had observed in the wards of an asylum in his home city of Philadelphia, where he saw "the insane, who have lost even the memory of hope, sit in rows, too dull to know despair, watched by attendants." And they were not the only victims of prolonged confinement. Their captors, the psychiatrists, had fallen into the same sort of paralysis: "The cloistral lives you lead give rise, we [neurologists] think, to certain mental peculiarities. . . . You [too] are cursed by that slow atrophy of the energizing faculties that is the very malaria of asylum life." Indeed, Mitchell concluded, "I cannot see how, with the lives you lead, it is possible for you to retain the wholesome balance of mental and moral faculties."[13]

Psychiatrists thus stood accused, and not for the first or the last time, of being nearly as mentally unstable as those they locked up on behalf of society. Many simply shrugged and, safe in their bureaucratic niches, waited for the storm to pass. But for the more ambitious among them, such passivity was intolerable, and the half-century following Mitchell's address saw these men embark on a steadily more extravagant series of therapeutic experiments on their captive audience in a desperate attempt to reclaim their identity through scientific work as medical men and as professionals who treated and cured their patients.[14] Their actions were made possible by the status of those confined in their institutions as people who were for all intents and purposes morally and legally dead: deprived of their selfhood, presumed to be lacking the capacity to make judgments about their own treatment, cut off from the larger world, and thus incapable of resistance.

The period between 1894 and 1945 marked in some ways a continuation of an earlier emphasis on the segregation of the mentally ill in total institutions. What was novel about this period, however, was the emergence of a whole host of treatments directed at what psychiatrists insisted was a disease like any other, a disease, that is, rooted in the body and thus to be attacked by somatic means. To be sure, there was a small group of dissenters operating for the most part outside the walls of asylums (or as they had come to be called by this point, mental hospitals) and mostly treating milder, less disturbed cases on an ambulatory basis. I will return to a consideration of these dissenters, who proclaimed madness had meaning and should be treated at the level of meaning by psychotherapeutics or "talk therapy." But it was the institutionalized patients, who numbered in the hundreds of thousands (American mental hospitals contained more than four hundred thousand patients by 1940, and a half million by 1950), who provided the bulk of psychiatric practice and occupied the time and efforts of the overwhelming majority of the profession, including, in these years, its most prominent figures. And for these patients, the routines of "moral" or milieu therapy that had been on offer in the nineteenth century (often on little more than a token basis) were now increasingly supplemented if not replaced by a gathering array of somatic interventions.

First came operations to sterilize: tying of the tubes for women, vasectomies for the men. These procedures, which were originally promoted by lay enthusiasts for eugenics as a means of restricting the breeding of the unfit,[15] were transformed in the hands of psychiatrists into something that purported to be of more direct therapeutic benefit to mental patients—an ideological move, as Joel Braslow has shown,[16] that was prompted by the discomfort many psychiatrists felt at the prospect of employing a "treatment" that seemingly benefited the community rather than the patients under their care.

But sterilization was pursued enthusiastically in only a handful of states, California and Virginia most notable among them. The operations always encountered religious and ethical objections, and in many jurisdictions this opposition proved decisive. Other therapeutic interventions, however, often spread much more widely, and they became central to psychiatry's efforts to re-emphasize its medical identity by insisting on the somatic roots of the disorders it treated. The early twentieth century was heir to the triumphs of Pasteur and Koch, and for a time the bacteriological model of disease swept all before it. Emil Kraepelin, a leading German psychiatrist, attempted to produce some order from the chaos that was madness via a new nosology that purported to be derived inductively from thousands of cases confined in German asylums, introducing the basic division between dementia praecox and manic depressive psychosis, a fundamental organizing tactic that would eventually have a major impact on the world stage.[17]

Kraepelin repeatedly voiced the opinion that dementia praecox had a toxic origin,[18] and this speculation found prominent supporters elsewhere. Ira Van Gieson, for example, who had been appointed the first director of the New York Pathological Institute, the research arm of the vast New York State mental hospital system (an institute set up in the aftermath of Silas Weir Mitchell's address explicitly to counter the complaint about the scientific backwardness of psychiatry), was equally convinced that infection caused insanity. Though Van Gieson was soon maneuvered from office, hurt by a premature announcement that he was on the brink of discovering the "germ of insanity," and even more by his visible contempt for the psychiatrists his institute was supposed to be serving, the basic hypothesis he was pursuing was one that drew considerable support.[19]

And soon there was a demonstration that substantial numbers of the mentally ill in asylums were indeed there because they had been infected. As many as 20 to 25 percent of male admissions (and a smaller fraction of the female population) were victims of general paralysis of the insane (GPI), a progressive disorder first diagnosed in France in the 1820s, and one of the few unambiguous diagnostic successes nineteenth-century psychiatrists could point to.[20] The increasing suspicions of many that GPI was the product of syphilitic infection was decisively confirmed in 1913 by Hideo Noguchi and J. W. Moore,[21] who observed syphilitic spirochetes in the brains of its victims.

As well as reinforcing the conviction of most psychiatrists that mental illness had a bodily origin, these findings led indirectly to further therapeutic experiments based on this hypothesis. In the United States, encouraged by the efforts of Henry Cotton[22] of the New Jersey State Mental Hospital at Trenton (who had trained, inter alia, under Kraepelin), and also independently in Britain, promoted by Thomas Chivers Graves,[23] head of the Birmingham mental hospitals—the results led to the claim that all mental illness was the product of hidden chronic infections, known as focal sepsis, which produced toxins that poisoned the brain and thus produced the symptoms of mental disturbance. The effect was to license a wide-ranging assault on the presumed sites where these infections lurked, a program of "surgical bacteriology" that began with the wholesale removal of the teeth and tonsils of mentally ill patients and extended in the United States to the excision of stomachs, spleens, colons, and other "unnecessary" organs. Though Cotton and Graves continued their surgical interventions for decades and were scarcely isolated figures, and though the notion of focal sepsis drew vocal support from such leading centers of advanced scientific medicine as John Hopkins and the Mayo Clinic (not to mention leading lights in British medicine and surgery), their vigorous proselytizing for this form of treatment never attracted more than a minority of their colleagues—perhaps fortunately, since the "beneficiaries" of their therapies were, it subsequently materialized, left maimed or dead.

By contrast, the other therapeutic intervention spawned by the discovery of the syphilitic origins of GPI enjoyed broad acceptance internationally and won for its inventor one of the only three Nobel Prizes that have ever been awarded to a psychiatrist. In the closing months of World War I, the Viennese psychiatrist Julius Wagner von Jauregg experimentally induced malaria in patients suffering from GPI. Earlier experiments with using other febrile agents to treat different forms of insanity had failed, but on this occasion, Jauregg announced he had achieved dramatic success in curing GPI, a condition regarded as uniformly fatal, and one that led to a particularly nasty end. After the war, despite Jauregg finishing on the losing side (and even being prosecuted for war crimes for his role in treating shell shock with painful electrical shocks), his new technique rapidly drew converts and spread internationally. Patients believed to be suffering from GPI were deliberately given malaria, either by using colonies of malarial mosquitoes or (more commonly) by injecting them with blood drawn from a malarial patient. The uncertain and intermittent course of GPI and the lack of any controlled trials of the procedure's efficacy make one wary of the extravagant claims of success that attended its use. But psychiatrists hailed it as a breakthrough, and the Nobel committee agreed with them in 1927.[24] More importantly, the advent of this therapy spurred on the search for other somatic interventions. In the absence of any check on experimentation on the captive populations in mental hospitals, and with the desperation psychiatrists felt to do anything that might improve the condition of their patients (and their own standing in the medical profession), a host of approaches were tried.

Many of these—experimenting with barbiturate-induced comas, injecting horse serum into the spinal canals of mental patients to induce meningitis, chilling patients down to temperatures barely consistent with life, heating them in sweat boxes, having patients breath pure carbon dioxide, injecting them with cyanide, among others[25]— have sunk into oblivion, but some came attached to extravagant claims of therapeutic success. It was alleged that 70 to 80 percent of schizophrenics were cured by treatments as diverse as creating comas by injecting the newly discovered insulin[26] and inducing grand mal seizures by injecting metrazol (a procedure that produced a feeling that one was about to die, followed by such severe fits that patients' spines and hip sockets were frequently fractured).[27] Most indelibly of all, there were large-scale experiments with severing portions of mental patients' frontal lobes (a technique introduced by the Portuguese neurologist Egas Moniz, who was awarded a Nobel Prize for the discovery in 1949, and popularized by his American disciple Walter Freeman in the mid-1930s)[28] and electroconvulsive therapy,[29] the latter of which is the only one of these innovations to still enjoy considerable professional approval today.

It goes without saying that none of these innovations produced the sorts of results their promoters claimed for them, a failure made manifest by the continued rapid upsurge in the mental hospital censuses through the middle of the twentieth century. For psychiatrists, however, these techniques provided the illusion that they were engaged in a therapeutic enterprise that involved treating sick bodies, just like the people they thought of as their colleagues, medical professionals at large. The therapies were accepted by most of the psychiatric profession as much for what they were not—psychotherapy, especially in its sexualized Freudian form—as for what they actually accomplished. Desperate patients (or more often, their families) clung to the notion that there might indeed be a medical breakthrough that would rescue their loved ones. And science journalists, ever susceptible to hype and always looking for a good story, were happy to relay reports of the latest miracle cure. Mental illness, mainstream psychiatrists repeatedly intoned, was a biological disorder and thus necessitated treatment by biological means.

It was Hitler and the exigencies of total war that shook up this consensus and for a quarter-century prompted American psychiatry to move in a completely contrary direction. Simultaneously, the war (and the ensuing Cold War) helped to create a rival profession, clinical psychology, with enduring effects on the mental health sector.[30] To be sure, psychologists, led by Robert Yerkes, had managed to make themselves useful to the military during World War I, and in the postwar period, further development of the IQ tests and other psychometric instruments that they had introduced had proceeded apace. Psychology had also enjoyed a growing stature in the industrial arena, persuading professional managers that it had instruments that could help with their tasks. And its psychometric technologies had also been mobilized in the new child-guidance clinics that had begun to proliferate with the support of the well-endowed foundations that emerged in this era, and in the identification and control of the "feeble-minded" and juvenile delinquents.[31] In carrying out the latter tasks, in particular, psychologists operated in clinical settings, rousing anxieties and opposition from psychiatrists, who resented any "trespassing" on what they insisted was an exclusively medical territory. There were pointed suggestions that any invocation of terms like "diagnosis," "treatment," and "clinical" on the part of psychologists would be viewed as an affront, for these were terms and tasks that were the preserve of the medically qualified. Intraprofessional tensions and hostility simmered beneath the surface right up to the outbreak of World War II, mitigated only by the fact that the largest group of applied psychologists busied themselves with nonclinical matters, while the continued dominance of the traditional mental hospital in the delivery of mental health services ensured the bureaucratic subordination of psychologists who had the temerity to express interest in clinical concerns.[32]

Freud himself had visited the United States briefly in 1909. Given the important place psychoanalysis came to occupy in the United States between 1945 and 1980, there has been a temptation retrospectively to assign more significance to the lectures he delivered at Clark University than is conceivably warranted by the modest impact they had at the time. Freud was only one of nearly thirty speakers on that occasion—the twentieth anniversary of the university's foundation—and he was far from being viewed as the most eminent or important of them. (The roster included two Nobel Prize winners, just for a start, and other speakers on psychological and psychiatric matters were more prominent than Freud and were paid more to attend.)[33] Mythology aside, however, Freud did succeed on this occasion in attracting a small and devoted following, a tiny bridgehead that had subsequently secured a following among some of the rich and chattering classes. His acolytes came partly from the ranks of psychiatry and partly from the neighboring profession of neurology, but the majority of both groups of specialists remained hostile to the claims of psychoanalysis, with neurologists preferring to concentrate on diagnostic and prognostic refinement in dealing with a host of mostly debilitating and usually fatal diseases that seemed more obviously organic in origin, and asylum psychiatrists dismissing talk therapy as useless when applied to their psychotic clientele and as actively threatening to their tenuous claims to an identity as medics.

Before the war, the Nazi persecution of the Jews, not yet as deadly as it would soon become, led many analysts to flee—Freud and his daughter to London, many others to New York and the Eastern Seaboard of the United States[34]—but while this somewhat augmented the numbers of psychoanalysts in America, particularly in New York, and created all sorts of complicated sectarian rivalries within the analytic community, it did little by itself to change the balance of power within psychiatry or the experience of most psychiatric patients.[35]

The war changed all that. Citing the epidemic of shell shock in World War I, American psychiatrists and psychologists succeeded in persuading the Washington powers that be that they should avoid a reprise of that wasteful and morale-sapping experience by screening all military recruits for signs of incipient mental instability.[36] (Robert Yerkes, who had directed the military's mental testing program in World War I, was particularly active in stressing the usefulness of psychometrics to this process.)[37] The examiners rejected as many as 1.75 million recruits on such grounds, only for breakdowns to occur among American troops at more than double the rate of the previous war.[38] Mechanized warfare and the maintenance of mental health turned out, not for the last time, to be incompatible in large numbers of cases.[39]

Painfully, the lesson that even the most stable of us is prone to mental collapse if put under sufficient stress was relearned, and doubt was thus cast on the portrait of mental illness as a purely biological event, one to which "normal" people were not prone. Wartime treatment, though it often took the form of tea (or coffee), cigarettes, and not too much sympathy, was generally what could be thought of as psychotherapy: if successful, it took the form of keeping the men close to the front lines, persuading them that they were just suffering from "combat exhaustion" and manipulating their sense of guilt at deserting their buddies in the platoon.[40] This bias in favor of psychodynamic explanations and interventions was reinforced from the very top, because the prior decision to appoint William Menninger from the family clinic in Topeka, Kansas, as brigadier general and chief army psychiatrist ensured that someone broadly embracing Freudian ideas headed what was a quintessentially top-down organization.[41]

The significance of the rise of military psychiatry was amplified by the dramatic rise it fueled in the number of those practicing on the mentally ill. In 1940, on the eve of the war, the American Psychiatric Association had only 2,295 members, virtually all of them employed in traditional mental hospitals, where they pursued their isolated and stigmatized careers. Psychiatric casualties among the armed forces were so numerous (over 25 percent of soldiers that saw combat exhibited serious symptomatology) that the demand for physicians to treat them greatly exceeded supply.[42] Doctors were drafted into the field and given a few weeks of emergency training before being let loose on the troops, and when even that didn't suffice, psychologists—previously members of a profession eschewing practical work and clinging to an identity as laboratory scientists—also found themselves called into the breach.[43] Both groups found the clinical experience engaging for the most part, and many of the more than two thousand army "trick cyclists" and their psychology counterparts sought to continue to practice in the field after the war finally came to a close.

The numbers of mentally disabled veterans provided one incentive for the federal government to invade the mental health territory— traditionally a purely state responsibility in the United States—and the extensive mobilization for total war had decisively broken down many of the objections that might formerly have been raised about states' rights. The size of the fiscal drain mental illness represented for state budgets—it was the largest single expenditure for many—was another motive for an expanded federal role. And soon enough, the outbreak of the Cold War prompted yet further efforts to enhance federal involvement in science and medicine—both in training new practitioners and in funding basic research. Before the war, there had been essentially no federal involvement in funding medical research or basic science; in its aftermath, with the formation of the National Science Foundation and the National Institutes of Health, the era of Big Medicine and Big Science had arrived. Expansion was the order of the day.[44]

Psychiatry, which had been enriched by funding from the Veterans' Administration at the war's end,[45] soon also saw major funding from the newly established National Institute for Mental Health.[46] The training programs funded by Washington fueled an extraordinarily rapid expansion in the numbers of psychiatrists and in academic psychiatry, while specialties such as neurology and neuropsychiatry declined. And the dramatic increase in the size of the profession was matched by an equally dramatic shift in its intellectual orientation and in the locus of psychiatric practice. The dominance of psychoanalytically oriented practitioners—intellectually, politically, and eventually numerically—was immediately signaled by the election of William Menninger as president of the American Psychiatric Association in 1948, triumphing over the candidate of the old guard, Charles Burlingame, superintendent of the ritzy private mental hospital the Institute of Living.[47]

Whereas virtually all psychiatrists practiced in mental hospitals in the 1930s, as early as 1947, a majority had moved to outpatient work, and by 1958, only 16 percent practiced their trade in traditional state hospitals. Numbers had grown from 2,200 before war to more than double that in 1948 and more than 27,000 by 1976.[48] Virtually every major medical school had placed a psychoanalyst or someone sympathetic to psychoanalysis at the head of its department of psychiatry, and virtually all the best students entering the profession undertook training analyses at the local Psychoanalytic Institute. The duds of the profession, and those who failed to complete a full residency, were left to colonize the increasingly unattractive and neglected mental hospital sector, where, alongside foreign-trained physicians who were otherwise ineligible to practice medicine in the United States, they practiced a form of psychiatry their superior brethren disdainfully referred to as "directive-organic psychiatry"—that is, a second-rate type of practice that continued to use some of the somatic therapies introduced earlier.[49]

The interest the war had stimulated among some psychologists in clinical work and the sheer size of the problems posed by mental illness encouraged the new federal bureaucracy to expand its subsidies for training clinicians to include psychologists.[50] Psychometrics, which had a long prewar history and enjoyed considerable legitimacy, attracted some of the available funding.[51] So far as clinical psychology was concerned, although there were one or two brief and somewhat feeble attempts to organize the new specialty along psychoanalytic lines, most notably at the Menninger Clinic, the fierce insistence of the Menningers and of other analysts on subordinating clinical psychologists rankled,[52] and soon enough those launching the new profession created an alternative model, one linked tightly to the newly emerging knowledge factories that were research universities and embracing the laboratory as the source of knowledge and legitimacy. A federally funded conference was organized in Boulder, Colorado, in 1949 to develop plans for training in clinical psychology. Consensus was soon reached among the participants on a plan that welded together training in academic psychology, statistics, research methodology, and clinical experience.[53]

The flow of federal dollars induced universities to embrace the new model, ensuring a rapid expansion of the whole psychological enterprise. Moreover, as government support of professional training was increasingly complemented by an exponentially increasing budget for research in an environment where the federal paymasters defined the knowledge "relevant" to the mental health problems of the nation extremely broadly and laxly, clinical psychologists were able to capture the lion's share of that money. The very nature of the psychoanalytic perspective on mental illness, and its practitioners' focus on the peculiarities of individual cases, made them strikingly unsuccessful in the grantsmanship game. Psychologists enjoyed an ever-increasing competitive advantage as they developed more elaborate research protocols and analytic techniques, and consolidated their membership on the relevant study sections. And they generated a series of short-term interventions (many of them sheltering under the rubric of cognitive behavioral therapy) that carried both the imprimatur of laboratory science and the statistical confirmation of their success in suppressing symptoms.[54]

In the army, and in hierarchical bureaucratic organizations like traditional mental hospitals, which were all headed by someone with a medical qualification, subordination of the social scientists could always be assured. But as the bulk of psychiatric practice moved outside these institutions, the competition between these two rival forms of psychotherapy— psychoanalysis and the very different version of psychotherapy developed by clinical psychologists—grew more heated. To be sure, psychoanalysts had the power and status that an MD degree conferred, but psychoanalysis, terminal and interminable, was directed at an astonishing array of psychological issues, and the analysts were ill-equipped to answer questions about the efficacy of their lengthy interventions with compelling data. Marginalized by their medical brethren, who saw talk as an odd sort of approach to the treatment of disease, their forms of psychotherapy were in some respects poorly placed to cope with the competition from their psychological colleagues, whose alternatives were more finite and more focused (and hence attractive to insurance companies, which increasingly were providing limited coverage for mental health problems), and whose prices (for theirs was a female-dominated and thus, as labor market economists would confirm, inevitably lower-paid profession) were distinctly cheaper. Psychoanalysts had elected to keep tight control over who was allowed to join their guild, but their decision to separate their training institutes from the legitimacy conferred by association with a university was a further handicap. So even as psychoanalytic psychiatry expanded, it did so on increasingly shaky foundations. It faced in clinical psychology a competitor for ambulatory and affluent patients—far more desirable than the indigent and grossly disturbed psychotic patients who had traditionally thronged the wards of mental hospitals—that constituted a growing threat.

And growing its rival most certainly was. Prior to World War II, not a single PhD-trained American psychologist would have identified as a clinical psychologist; the set was essentially an empty one. By the war's end, membership in the American Psychological Association had risen only slightly, from 2,739 in 1940 to 4,173 in 1945. But fifteen years later, it had shot up to 18,215, and a National Science Foundation survey taken just four years after that suggested that more than two-thirds of psychologists with a doctorate were working in the mental health field. The clinical tail was wagging the academic dog, a problem that had plagued psychiatry in an earlier era. By 1990, there were 63,000 clinical psychologists in practice, a number that has since doubled again.

These were ominous developments for psychiatry, but the threat they posed has largely been alleviated by the third major shift in the profession's ideological foundations: the virtual abandonment of psychotherapeutics by psychiatrists within a quite remarkably short space of time, and the resort instead to drug-based treatments. That changed orientation was, I will suggest, only partially driven by concerns about competition from clinical psychology, though it did a great deal to nullify or at least sharply mitigate that concern. And ironically, it has proved so successful that it has forced some segments of organized clinical psychology to attempt to breach one of the most entrenched monopolies our society has granted to a single group of professionals: sole control over the right to authorize the use of prescription drugs. These psychologists contend that they, too, ought to be licensed to prescribe psychotropic medications.[55]

Both directly and indirectly, innovations in drug treatment for mental illnesses were one of the crucial sources of changed perspectives on the psychiatric patient's treatment. But as the timing of the intellectual revolution demonstrates, there was nothing automatic about its arrival. The advent of the psychopharmaceutical revolution, after all, dates back to the approval by the FDA of Dilantin for the control of epileptic seizures in 1953 and of the first so-called antipsychotic medication, Thorazine, in 1954, just over a quarter-century before psychoanalytic hegemony abruptly collapsed. Millions of patients were taking the new magic potions, which were soon joined by such "minor" tranquillizers as Miltown and Valium, during the very decades when psychoanalysis enjoyed unparalleled dominance within the psychiatric profession. Drugs and talk therapy somehow coexisted for years. And then they didn't.

The initial response of many psychoanalysts to the new compounds was to reject them, just as they had rejected the symptomatic treatments proffered by the clinical psychologists; they were both Band-Aids that treated surface symptomatology while leaving the deeper personality disorders that allegedly underlay mental distress untouched. Since psychoanalysts did not have major clinical responsibilities for the institutionalized psychotic patients, this was a stance that endured for a time, but as the drugs made further inroads, an alternative tack became popular: drugs were a useful adjunct, a way of reducing florid symptomatology so that the "real work" of analysis could proceed.[56] It was a conceit that worked for a time, but it was inherently unstable.

Problems arose on a number of levels. One of the most serious was something the psychoanalysts were reluctant to take seriously because in their worldview it scarcely mattered, but it became increasingly hard to ignore in the late 1960s and early 1970s: the question of diagnosis.

Focused as they were on what they saw as the precise psychodynamics of individual cases, analysts viewed diagnostic labels as essentially an irrelevance, artificial creations that added nothing of substance to the understanding of a patient's problems or to the treatment process. Karl Menninger had even taken this skepticism to its logical conclusion, calling for the abolition of diagnosis in psychiatry altogether on the grounds not just that it was a charade but that it actively harmed patients by labeling them.[57] Among analysts, it probably didn't help matters that the dominant nosology to that point derived mostly from the work of Emil Kraepelin, someone Freud had regarded with contempt and referred to scornfully as "the Great Pope of psychiatry." To be sure, there was an official guide to diagnosis, which had appeared in two editions, in 1952 and 1968. They were slight documents, barely over a hundred pages long, and contained around the same number of separate diagnoses, each with a purported psychodynamic etiology attached. Beyond a broad distinction between psychoses and neuroses, there was little attempt at precision or operationalizability, and the manuals were lightly regarded and seldom consulted. When efforts were made, as by the Philadelphia psychiatrist Aaron Beck,[58] to examine the reliability of professional diagnosis using this template, the results showed that psychiatrists regularly disagreed among themselves to a quite extraordinary extent. A systematic cross-national study comparing diagnostic practices and labels in Britain and the United States by J. E. Cooper and associates appeared in 1972 and made the point much more forcefully.[59] Schizophrenia was diagnosed far more frequently in the United States, whereas manic-depressive psychosis was diagnosed more often in Britain, and compelling evidence demonstrated that this outcome was the artifact of two very different psychiatric cultures. American psychiatrists "saw" schizophrenia, while their British counterparts were convinced the problem was manic-depressive illness.

What was one to make of diagnostic practices that produced such contradictory results? How could one have confidence in the scientific legitimacy of a profession so demonstrably unable to agree on what was wrong in an individual case or indeed whether anything at all was amiss? The threat to psychiatry's legitimacy was patent and soon became much worse. In 1973, a Stanford psychologist, David Rosenhan, allegedly conceived of a novel way to dramatize psychiatry's diagnostic incapacity: he sent a series of pseudopatients to twelve different local mental hospitals with instructions to report limited auditory hallucinations but otherwise behave completely normally.[60] All were diagnosed as either schizophrenic or manic depressive, and all were admitted and medicated. Although they behaved normally thereafter, it took between seven and fifty-two days for them to be released, which took place only after they admitted being ill. Rosenhan published his findings in *Science* and concluded that they were an indictment of psychiatry's failings. The study drew enormous media attention and, fierce rejoinders from some psychiatrists notwithstanding, contributed to public cynicism about the profession's scientific standing. That the study may well have been fraudulent, as Susannah Cahalan shows,[61] does not alter the profound impact it had at the time.

Soon, criticisms of psychiatry's competence were not confined to the court of public opinion. The civil rights movement of the 1960s had helped bring into being a cohort of public interest lawyers interested in rights issues, and in the 1970s, some of these lawyers became active in mental health issues, suing for patients' rights to treatment, then for the right to refuse treatment; for the abolition of "institutional peonage" (using patients to perform hospital labor without pay, under the guise of "work therapy"); and for the right to challenge involuntary commitments for mental illness in court. The profession's diagnostic incompetence was regularly cited as a way to impeach psychiatrists' claims to expertise, with one law review article comparing the reliability of their testimony to "flipping coins."[62]

Pressures to amend this unsatisfactory situation were emerging from another quarter as well—from the ranks of the pharmaceutical houses that were anxious to expand the market for drugs for psychiatric disorders, which had proved enormously lucrative. Bringing new drugs to market required data from controlled clinical trials, and both these studies and attempts to segment the market (to find a use for new pills that failed to work universally but appeared to have some efficacy in a subset of cases) depended on being able to distinguish among mental patients in some reliable fashion. Without stable diagnoses, moreover, it was difficult, and often impossible, to replicate prior findings. And if the range of mental disturbances could be carved up, drug companies would have a whole series of targets to aim at when trying to demonstrate the value of new compounds, and psychiatrists would have some sort of rationale for the prescriptions they wrote. Looming in the background was the knowledge that a new version of the *International Classification of Diseases, ICD 9*, was being prepared under the auspices of the World Health Organization, prompting concerned bureaucrats at the American Psychiatric Association to worry about harmonizing American diagnostic practices with this document.[63] (As it turned out, the versions of the *DSM* from *DSM III* onward, with the power of the pharmaceutical industry behind them, became the hegemonic documents in most of the world.)

The move to create more reliable diagnoses was thus overdetermined. That did not mean that most psychoanalysts embraced it. Instead, they largely ignored the task force that the American Psychiatric Association assembled to address the issue. Only one of their number, John Frosch, joined the process, and, quickly marginalized, he stopped attending. The revamping of the diagnostic schema thus fell by default into the hands of biologically inclined psychiatrists, led by Robert Spitzer of Columbia University. The upshot, ratified after a brief struggle in which Spitzer and his allies comprehensively outmaneuvered the analysts, was a vastly expanded new edition of the *DSM*. Gone were all the speculative psychodynamic etiologies for the comparatively small number of mental disorders the first and second editions had recognized. Gone was the distinction between neuroses and psychoses, as well as such illnesses as "hysteria" that had hitherto formed the bread and butter of psychoanalytic practice. Protests from the analysts led to some minor modifications to the scheme (parenthetical references to alternative labels preferred by the Freudian fraternity were added), but these were purely tactical concessions to quiet the critics and were rapidly abandoned in subsequent editions of the manual. (Interestingly, the decision by mainstream psychiatry to abandon the word "hysteria" was not echoed elsewhere. The category persisted, for example, in psychometrics, with technologies like the Minnesota Multiphasic Personality Inventory maintaining references to it.)

Treatment of symptoms had been scorned by psychoanalysts as beside the point: symptoms were just the visible sign of the underlying disorders of the personality that needed attention. Treating them, they insisted, was like playing whack-a-mole so long as the underlying defects of personality were left untouched. Now, on the contrary, they became the very markers of disease, the key to deciding what ailed the patient one was confronting.

Unable to demonstrate convincing chains of causation for any major form of mental disorder, Spitzer and his team opted to abandon any pretense of doing so. Instead, they devised ways of maximizing inter-rater reliability, creating a tick-the-boxes approach to diagnosis that ensured that psychiatrists examining a particular case would agree on what was wrong. Facing a new patient, the practitioner would record the presence or absence of a given set of symptoms, and once a certain threshold had been reached (six out of ten symptoms in the case of schizophrenia), a diagnostic label was applied, with comorbidity invoked to explain cases where a patient qualified for more than one diagnosis.

Disputes about what belonged in the manual were resolved by committee vote, as was the arbitrary decision about where to situate cut-off points—that is, how many of a laundry list of symptoms a patient had to have before he or she was declared to be suffering from a particular form of psychiatric illness. Questions of validity were simply set to the side. If diagnoses could be rendered mechanical and predictable, consistent and replicable, that would suffice. Latent in this approach was the possibility, soon realized, of a vast increase in the range of conditions that could be redefined as pathology and thus brought within the ambit of psychiatric intervention.

Despite the obvious flaws that marked the enterprise from the outset, *DSM III* was a political and "technological" triumph. Its publication in 1980 marks the third and final shift in the orientation of psychiatry, and it is one that persists today, despite growing signs of strain.[64] The appearance of *DSM III* led to a conceptualization of mental illnesses, by the profession and public alike, as specific, identifiably different diseases, each amenable to treatment with different drugs. Despite the absence of any plausible claim to link the labels assigned in *DSM III* to physical phenomena, the artificially created stability of its categories was invoked to render them into "facts" about the world, features of nature itself, and to suggest that such stable categories must rest on biological foundations. Neo-Kraepelinian psychiatry, as this new approach soon labeled itself, was biologically reductionist, a point made forcibly when President George H. W. Bush proclaimed the 1990s "the decade of the brain."[65] With quite remarkable rapidity, psychoanalysis was cast aside, defenestrated from its privileged position in departments of psychiatry, where neuroscientists and psychopharmacologists replaced its acolytes.

The rapid triumph of the new approach was crucially aided, I suggest, by two major factors besides the fact that it provided a "solution" to a source of profound professional embarrassment. For one thing, it proved immensely attractive to the ends of the commercial insurance industry, providing stable guidelines to a new territory the industry was beginning to cover, the uncertain boundaries and therapeutic miasma of which had hitherto proved profoundly threatening. If the means for regularizing the diagnosis of mental illnesses could be linked to standardized patterns of treatment, then uncertainty could be replaced by predictability and finite limits to insurance coverage set, an important objective from the insurers' point of view. Very quickly, therefore, reimbursement for psychiatric care came to be tied to use of the *DSM*'s categories: no diagnosis, no payment. The *DSM* thus became a technology impossible to ignore and impossible not to validate, even if only by employing its categories. Moreover, as the manual passed through subsequent revisions, always expanding in size and in the range of conditions alleged to constitute medical conditions, another subtle shift occurred, one underlining the importance of the second factor that underlay the triumph of the neo-Kraepelinians. For where once the disease had led to the treatment, now the treatment led to the disease. If only a subset of patients responded to a particular form of treatment, why, they must be suffering from a separate kind of mental disorder, and thus new "illnesses" emerged, created in the marketing departments of Big Pharma.[66]

The other force behind the stabilization of the psychiatric profession around *DSM III* and its successors was the collection of intimate links that developed between specific diagnostic categories and specific forms of drug treatment. That patients (allegedly, and sometimes in reality) responded to particular classes of drugs was cited as "proof" that they suffered from a particular form of illness. And that the drugs had effects on the course of mental illness was simultaneously "proof" that mental illness was rooted in the brain. Why else would the pills work, if they were not manufacturing normal brains? After the fact, therefore, accounts were constructed about why particular classes of drugs worked: phenothiazines combated schizophrenia because they affected dopamine levels in the brain; Prozac and other selective serotonin reuptake inhibitors (SSRIs) relieved depression because they combatted a shortage of serotonin in the brain. These were scientific fairy tales and were swiftly discredited. But they were retailed to the public by professionals and science journalists alike so plausibly and repeatedly that many embraced the portrait of mental illnesses as biologically rooted events that were probably dependent on disturbances in brain biochemistry.

Furthermore, for the families of the mentally ill, who the psychoanalysts had implied bore primary responsibility for the disorders of their offspring (refrigerator mothers being particularly at fault), the neutral language of biology provided a welcome alternative. Newly formed pressure groups like NAMI (the National Alliance on Mental Illness) became fierce proponents of the new orthodoxy, their value recognized in very tangible form by the pharmaceutical industry, which provided them with large hidden financial subsidies. In 1999, for example, *Mother Jones* reported that eighteen drug companies had given NAMI a total of $11.72 million between 1996 and 1999. Eli Lilly, which had contributed $2.87 million during that period, gave $1.1 million in 1999 alone. In addition, it "loaned" NAMI one of its executives, Jerry Radke, to provide the group with advice on "strategic planning."[67] Eight years later, the *Wall Street Journal* indicated that Eli Lilly continued to fund NAMI to the tune of $544,500 in 2007 and that GlaxoSmithKline had given more than $12 million to similar groups in Europe.[68]

The assertion that psychoses represent forms of brain disease persists, though its evidentiary basis is weak and rests more on programmatic claims and plausible hunches than on demonstrable evidence. Baldessarini's conclusion from almost two decades ago still summarizes the basic state of play:

> Despite more than a century of searching, the idiopathic psychotic and major mood disorders lack a convincing and consistent neuropathology or coherent metabolic pathophysiology. . . . Evidence of excessive activity of dopamine as a neurotransmitter in psychotic or manic patients is highly inconsistent. . . . Although proposed actions of drugs effective in the treatment of major psychiatric disorders are obviously important pharmacologically, and although some predicted metabolic changes can be gleaned as additional *descriptors* of psychopathological states of psychiatric patients, proof that such findings or activities are primary or causal in psychotic or major affective disorders remains elusive. . . . It seems risky to construct hypotheses of the pathogenesis of psychiatric disorders based actions of drugs that affect relatively nonspecific central autonomic systems mediating arousal, activity, and homeostatic and alarm responses, because their clinical benefits may be relatively nonspecific and indirect.[69]

The tight linkages formed between the new version of psychiatric knowl-edge and the pharmaceutical industry reflected the mutually beneficial out-comes this provided for both professionals and industry. Psychoanalysts had a terrible track record of attracting large external funding. Less than 5 percent of the National Institute of Mental Health research budget came their way, even during the period of their hegemony. They were not trained as grantsmen, and they scorned the large-scale research enterprises that the federal bureaucrats preferred. But in the era of Big Science and Big Medicine, research universities became addicted to the flow of research funding—indeed their very existence depended on these vast new sources of money, from Washington and elsewhere. Psychoanalysts were already sus-pect for their emphasis on sex and talk. But academic psychiatrists with psychoanalytic inclinations were doubly marginalized in the knowledge fac-tories because they failed to bring in the coin of the realm: research dollars. By contrast, the new biologically oriented, pharmacologically entranced type of psychiatrists soon became the darlings of medical school deans, for they attracted large sums of grant money to underwrite their work. And those sums materialized because drugs for psychiatric conditions were among the most profitable products Big Pharma manufactured.

Prozac, the first of the blockbuster SSRIs, reached the American mar-ket for the first time in December 1987. In its first full year on the market, it had sales of $125 million, rising to $350 million in 1989—and this expo-nential growth pattern spread throughout the entire market for psycho-tropic medications. Between 1986 and 1991, world sales of these medica-tions rose from $2 billion to $4.4 billion. By 2001, three of the top ten drugs in the United States, by far the most lucrative drug market in the world, were SSRIs—Zoloft, Paxil, and Prozac. And sales continued to grow apace, though the "science" that underpinned their popularity was by now thoroughly discredited, the symptomatic relief they provided increasingly doubtful, and the side effects of taking such pills a source of growing concern. Yet the antidepressant market—largely a market for SSRIs—continued to boom, with sales rising from $5.1 billion in 1997 to $12.1 billion only five years later.[70]

More generally, the neo-Kraepelinian synthesis provided a new ground-ing for psychiatric authority and a less time-consuming and more lucrative foundation for psychiatric practice. It was far easier and more rewarding to spend five minutes prescribing pills than an hour providing psycho-therapy. The result has been a rapid abandonment of what had been the lynchpin of out-patient psychiatric practice and the ceding of that portion of the marketplace to the cheaper competition: clinical psychologists and psychiatric social workers. Psychiatric training has de-emphasized psy-chotherapeutics, and little remains of an earlier form of office-based psychiatric practice.[71] Though this has opened up a large space for the psychologists to colonize, they have done so under the shadow of the enor-mous influence of the *DSM*, whose categories they have been forced to embrace in order to get paid, though it is their competitors, the psychia-trists, who uniquely control this instrument. In parallel fashion, psychia-trists outside North America have also found themselves constrained to adopt the *DSM*'s ways of categorizing the patients they treat, such is its hegemonic power, not least because of the tight linkages between its cat-egories and the drugs the profession now depends on. For psychologists and clinical social workers, moreover, the links to pharmacology highlight still another concern: to the extent hoi polloi have come to embrace the notion that mental illnesses are ultimately biological phenomena—the product of faults in the brain, and more specifically faults in its biochemistry—they have also absorbed the lesson that the weapons of choice in battling the depredations of these diseases must accordingly be chemicals that purport to rectify such imbalances. Yet medics monopolize the power to prescribe such potions, which reveals yet another way in which psychologists subtly find themselves relegated to a second-class, subordinate status in the psy-complex.

Thus instead of living in an era of what Philip Rieff once called "the triumph of the therapeutic,"[72] we seem to be in an epoch in which wholly new values and forms of knowledge have come to the fore. In the after-math of the psychopharmacological revolution and the immense wealth it spawned, modern laboratory science has helped to hide the banality of the intellectual foundations on which this whole complex edifice rests, a set of political fudges and compromises hatched in committees and presented to the outside world as *wie die Dinge sind,* how things are. But that founda-tion is not just banal, it is a ramshackle Rube Goldberg apparatus, one threatened with collapse from two directions.

The drugs revolution has been vastly oversold. The problem is not only that antipsychotics and antidepressants are not psychiatric penicillin but also that the symptomatic relief that these drugs provide to some (very far from all) of those to whom they are prescribed often comes at a very heavy price indeed. It took psychiatry over two decades to acknowledge the iatrogenic price schizophrenics paid in return for whatever benefits flowed from taking phenothiazines like Thorazine (and for many psychotics, the "benefits" were wholly illusory).[73] And despite decades of research, attempts to ward off or treat such stigmatizing and distressing iatrogenic disorders as tardive dyskinesia and motor control problems have proved fruitless. That, plus the desire of drug companies to reap monopoly profits from a new generation of drugs, so-called atypical antipsychotics like Olanzapine, Risperdal, Clozaril, and Zyprexa, has prompted shifts in pre-scribing practices and some associated changes in the typical side effects patients experience toward heightened risks of metabolic disorders, rapid weight gain, diabetes, heart disease, and premature death (which is not to say that neurological complications disappear when the new drugs are substituted for first-generation drugs). As a recent commentary in *The Lancet* put it, "As a group they are no more efficacious, do not improve specific symptoms, have no clearly different side effect profiles than the first-generation anti-psychotics, and are less cost effective. The spurious invention of the atypicals can now be regarded as invention only, cleverly manipulated by the drug industry for marketing purposes and only now being exposed."[74]

Similarly, SSRIs like Prozac, initially hailed as making depressed patients "better than well," are now facing mounting questions about their efficacy and the range and seriousness of the side effects associated with their use. Their supposed mechanism of action has long been exploded (drugs that lower levels of serotonin in the brain have been shown to be as efficacious as those that raise it, for instance). And over the past two dec-ades, very serious questions have been raised about the "science" on which the approval of these drugs was based. Drug companies now "own" the data on clinical trials, and there is mounting evidence that they suppress the trials that produce results they don't like and manipulate the data that do see the light of day in disreputable fashion.[75]

Articles in major and minor peer-reviewed journals are often ghost-written by Big Pharma employees, while the names of major academics appear on the relevant papers.[76] Evidence-based medicine turns out to rest on evidence not worthy of the name. And once a drug has secured regulatory approval as useful for one type of illness, the pharmaceutical industry has directly and indirectly conspired to expand its markets by encouraging "off-label" uses—prescribing the drug as useful for other disorders when no solid scientific evidence exists that this is the case.[77] As class action lawsuits have led to the release of documents that demonstrate just how routine these practices have become,[78] and as some of the newly released data have shown that, perversely, so-called antidepressants may heighten the incidence of suicidal behavior, questions have arisen, not just about the rapacity of the industry but also about the ethics of a profession that has collaborated in these behaviors.[79]

The bulk of the published literature on antipsychotics and antidepressants is useless when it comes to assessing the risks of serious adverse effects associated with taking these drugs. The reason for this is quite simple: Randomized controlled trials are typically designed to measure whether a given drug can be shown to represent a therapeutic intervention that is superior to either a placebo or (more commonly) an existing treatment. What generally suffices here is a demonstration of a statistically significant (as opposed to clinically significant) advantage for the drug under study, since two such studies suffice to secure access to the marketplace. As we have just seen, even with this narrow barrier to surmount, there are good reasons to be skeptical about these sorts of results. But when it comes to assessing the side effect profile of antidepressants and antipsychotics, these studies suffer from other problems. The size of the patient groups studied and the short-term nature of the trials themselves mean that they are of relatively little use in assessing the prevalence and significance of adverse effects. Adverse effects emerge and intensify over time and are more likely when patients are prescribed more than one drug. Polypharmacy is common in clinical practice as psychiatrists search for a drug cocktail that will influence the course of a patient's serious mental disturbance,[80] and it is known to heighten the risk of adverse neurological, metabolic, and cardiac side effects, as well as sedation and sexual dysfunction.

Since psychoactive drugs are typically prescribed for long-term use, the dearth of careful studies of their long-term effects on health and well-being is itself a remarkable commentary on contemporary psychiatry. But long-term observational studies do exist, and a recent systematic review of the more reputable and well-conducted research of this sort conducted on patients receiving extended treatment with antipsychotics reached some sobering conclusions. "Adverse effects," the authors concluded, "are diverse and frequently experienced, but are not often systematically assessed." The profession's neglect of this situation is, in their words, "remarkable." The "findings confirm that the AE [adverse effects] of the newer antipsychotics are as worrying as the older equivalents for the patient's long-term physical health." There has been "a false dawn of therapeutic optimism," and the data on long-term side effects is the more concerning given what we know about "the premature mortality of those with serious mental disorder."[81]

If the links to psychopharmacology are now proving a double-edged sword, the construction of the nosological bible is also coming under increased criticism. The very arbitrariness of the foundations on which it was built put no obvious obstacles in the path of revising it, and pressures to do so come from many quarters. One significant sort of pressure will be familiar to students of psychiatric history: the tendency of the profession to widen the range of behaviors that fall within its ambit. Various forces drive this process. To cite just a few: demands from potential patients or their families who are seeking relief from problems and see medical labels as the route to resources (something that plagues those professionals who subsequently attempt to reign in diagnostic imperialism because that threatens to curtail resources flowing in particular directions); the attractions of expanding professional markets and perhaps, by including more marginal cases, finding more readily treatable patients; and the constant efforts by the drug industry to pathologize behaviors and expand demand for lucrative new products.[82]

Every few years, therefore, we have seen revisions to the *DSM*, each presented as "fixing" the flaws of the previous edition and incorporating new layers of understanding. The upshot is a manual that has expanded like the Yellow Pages of old on steroids, from the 104 pages of *DSM I* to the 992 pages of *DSM IV TR* (text revision). *DSM III*, published in 1980, became *DSM III R* (revised) in 1987, which in turn begat *DSM IV* in 1994, and *DSM IV TR* in 2000. Not only has the range and variety of "illnesses" one can potentially suffer from grown dramatically with each version, but the definitions of particular disorders have shifted dramatically over time, and often in ways that have produced soaring increases in the numbers of those "suffering" from a particular condition. Following changes to the definition of juvenile bipolar disorder in 1994, the number of patients with this diagnosis grew up to fortyfold in a decade.[83] After the definition of autism was revised in *DSM IV,* an autism epidemic broke out, and this previously rare condition, seen in only one in every five hundred children in 1994, was found in one in every ninety children only ten years later. Diagnoses of hyperactivity have similarly seen an explosive growth in numbers, and there has been an associated skyrocketing in the prescribing of drugs that purport to control it. One in every seventy-six adult Americans qualified for welfare payments based on mental disability in 2007. After a certain point, such data begin to strain credulity.

If psychiatrists' inability to agree among themselves on diagnoses threatened to make them a laughingstock in the 1970s, the relabeling of a host of ordinary life events as psychiatric pathology now seems to promise more of the same; oppositional defiant disorder, school phobia, and narcissistic and borderline personality disorder seem poised to be joined by such things as pathological gambling, binge eating disorder, hypersexuality disorder, temper dysregulation disorder, mixed anxiety depressive disorder, minor neurocognitive disorder, and attenuated psychotic symptoms disorder. That these diagnoses provide lucrative new markets for psychopharmacology's products raises questions in many minds about whether commercial ends are illegitimately driving the expansion of psychiatric means—a concern that is scarcely allayed when one recalls that the great majority of the members of the two most recent *DSM* Task Forces were recipients of drug company largesse.

Increasingly, the vast enterprise that is descriptive psychiatry seems to survive only by a thread. The frailty of the foundations of much that passes for the science and medicine of mind and brains has become ever more exposed, and the many professions involved confront, as they have in the past, profound questions about their legitimacy and future.

PART IV Neuroscience and the
Biological Turn

13 Trauma

David Morris served as an officer in the United States Marine Corps between 1994 and 1998, thus by luck rather than by choice escaping any involvement in combat. He describes his time in the armed forces as routine, boring even. Dividing his time between Camp Pendleton in Southern California and the United States military base in Okinawa, he spent four years playing war games and waiting. And waiting. By his own account, he was only a middling officer, and he left the service "feeling vaguely disappointed, incomplete, as if some secret in me had been left unrevealed."[1] No military adventures for him.

All that changed with the outbreak of the Second Iraq War. In graduate school when the 9/11 terrorists struck, Morris sensed an opportunity to experience what he had missed—this time as a war correspondent, not a soldier. He made several trips to Iraq to observe the fighting. One day in October 2007, he was out on patrol in a Humvee with a unit from the First Infantry Division in a Sunni neighborhood west of Baghdad. His presence on this occasion caused not a little resentment. One member of the platoon confronted him directly, wondering aloud what would prompt any sane person to put himself in harm's way like this. As a soldier, he spat, he had no choice. It was poverty, not love of country, that had prompted him to volunteer for service. The military was his only way out of a dead-end existence, and look where it had landed him. But though he could not help being stuck in this hellish environment, what the hell was wrong with Morris that he had *chosen* to come to Iraq? The young man obviously found such a decision completely unfathomable.

Soldiers are often a superstitious lot. Knowing that their lives could end at any moment or that they could end up badly wounded, maimed for life, men and women on active duty learn to ignore the obvious and to engage in various forms of magical thinking. It is an unspoken rule not to push one's luck by speaking of possible impending doom. So, when one of the other soldiers turned and casually asked Morris, "Have you ever been blown up before, sir?"[2] it was obvious what would soon happen, and it did. Following a Bradley tank into a burning neighborhood and finding the Humvee trapped in a pall of black smoke, the driver attempted to reverse and turn around. A hidden IED detonated under the vehicle.

The crippled Humvee, its right rear wheel all but destroyed, somehow limped back to base. By some miracle, all its occupants had survived, though the driver's eardrums had been blown out. A week later, Morris was back in California. A lucky man. But a damaged man, damaged in ways he did not yet comprehend. Greeted at LAX by his girlfriend, Erica, he set out to resume a "normal" civilian life. Postwar bliss beckoned. But not for long. Morris had nightmares. The two went to the cinema to see an action movie, replete with explosions. Morris blacked out, and when he came to he found himself outside the theater (he had run out in a panic but had no memory of doing so). He went back in and sat down next to Erica. Almost insupportable fears overwhelmed him at unexpected moments: when he encountered turbulence on a plane, or when he got three parking tickets in a week. His angry fits, which were frequent, were explosive and frightening. One day, Erica simply left. She had had enough. So had Morris, but his demons could not be so easily cast aside.

The autobiographical portions of *The Evil Hours* puts on display, in an often moving and revealing fashion, the author's own struggles with his mental disorder and his reactions to being treated by therapists at his local VA hospital (not ten minutes from where I live) like a clinical specimen to be dissected and remade rather than a suffering human being. But Morris has also read extensively about the history of military trauma and looked broadly at the medical literature on its etiology and treatment. He is a bit defensive at times about the whole exercise. He says, "I hate the idea of turning writing into therapy, and I did not conceive of this book as a therapeutic project"—though in the very next breath, he concedes that "delving into the history and literature of PTSD has, in fact, been extraordinarily useful."[3] And not just to him. One of the things that give the book its impact is precisely Morris's ability to place private troubles in a larger social, cultural, and historical context, and in this, he has done his homework well. The historical sections of this book have real bite.

The shell shock crisis of World War I provided for some the first inkling that modern industrialized warfare was not ideally suited to the maintenance of mental health among the troops. Within months of the start of the fighting, a military stalemate had ensued. Trapped in the Flanders mud, soldiers in trenches waited for death—from high-explosive shells, from flesh-tearing bayonets, from machine gun bullets, from poison gas. No army was spared the epidemic of nervous disorders that followed. By the thousands and tens of thousands, soldiers were struck dumb, lost their sight, became paralyzed or incapable of normal motion, wept, screamed uncontrollably, lost their memories, hallucinated, were rendered sleepless and incapable of fighting. As the very name shell shock suggests, many military psychiatrists initially thought, in keeping with the somatic theories that still were the ruling orthodoxy of their profession, that the disorder was the manifestation of real damage to the nervous system produced by blasts from high explosives. But such claims seemed increasingly implausible and even untenable. Soldiers who had not even reached the front lines became symptomatic. Those who were taken prisoners of war, and thus not exposed to the tensions of life in the trenches, never did. The military high command on both sides of the fighting saw in these findings evidence that the victims were simply cowardly malingerers, and some of the sadistic treatments meted out by physicians—electric currents applied to tongues and genitals, for instance—seem to have reflected a similar hostility on the part of therapists, or a simple determination to force these soldiers back into the fighting. But the preternatural tenacity with which shell shock victims clung to their symptoms made claims of simple malingering hard to sustain. The Germans adopted the label *Schreckneurose*, or terror neurosis. Trauma and psychological stress, it seemed, could cause even the apparently stable to break down and become maddened with fear, disgust, and horror.

Actually, had anyone been paying attention, the extraordinary bloodletting that marked the American Civil War had provided a preview of those early twentieth-century traumas and their impact. American neurology emerged as a specialism from the experience of treating men with brain injuries, lost limbs that gave rise to phantom pain, and damage to their central nervous systems. But the waiting rooms of the postwar nerve doctors were crowded with veterans whose wounds were of a less obvious, less visible sort. Morris tells us that at the war's end, 8 percent of the Union Army alone, some 175,000 men, were listed as suffering from "nostalgia" (usually a synonym for depression or panic), from a variety of nervous complaints, or from simple insanity. And the war's aftermath was marked by an upsurge in criminal violence, the racialized atrocities of the Ku Klux Klan, and genocidal campaigns against native American tribes, outcomes Morris suggests were not unconnected to the trauma of war: "Violence changes people in mysterious ways, and when normal human prohibitions against murder and cruelty are lifted on a wide scale, it unleashes violent impulses that are not easily controlled."[4]

World War II was, of course, the "good war," one fought by the greatest generation against the horrors of Hitler and Hirohito. As the nation entered the war, America's psychiatrists promised to screen out the mentally unfit, and they did so to the tune of rejecting nearly two million men from military service, but to no avail. After the war, America had more than fifty thousand mentally broken military men confined in veterans' hospitals, and another half million were receiving pensions in 1947 for psychiatric disabilities linked to their military service. They called it combat exhaustion or combat neurosis this time around, but just like the code of silence embraced by those who had endured the Great Depression and the stigma that wrapped its tentacles tightly around anything that smacked of mental illness, it was an epidemic endured largely in silence. These troubles would only acquire their current name and public visibility after still another war, this time the bad war and the defeat that was Vietnam.

Post-traumatic stress disorder, or PTSD, was the brainchild of a handful of disgruntled Vietnam veterans and two sympathetic psychiatrists, Robert J. Lifton and Chaim Shatan. (Nixon would have probably preferred it if the latter had dropped the *h.*) Meeting with members of the fledgling organization Vietnam Veterans against the War, Lifton and Shatan shared their feeling that the war was an abomination, a crime against humanity, and sympathized with these men's struggles to develop some insight into the mental turmoil that threatened to engulf them. The Pentagon was busy assuring America that the rate of psychiatric casualties in Vietnam was lower than in any previous war. The angry veterans knew better. Borrowing from the "consciousness-raising" meetings of the fledgling women's movement and the therapeutic communities found among recovering alcoholics and addicts, they and their psychiatric allies set up rap sessions and gradually began to speak of a "post-Vietnam syndrome," a concept Shatan introduced to the wider world via an op-ed piece in the *New York Times.* Veterans, he claimed, suffered from a variety of psychic ills: depression, emotional numbness, unpredictable episodes of anger and of terror, and a sense of disorientation and disaffection. In the face of fierce resistance from the US Department of Veterans Affairs (VA) and its staff doctors, these veterans stubbornly insisted on the reality of their suffering.

Typical of the era, the veterans' allies were psychoanalysts (Lifton held an appointment at Harvard; and Shatan, at Columbia). Psychoanalysis was a perspective on mental illness that had dominated American psychiatry from 1945 into the 1970s, but it was an approach that, unbeknownst to all sides, was about to be eclipsed and replaced by a resurgent biological reductionism and by a renewed emphasis on precise labels for psychiatric disorders (or at least labels that trained psychiatrists could reliably assign on command).

Morris astutely describes this revolution, which was inspired by the Columbia psychiatrist Robert Spitzer, whom the American Psychiatric Association (APA) had charged with devising an improved system of psychiatric classification, the result being the *DSM.* Spitzer had the passion of a true believer and political skills to match. He and his task force insisted that they were data-oriented persons and had little time or sympathy for what they saw as psychoanalytic nonsense. When Lifton and Shatan approached Spitzer to seek inclusion of "post-combat reaction" in the new manual, they were scornfully turned away. "You don't have any evidence. You don't have any figures. You don't have any research," Spitzer told them.

The biological psychiatrists who had Spitzer's ear were equally dismissive. Lee Robbins from Washington University in St. Louis was unsparing in his assessment: "These guys are all character disorders. They came from rotten backgrounds. They were going to be malcontents and dysfunctional anyway. . . . Vietnam is not the cause of their problems. They're alcoholics and drug addicts."[5] (Such ideas were also commonplace among many medical men seeking to explain shell shock in World War I. Drawing on then current psychiatric theory, they had dismissed such casualties as degenerates, whose preexisting mental frailties explained their symptoms.)

But Spitzer's claimed scientific objectivity was a pose, an ideological proclamation that was sharply at odds with how the *DSM* Task Force he led actually conducted its business and reached its conclusions. He had previously overseen the process by which homosexuality, long dismissed by psychiatrists as a form of mental illness, had been depathologized in the face of an overtly political campaign by the National Gay and Lesbian Taskforce. Pressured by what Morris characterizes as a relentless, almost military campaign, the APA voted to reverse itself and disavowed its earlier assertion that homosexuality was a mental disorder. Behind the scenes, Spitzer's task force routinely engaged in similar political decision-making, such as voting on how many of a long list of symptoms a patient had to have to be diagnosed as schizophrenic, and on what other psychiatric "illnesses" to recognize and under what names. By 1975, Shatan and his allies had cobbled together the "evidence" Spitzer had demanded, and the latter relented, though he insisted that their proposed "post-catastrophic stress disorder" be relabeled "post-traumatic stress disorder" and eliminated any reference to Vietnam. Once launched into the world, PTSD soon extended itself beyond the ranks of traumatized soldiers to include victims of such things as natural disasters and (a topic to which Morris directs only a limited amount of attention) the victims of sexual violence. And as war has become more of a technological exercise, with death and destruction visited on unsuspecting humans at the push of a button controlling an unmanned drone, it turns out that even those experiencing the trauma of war at a "safe" distance can succumb to the psychological effects of their work.

The publication of the third edition of the *DSM* in 1980 provided an official seal of approval for PTSD. It also marked the moment when the psychoanalytical dominance of the profession entered its death throes. Within less than a decade, analysts had been ejected from their positions at the head of university departments of psychiatry, and their institutes were scrambling for recruits, causing them to eventually abandon their long-held insistence that only medics could become analysts. Whether rightly or wrongly, mainstream psychiatry now saw Freud as a corpse. Biology was back with a vengeance, and the future appeared to belong to drugs and to neuroscience. If the proponents of the PTSD diagnosis, Lifton and Shatan, had been convinced that they were dealing with a psychological, not a biological, disorder, the newly reshaped discipline of psychiatry was no longer disposed to agree. "Accordingly," Morris notes, "the global research agenda for PTSD, heavily influenced by the budget priorities of the US Veterans Administration and the Department of Defense, has tended to favor exploring the neurological and biological foundations of PTSD rather than the psychoanalytic, cultural, and cross-cultural aspects of the condition."[6] Like a drunk looking for his lost watch under a lamppost, that is where much of the research effort has been expended, for that is where the money is, and thus academic medics build their careers not on politics or psychic conflict but on stress hormones and the chemical soup that bathes brain cells. Veterans have often been tempted to embrace this narrative, for, like comparable myths about the chemical origins of depression, it makes the disorder unambiguously "real" and medical, and perhaps thereby helps to diffuse the stigma so often attached to it. In the process, mere "subjective" experience is dismissed, and neuroscience is portrayed as the only rubric for understanding human experience. It would be a clinical culture with which the traumatized David Morris would become intimately familiar, not always to his advantage.

It is Morris's account of his encounter with the VA bureaucracy and his reactions to the therapies it doled out that I found most memorable. In keeping with the dominant approach to most forms of mental illness, PTSD has been the target of the magic bullets provided by modern psychopharmacology. But as with depression, bipolar disorder, and schizophrenia, those bullets, when shot at PTSD, turn out to be less than magical after all. With little or no systematic research to underpin their use, SSRIs (selective serotonin reuptake inhibitors) like Zoloft, Paxil, and

Prozac began to be prescribed for PTSD patients. The first systematic studies claiming that these drugs provided a measure of symptomatic relief for sufferers from the condition weren't published until 2002, and they were judged sufficient by the Food and Drug Administration to license this class of drugs for the treatment of PTSD, an approach officially endorsed by the APA two years later. In reality, however, the data never provided solid support for their use on the affected veterans, and in 2008, the prestigious Institute of Medicine reached that conclusion. The organization released a report "that officially recognized what many researchers already knew: there was no evidence that any drug actually treated PTSD across the board, SSRIs included."[7] At best, the VA now concluded, existing drugs played a role as an adjunctive therapy. They were not the gold standard of treatment they had once been held to be. Still, the fact that they were being prescribed to patients with PTSD had other consequences in the scientific community: a lack of interest in listening to survivors' stories, "experiences that are difficult to listen to and do not easily lend themselves to scientific measurement"; and a disposition to treat "brain-imaging technologies . . . not . . . as useful instruments in the larger toolkit but as actual windows into the mind"—a transparently delusional belief.[8]

If drugs are no more than palliative much of the time (though Morris does suggest that "in many cases Zoloft and other similar drugs have been one of the only things that have kept some trauma survivors from killing themselves"[9]), the attempt to provide a biological account of PTSD has likewise run into the sand. Morris's traipse through the literature and his own encounters with leading PTSD researchers have convinced him of "the utter lack of a coherent neurobiological model" of the disorder: "PTSD remains a cultural and existential problem, a condition with no cure and little biological grounding." It is a situation he finds profoundly frustrating and disheartening.

If not drugs, then what? Certainly not psychoanalysis. In its place, the VA turned to forms of psychotherapy that purported to be grounded in science and in the authority of controlled laboratory trials. Morris was never assigned to a period of drug therapy, though he came close on a couple of occasions and, on his own account, self-medicated with alcohol. Perhaps that explains his (uncharacteristic) willingness to accept professional assurances that Prozac and its ilk are safe and largely free of side effects. Instead, Morris was assigned to some of the "tried and true" forms of psychotherapy.

Trips to the La Jolla VA Hospital became like traveling to "a morbid version of Disneyland." Bright-eyed and bushy-tailed young researchers arrived with clipboards to conduct intake interviews and see whether Morris qualified for the particular variant of psychotherapy their bosses were studying. There were twenty studies running at the time, and Morris learned that volunteering for one of them was the quickest way to circumvent the interminable waiting that the system uses to ration veterans' care. Mark, a young technician, arrived to supervise Morris's induction into this new world. He informed Morris that his boss, the author of the study, was a rock star, with "a résumé that is thirty-six pages long"! How fortunate Morris was to be selected to take part in an investigation into a marvelous new therapy, prolonged exposure (PE), which "works in about 85 percent of people."[10] (Talk about creating a placebo effect.)

Mark passed him on to Sarah, who had a thick binder to go through to make sure he was eligible for the study. A lengthy series of questions were posed, to be rated on a four-point scale. The whole traumatic experience of Iraq, lasting many months, was supposed to be boiled down into one or two incidents, and those incidents reduced to numbers on a simple scale. But Morris couldn't conform to this twisted logic. He recalled more than the requested one or two traumas. Sarah stared into space, ignored his wanderings, and waited until she could reinsert him into the Procrustean bed she had prepared for him. "When I looked back at her," Morris recalled, "her face was blank, as if she had been waiting for me to finish. Her pencil, I noticed, was not moving."[11] Drug pushers, it turns out, are not the only psychiatric technicians who stop listening.

A week later, Morris got bad news. He had reported at one point that he had occasionally had more than three drinks in a day. That disqualified him from the study. Not to worry, said the cheery Mark, there were plenty of other promising studies to which they could assign him. Unfortunately, however, he would have to go through the mechanical rating process to get into them, and he must not forget to mention his drinking, for these studies needed veterans who drank. So he was eventually assigned to sessions with a trainee clinical psychologist, a nice and enthusiastic young man who, like his counterparts whom Morris would later encounter, seemed blissfully ignorant and illiterate about the War on Terror.

Those who pay even a modicum of attention to the news will be aware that a certain amount of fuss has arisen about the side effects of psycho-pharmacological substances, such as the tardive dyskinesia and the diabetes that so often accompany the administration of antipsychotics; and the impotence and the heightened suicidal ideation that can affect users of SSRIs. But as Morris was about to discover, drugs are not the only psychiatric treatments with side effects. His encounter with a revised version of PE left him shaken and shaking. The idea was to flood him with memories like the ones that had traumatized him, albeit in the safety of the therapist's office, and thus over time desensitize him, wean him from the trauma-induced bad behaviors and transform the original horrors into something like fiction. There was to be no deviation from the script. Ninety minutes each week of recalling the same terror. No wandering off point. No elaboration or free association. Repeat, repeat. "A therapy, in other words, whose results were designed by researchers for researchers, a therapy designed to be touted by medical administrators as being 'efficacious' and scientifically tested."[12] Punitive. Excruciating. It made Morris steadily worse, until one afternoon he turned violent, fortunately within the confines of his apartment, smashing his furniture, stabbing his cell phone, raging, and screaming until his neighbors contemplated calling the police. Morris must have been one of the 15 percent not cured by this therapeutic magic. Or perhaps the statistics were as bogus as those promulgated by Big Pharma about their magic potions. Perhaps, after all, subjecting deeply traumatized people to more trauma might not be the best idea. Perhaps a treatment designed originally for simple phobias was a poor match for people who had gone through psychic hell.

In 2008, an Israeli study of army veterans suffering PTSD in the aftermath of the intifada reported an increase in the extent and severity of their psychotic symptoms post flooding. Undeterred, the VA ploughed ahead with its new "gold standard." Clinicians and patients protested, one of the former calling the use of the therapy "unconscionable." Morris interviewed a rape victim who had also been given the treatment. "Flooding. That's about right," she told him. "I am once again flooded by fear and paranoia."[13] Such reports were dismissed by the bureaucrats as mere anecdotes, carrying no weight compared to their quantified, statistically significant measures. Here, their bosses assured them, was an efficient, assembly-line therapy that was cheap and easily mass-produced. It only required that they follow the prescribed protocol, and there was a very limited place for initiative on the part of the therapist. Small wonder that those conducting the treatment tuned out the discordant voices.

Morris had had enough. He became what the VA called a "non-compliant patient." He explained to the polite young therapist, through clenched teeth, that urging him to continue with a therapy that was making him violent was "completely insane." What is it, he wondered, about PTSD "that makes such sadistic methods seem reasonable"?

But the VA was not done with him yet, nor was he done with the VA. He felt immediately better after quitting PE, and he continued to improve for a few weeks. But he was far from cured. He approached the hospital to learn about other options and was referred to the other "gold standard therapy," cognitive processing therapy, or CPT, a group treatment designed to teach patients how to avoid extreme thoughts. CPT has no interest in the past and, once again, is intentionally designed to minimize the role of the individual therapist (it is a mass therapy after all). Undergirding the therapy is the belief that patients haunted by murdered memories (and memories of murder) must find ways to forget. It's a matter of ABCs. Morris was told by his sweet young therapist to write a list of things that bothered him:

A. The government lies.
B. People in power are liars and their lies killed friends of mine.
C. I feel sick and helpless about it.

To this, the naive therapist replied, innocently, and like most of us who know nothing of the war in question would, "Shouldn't you investigate whether your second belief is 100 percent realistic?"[14]

Yes, Morris concludes, it is. Bush, Cheney, and their ilk escaped all accountability for their crimes. They lied to justify the war. Their minions covered up friendly fire incidents. They sent far too few troops to pacify Iraq once it had been conquered. They overruled the judgments of their commanders. They insisted the Sunni insurgency was in its last throes even as conditions steadily worsened. They boasted that the surge they had devised to pull the fat out of the fire was working, and that Iraqi troops were well on their way to assuming responsibility for maintaining order, when in fact the Iraqi troops the augmented American forces had trained crumbled and collapsed at the first hint of opposition. They ordered and condoned torture. They presided over and excused the stain that was Abu Ghraib. And what price had they paid for all the death and destruction they had wrought? Morris decided that his disgust was warranted, and he reminds us that Siegfried Sassoon, a fantastically brave World War I officer who was known as "Mad Jack" for his exploits, had voiced a similar contempt at the conclusion of World War I: "In the name of civilization these soldiers had been martyred, and it remained for civilization to prove that their martyrdom wasn't a dirty swindle"[15]—an urgent necessity that didn't disappear because a dirty swindle was the least of it.

In the end, the CPT helped Morris a bit. It gave him a method that on occasion allowed him to cope with his symptoms. But fundamentally it was a superficial Band-Aid; it didn't salve his inner wounds. "Never was I invited to think of how my experiences might be converted into a kind of wisdom or moral insight," he writes. "When I did so on my own initiative, I was admonished for 'intellectualizing' and for straying from the strictures of the therapeutic regime."[16]

One of the things that may shock readers of *The Evil Hours* are passages where Morris recounts the attitudes some of the soldiers with whom he was embedded had toward the country they were allegedly sent to defend. Take the views held by one member of the platoon in the Humvee even before they were all blown up. The Reaper, as Morris nicknamed him, had been posted to Iraq for what felt like an eternity, thirteen months straight. His disaffection with his fellow countrymen was palpable: "I'm serious, sir, I can't stand Americans."[17] It was a sentiment Morris came to share. The willful ignorance of his fellow citizens angered him. Their careless lack of attention to the horrors experienced and inflicted in their name "was an obscenity surpassed only by the obscenity of the war itself. . . . Coming home and feeling the dullness of the people, the pride they took in their ignorance. . . . How could this be allowed to happen? In time, I resolved to hate the country I had once served: the fat, sheltered land with its surplus of riches, its helicopter moms and real estate agents—narrow-minded, smug, and only dimly aware of any lives other than their own."[18]

At the very end of the book, Morris returns to this theme. Years after leaving Iraq, he came across a poem by Siegfried Sassoon. Sassoon was diagnosed with shell shock shortly after he had denounced the war as a serving officer on active duty. He was treated in a mental hospital he called Dottyville, and he then returned to fight, unable to abandon his men to their fate. He fought still more recklessly than before but somehow survived.

Sassoon remained a fierce critic of the venal politicians and the con- scienceless generals who had sent his whole generation to die in the mud and the muck of the trenches. He had a visceral contempt, too, for the blimpish civilians who prattled emptily about the glories of war and turned on anyone who "shirked their duty"—not to mention for the yellow journalists who had hyped up nationalist feelings and sanitized the slaughter. The hero had grown to loathe them all. In "Fight to a Finish," he indulges in a fantasy in which he and his men wreak their revenge.

In the poem, the soldiers are invited to take part in a victory march down Whitehall in London. The streets are lined with the smug, safe jour- nalists who had exploited the courage of the troops and helped send the soldiers' mates to their deaths, building their own journalistic fortunes in the process (*plus ça change . . .*). Suddenly, one group of soldiers, bayonets fixed, breaks ranks and rushes the journalists, who scream like pigs as they are stabbed to death. In the meantime, Sassoon and his men peel off and charge into Parliament, grenades at the ready. The politicians who launched the war are about to have its realities brought home to them, if only for the few, terror-filled seconds before they meet their fate.

"Fight to a Finish" is a brutal and sadistic poem, but one whose emo- tions Morris acknowledges that he completely understands: "I recognized the anger, the feelings beneath it, feelings so potent you never spoke of them, even to friends. Even to lovers. Even to yourself most of the time."[19] One wonders how many young soldiers feel like this on their return from combat?

It is a disturbing thought. Perhaps it ought to give those of us fortunate to have been spared the traumas of the battlefield nightmares of our own. What other horrors may we yet prove to have wrought?

14 Empathy

The images seem so seductive. Reproduced in vivid Technicolor, they show our brains in action, different regions lighting up as our thoughts and emotions fluctuate. Here's an angry brain. There's one bent on seduction. And compare these two: the brain of someone blessed with a strong empathy instinct and a psychopathic brain, whose empathy circuits remain dark and unilluminated even when confronted with sights one might assume would melt the coldest of hearts. What wonders modern functional magnetic resonance imaging (fMRI) can reveal. Why, we can watch in real time as someone's brain morphs from one state to another. Our Victorian forebears were entranced by the old pseudoscience of phrenology, which extrapolated from the external lumps and bumps of the skull to reveal the character that lay beneath: benevolent or miserly; loving or hostile; irascible or placid. But now we have real science at our disposal. The advances of modern imaging technology mean that we no longer have to guess what the brain is up to. Look! Our innermost thoughts and character can be put on display, and these scans lay bare who has lots of empathy and who has none, who lies and who is a truth-teller, whom we should trust and welcome as a friend, and whom we should shy away from. Thanks to modern neuroscience, claims British television executive

Peter Bazalgette in his book *The Empathy Instinct: How to Create a More Civil Society* (2017), we can begin to piece together, for example, how we might "improve our society by harnessing the extraordinary positive force of empathy."[1] Since "neuroscientists, psychologists and geneticists now know which parts of the brain are specifically linked to empathy and compassion," we should be "considering how we can enhance these abilities. . . . The empathy instinct is an idea whose time has come."[2]

Harnessing this new technology, Bazalgette tells us, would allow us to create a more civil society. That may seem an odd sort of promise for someone who did so much to debase popular taste through his role in developing modern "reality" television, but when all is said and done, prodigal sons are always welcome. Bazalgette assures us we can work with the "profound insights into the human mind" that "the mapping of our emotions using functional brain imaging" has made possible, and all sorts of improvements will then follow. His particular hero is the Cambridge academic Simon Baron-Cohen, whose pioneering work he repeatedly draws on and praises.

What exactly is it that the fMRI scans show us about the brain? Crudely, and with a lag, they measure blood flow in the brain and thus can trace levels of activity in particular regions of the brain in limited but potentially scientifically interesting ways. The digital data that fMRI machines produce can, through careful manipulation, be transformed into pictures, and those images can be produced or manipulated to appear in color so as to highlight patterns to which we wish to draw attention.

Few will be surprised to learn that our thoughts and feelings are associated with physical changes in our brains. Note well, however, that the observed patterns differ from individual to individual, and from experimenter to experimenter. Moreover, statistical averages derived from the gross changes in brain function in large experimental groups—themselves derived from simple simulated experiments that in no way capture the intricacies of everyday social situations—present enormous difficulties when we attempt to interpret them at the level of the individual subject. Correlations of this sort, even if they were more robust and replicable than many of them appear to be, prove nothing about the causal processes involved, and more seriously still, we possess no way to translate "heightened activity" into the contents of people's thoughts. And we have no prospect of making such translations. As if these problems are not serious enough, it is wrong to think that empathy (or other forms of thinking, feeling, and remembering, come to that) is localized in particular regions of the brain or is the property of individual neurons. On the contrary, it is the product of complex networks and interconnections that form in the brain as we mature. Functional MRI images don't allow us to "see" an "empathy instinct" (or a property instinct, a justice instinct, or a democratic instinct—all of which have purportedly been discovered by some of the neuroscience crowd). These are problems to which I will return shortly.

Let us pretend for a moment, though, that we can accept Bazalgette's claims about the digital mapping of the empathy instinct. He then invites us to consider how differently the history of the twentieth century might have been if only this new knowledge had arrived a few decades sooner. Hitler, Stalin, and Mao liquidated a hundred million of our fellow human beings. "Had we the benefit of today's diagnostic tools, chiefly MRI scanners," Bazalgette suggests, "we might have seen some serious abnormalities in the three dictators' brain functions."[3] (Or not, as the case may be.)

Just how the existence of these images might have prevented the horrors of mass exterminations is left wholly unclear. The difficulty deepens when Bazalgette goes on to acknowledge the mass involvement of Germans in the killing of Jews, and of Turks in the massacre of Armenians. According to the account he offers in the remainder of his book, we all possess an empathy instinct to a greater or lesser degree, and it is this "instinct" that underlies our ability to counter "religious conflict and racism, [to fight for] decent health and social care, effective and humane criminal justice," and human rights more generally.[4] Like Hitler, Stalin, and Mao, all those Germans and Turks must have misplaced their empathy instinct temporarily, allowing a civilized society to behave collectively in such a barbarous fashion. Unblushingly, this is basically the intellectual move Bazalgette promptly makes: Why did these "terrible events" occur? "Whole communities switched off their empathy to do cruel things to their fellow citizens."[5] So here we have an "explanation"—an "instinct"—that can conveniently be invoked in an ad hoc and frivolous fashion to explain whatever one observes, because whenever the evidence contradicts what the instinct theory would lead one to suggest, why, the people in question must have just switched off their empathy. QED. Or not.

Where does this empathy instinct come from? From our genes, Bazalgette suggests. It is a quality we inherit (in varying quantities, to be sure). Simon Baron-Cohen is again invoked as the authority here. Those with "borderline personality disorder," the Cambridge professor informs us, make up perhaps 30 percent of suicides and half of the people who are addicted to drugs. The provenance of these statistics is, to put it charitably, murky in the extreme. Baron-Cohen then adds an even more far-fetched estimate that this condition is 70 per cent heritable and 30 per cent the result of abuse and neglect in childhood.[6] It is reassuring to know that the nature versus nurture debate, at least in this instance, has been so decisively solved—except that the "solution" relies on bluster, bad science, and speculation rather than evidence. Whether one is trying to explain schizophrenia, depression, homosexuality, or (as in this case) empathy, claims to have discovered genes that give rise to and shape complex human behaviors have evaporated when put to the test.

And why do we possess an empathy gene? Because of our evolutionary history, of course. Here, Bazalgette retells the fairy stories evolutionary psychologists have constructed to explain why various social and cultural constructs have arisen and persist. We have been here many times before. Victorian brain scientists, for example, invoked "the facts of physiology" to explain that the existing gendered social and moral order was rooted in the inescapable realities of the natural world. Males and females had evolved differently. There were male brains and female brains, and the sorting of roles and activities along gendered lines neatly corresponded to underlying biological differences. The biology of women made them empathetic, nurturing creatures, suited primarily to serve as wives and mothers. Men were the strong, rational risk-takers.

We are inclined to laugh these days at such transparently self-serving attempts to justify male privilege and the exclusion of women from higher education and the public sphere by invoking the ineluctable realities of biological "science." The contention that allowing women to get a university education, enter the professions, and compete alongside men would invite "race suicide" is treated with the scorn it deserves, refuted by over a century of progress toward the emancipation of the "second sex." But here they are trotted out again in the guise of modern neuroscience. As Professor Baron-Cohen would have it (and he is echoed by his slavish disciple Peter Bazalgette), there are male and female brains. Female brains have evolved to be better at empathizing and communicating and are hardwired for empathy. Male brains are more suited to rational under-standing and system-building—from making machines and writing soft-ware to engaging in abstract thought, writing music, playing at politics, or theorizing about the fundamental foundations of physics.[7] As Yogi Berra would say, it's déjà vu all over again.

Bazalgette's worship of Baron-Cohen is scarcely surprising, since empa-thy and its absence have long been a source of fascination for the Cambridge neuroscientist. One of Baron-Cohen's more extended forays into this territory was published nearly a decade ago. In *Zero Degrees of Empathy: A New Theory of Human Cruelty* (2011), he seeks to give an explanation of the human capacity for cruelty and to provide a neurosci-entific account of those who appeared to lack this crucial human capacity. He begins to tackle this important question by recounting some familiar and highly distressing images of the sorts of evil human beings have proved themselves capable of engaging in.

We are invited to contemplate the case of Josef Fritzl, the Austrian who confined his daughter in the cellar of his house for twenty-four years, repeatedly raping her and fathering seven children in the process, three of them left to share their mother's confinement. On a broader scale, he reminds us of the Armenian Genocide of 1915 at the hands of the Turks, who to this day deny the overwhelming evidence of what occurred. Or we might consider a case in which rebel Ugandan soldiers arrived at the vil-lage of Pajong in 2002, proceeded to kick one two-year-old to death, and then, on the orders of their female commander, who had presumably enjoyed the spectacle, forced all the mothers present to pick up their chil-dren and smash them against veranda poles, beating the women if they failed to batter their children to death fast enough. Even if we confined ourselves to the horrors of the past century, most of us could readily expand on this catalogue of horrors.

What are we to make of all this? How are we to account for the barba-rism, the ability of some of us to commit the most appalling sorts of cru-elty? As a neuroscientist, Baron-Cohen is disposed to seek the answer by examining people's brains. Differences in the way we are wired, he claims, underpin our differential propensity to engage in these behaviors. We need, he suggests, to abandon "the unscientific term 'evil'" as an explanatory move. (I had thought that "evil" was intended as a moral description of such actions, not an explanation of them, but let that pass for the moment.) Baron-Cohen urges us to substitute "the scientific term 'empathy.'"[8] Some people behave horribly, he argues, because they lack empathy and hence have no compunction about treating other human beings as objects. And empathy can be measured by means of questionnaires and visualized in the brain via the use of fMRI. Using this relatively novel technology, we can map what he calls "empathy circuits" in the brain.[9]

Cruel people, it turns out, suffer from "empathy erosion."[10] The relevant circuits in their brains fail to light up, or glow only dimly, when they are subjected to experiments designed to elicit empathy while the cruel folk are confined in an fMRI machine. And the deficits they display correspond to low scores on questionnaires that Baron-Cohen and his team devised to assign an "Empathy Quotient," or EQ. Readers are invited to score themselves on this "scientific measurement device," which is reprinted in an appendix.[11] (There is even a modified test you can use to discover your child's score.) Do you hog conversations? Are you bothered by being late to meet a friend? Are you upset when you see people cry? Answering forty questions of this sort will give you an EQ, and we are informed that scores for the population at large approximate a normal distribution, with small numbers of people possessing either zero degrees of empathy or extraordinarily high levels of empathy, dubbed level six, and most of the rest of us falling somewhere in between. (Baron-Cohen is insistent that there are six degrees of empathy—seven really, counting the zeros—but never gets around to telling us how he arrived at that number rather than, say, four, eight, or ten.)

Those at the bottom end of the curve, the zeros, are, he claims, the source of trouble in the world. There are, he suggests, three types of zeros: zero-negative type B, zero-negative type P, and zero-negative type N—or, if you prefer, borderlines, psychopaths, and narcissists. And then there are the zero-positives—the rigidly rule-bound, socially inept sorts who often display brilliance across a limited spectrum of skills and find themselves labeled more conventionally as people with Asperger's syndrome or autism spectrum disorder. The zero-positives are super-moral, not amoral. But the zero-negatives are in varying ways highly dangerous individuals, and these differences are rooted in their biology. These variations in their "empathy circuits" are largely fixed, immutable features of their brains: their ventromedial frontal cortex and their orbitofrontal cortex are under-active, while their ventral striatum and their amygdala are overactive, and problems lurk elsewhere as well.

But how do we explain the occasional cruelties of the rest of us, our lapses into schadenfreude, our selfishness? Why, Baron-Cohen tells us, those things happen when our empathy circuit has been temporarily turned off. And how do we know that's what's going on? Why, because we temporarily treated another human being as an object. QED.

Next, Baron-Cohen asks: Why do people with zero degrees of empathy exist? Why are some type B, others type P, and still others type N? And why are there people at level 1, level 4, or level 6 (Desmond Tutu, he suggests, is one such person)? Perhaps because of their genetics. (Baron-Cohen assures us that "there are *genes for empathy*.")[12] Perhaps because of their upbring-ing. Or perhaps because of other aspects of their environment. Children raised without love, for example, are emotionally scarred; they don't have what Baron-Cohen dubs the "*internal pot of gold*" that those raised in "nor-mal" families get and can make use of when life gets tough.[13] Their brains, which continue to evolve in early childhood, have developed in dysfunc-tional ways. Baron-Cohen is happy to draw on any and all of these ad hoc factors to account for the actions of his deviant subjects, depending on which can plausibly be invoked in a given case. Decent folk, on the other hand, are the way they are because they have decent brains—that is, ones with a reasonable amount of empathy. They have been lucky in the genetic lottery, or in their choice of parents. For, as neuroscience has now shown, "which band we are in is broadly fixed."[14]

It would appear, then, that once we accept the alleged findings of neu-roscience, the problem of evil vanishes, or gets put into its proper scien-tific context: "Back to the key question behind this book. Does Zero Negative explain human cruelty? . . . Not all the data are yet in to answer this question, but the claim is exactly this. . . . We can assume that what-ever the nature of the act (be it physical unempathetic acts—physical vio-lence, murder, torture, rape, committing genocide, etc.—or non-physical unempathetic acts—deception, mockery, verbal abuse, etc.), at the very moment of the act, the empathy circuit 'goes down.'"[15] Notice the elision of moral failings of vastly different sorts; notice that the "empathy circuit" allegedly displays the same patterns when people commit war crimes or other heinous forms of cruelty as when they snub someone else or treat them with disdain or insufficient consideration. These all may represent lapses from ideal ways of behaving (though some people, and some arguments, I would contend, merit disdain).

A set of "findings" about the brain that lumps together such wildly discrepant actions and yet claims to provide a new account of the origins of evil ought not, I suggest, to carry much weight. But this is just one of many problems with Baron-Cohen's argument.

Take, for example, the instrument used to assign an EQ to individual subjects. Responses to a self-report questionnaire of the sort that regularly appears in pop psychology magazines and potboiler self-help guides might not seem a terribly reliable way of getting at fundamental human traits. To this line of criticism, Baron-Cohen has two forms of defense. First, he argues that "worries about whether some people might not fill out their EQ accurately are probably unimportant because when you have large samples of data, occasional inaccuracies are cancelled out."[16] But why should the "inaccuracies" be occasional or random? Psychopaths and narcissists can readily work out the "preferred" answers to such a test and, by definition, have no scruples about gaming it. Baron-Cohen then falls back on the results of brain scans. Even some of those psychopaths who have killed without remorse have been persuaded to climb into an fMRI scanner, and as a result, he asserts, we now understand "the neural basis of empathy and of its absence."[17]

Throughout *Zero Degrees of Empathy*, there are claims that we have the ability to peer into the brain, to see what is happening in various regions of the brain, to make a connection, through the miracles of fMRI technology, between brain and behavior. This is, let me be blunt, nonsense. Despite important advances in neuroscience, we are very far indeed from being able to connect even very simple human actions to the underlying structure and functioning of people's brains. We are decades away from successfully mapping the brain of the fruit fly, let alone successfully tackling the infinitely more complex task of unraveling the billions on billions of connections that make up our own brains. For all the talk of an "empathizing mechanism," nothing of the sort has been demonstrated.

Magnetic resonance imaging is a remarkable scientific advance. It has allowed us to penetrate solid tissue and to generate extraordinary images of the human body, and these have proved to be of enormous clinical use in medicine, not least because they can be obtained without the use of damaging ionizing radiation. Functional MRIs, developed in the early 1990s, give us the ability to measure variations in blood flow in the brain, which to some degree are correlated with increases in neural activity. How this is accomplished remains a mystery to noninitiates, the very people to whom Baron-Cohen's book is addressed. It's all a bit of modern scientific magic, and if the scientists assure us that they are measuring the passage of thoughts and emotions in the brain, there is a strong temptation to believe them. Hence the rise of fMRIs has coincided with a greatly enhanced estimate of the capacities of neuroscientists and a spread in popular culture of reductionist accounts of human behavior supposedly rooted in hard scientific findings, like those advanced by Peter Bazalgette.

But much of this faith is misplaced. Correlation is not cause, so finding (rather crude) patterns of activity in the brain is far from demonstrating how we think—not to mention that the same regions of the brain "light up" under very different circumstances. Human brains are interconnected to an almost unfathomable degree, and complex human actions are infinitely removed from the simple stimuli presented in Baron-Cohen's work and other laboratory experiments, which by their very nature cannot capture how our brains function under these circumstances. Moreover, it is unclear whether the extremely indirect and temporally compromised signals that are used to construct fMRI images provide more than the most simplistic look at what is taking place. Since millions of neurons must be active to register on the scan, for example, much is necessarily not being recorded by the instrument. And so on, and so on.

It should therefore come as no surprise that although Baron-Cohen speaks on crucial occasions as if his claims rested on solid and indisputable scientific findings, elsewhere the attentive reader will detect a rather different tone. "There is some evidence that fits the idea" is accompanied by a plethora of "is consistent withs," "mays," and "perhapses." "These steps are still to be clarified" marches hand in hand with the belated acknowledgement that "it is a big jump from finding genes to understanding how their functions have an impact on empathy."[18] Yet such apparent concessions are immediately countered by the truculent insistence that "a start is a start."[19] But is it? What if it is a false start?

The difficulty, as always, is the vast gap between the simple simulated experiments using fMRI machines and crude stimuli (such as pictures of someone being pricked with a pin) and the world of soldiers committing heinous war crimes, of Josef Mengele conducting "experiments" on children in concentration camps, and of Turks disposing of more than a million Armenians. We are quite incapable of translating heightened activity in certain regions of the brain into the contents of people's thoughts, let alone their behaviors. Even framing things in this fashion is to assume, of course, something potentially of greater significance still, something that Baron-Cohen never bothers to argue for: that our thoughts are the simple product of neural activity in the brain. Might it not be the other way around? What scientific finding, rather than a priori metaphysical assumption, allows us to conclude that human decision-making is a mechanical process, wholly determined by previous mechanical processes? And were we indeed to be mechanical inhabitants of such a universe, why would someone like Baron-Cohen attempt to influence us by rational argument? Surely such an enterprise would be intellectually incoherent, not to mention redundant.

Baron-Cohen ends his brief book with a paean to empathy, that "universal solvent": "Each drop of empathy," he solemnly assures us, "waters the flower of peace."[20] One way to view these final passages is as an extended riff on a variant of the Beatles' bathetic claim that "all you need is love." Israel and the Palestinians, Baron-Cohen reminds us, presumably to cement his case, have been at war for more than six decades: "Remarkably, just one day after the State of Israel was founded in 1948, it was invaded by its Arab neighbours. Why?" (There are, of course, some rather obvious rejoinders.) "Whatever the original cause, the result has been sixty years of Palestinian bombers and Israeli tanks in a cycle of tit-for-tat attacks, leading to ever more human suffering."[21] All together now: "All you need is . . . empathy." That'll fix things.

Luckily enough, "empathy is free. And, unlike religion, empathy cannot, by definition, oppress anyone."[22] No more zeros, please. And no more evil either. With apologies to the late John Lennon and, (in a very different way,) to those whose taste in political analysis extends beyond such empty platitudes: imagine.

Both Simon Baron-Cohen and his disciple Peter Bazalgette assume that empathy is a "good thing." Indeed, the dust jacket of Bazalgette's book is adorned with a quotation from Barack Obama that has rapidly become a cliché: "If we are going to meet the moral test of our times, then I think we are going to have to talk more about The Empathy Deficit. The ability to put ourselves in somebody else's shoes, to see the world through somebody else's eyes." It is a shibboleth the Yale psychologist and neuroscientist Paul Bloom aims to bury. In *Against Empathy: The Case for Rational Compassion* (2016), he seeks to persuade us that empathy is something that can lead us down some very dubious moral pathways and is not to be trusted as a guide for how to conduct ourselves.

It is at first blush an arresting intellectual move, one guaranteed to stir up controversy and (Bloom surely hopes) sell his book. Lest this seem a trifle cynical on my part, note that Bloom jabs at Stephen Asma for the title of *his* book, *Against Fairness* (2012): "Not to pick on Asma here, but can you *imagine* a more obnoxious title?"[23] I am sorely tempted to reply that *Against Empathy* is surely in the running.

So, what is it about empathy that draws Bloom's ire? Before we can address this question, it helps to be clear about what we mean by the term. The basic sense in which most of us use the word "empathy" is analogous to the way Adam Smith defines "sympathy": the capacity we possess (or can develop) to see the world through the eyes of another, to "place ourselves in his situation . . . and become in some measure the same person with him, and thence from some idea of his sensations, and even feel something which, though weaker in degree, is not altogether unlike them."[24] Bloom quotes this passage with approval and indicates that this is the sense he will use to approach the subject.

In making moral choices, many would claim that empathy in this sense makes us more likely to care about others and to consider their interests when choosing our own course of action. Siep Stuurman, for instance, whose massive new tome *The Invention of Humanity: Equality and Cultural Difference in World History* (2017) I will turn to shortly, sees the emergence of a sense of common humanity and the widening and deepening of a discourse of human rights as depending on long processes of cultural change and intellectual argument whereby the deeply ingrained ethnocentrism that was omnipresent at the dawn of history has been increasingly modified and left behind, moving toward (though never entirely realizing) a changed mental universe where "people believe that all people are fellow humans, or even equals."[25]

Whereas Stuurman, looking at the *longue durée*, sees the empathetic circle gradually widening and the discourses of otherness and inequality ceding ground to notions of common humanity, Bloom is inclined to focus on the limits to our ability to overcome particularism and bias. Going further, he suggests that much of the time, empathy can reinforce rather than mitigate our biases. It's easier, he suggests, to feel sympathy for those most like us, so as a guide to action, "empathy distorts our moral judgments in pretty much the same way that prejudice does."[26] Moreover, empathy focuses on small numbers of people. We cannot, Bloom argues, feel everyone's pain. We necessarily focus on some small subset of individuals, and this often sways our choices toward these people, although doing so damages the interests of a far larger group that remains an anonymous statistical mass. Bloom also notes that achieving long-term goals often involves inflicting short-term pain. Consider a parent raising a child. Of necessity, the parent "often has to make a child do something, or stop doing something, in a way that causes the child immediate unhappiness but is better for him or her in the future." Or consider a physician empathizing excessively with the patient's pain and suffering; such an individual is unlikely to act in the disinterested rational fashion that would best serve the patient.

For Bloom, "Empathy is biased and parochial; it focuses you on certain people at the expense of others; and it is innumerate, so it distorts our moral and policy decisions in ways that cause suffering instead of relieving it."[27] As if that were not bad enough, Bloom contends that a still worse set of consequences flows from another, more restricted sense of empathy, what he and others have called "cognitive empathy." One can mirror another's feelings, after all, in the sense of grasping what they are, without this leading to treating that person better. The best torturers, for instance, are those who can anticipate and intuit what their victims most fear and tailor their actions accordingly. Here, Bloom effectively invokes the case of Winston Smith's torturer O'Brien in Orwell's *1984*, who is able to divine the former's greatest dread, his fear of rats, and then use it to destroy him.

As his subtitle indicates, Bloom wants to substitute what he calls "rational compassion" for this fuzzy thing called empathy, an emotion he argues is all too likely to lead us astray. His is a utilitarian ethics, and one that suggests that attending to empathy alone is often likely to lead us in morally dubious directions. Fair enough, and his astringent and often witty prose in many places successfully skewers the kind of mawkish nonsense memorably encapsulated in Bill Clinton's statement, "I feel your pain," and gracing the covers of the myriad books that can be purchased on Amazon touting the merits of a soppy sort of empathy (there are fifteen hundred with "empathy" in their titles, by Bloom's recent count). Other passages, however, suggest to me that Bloom actually has a soft spot for empathy and the kindness and regard for others that can flow in its wake—provided only that we temper our emotional responses with a strong dash of reason and an attention to the broader consequences of our decisions. And that, I think, is a more defensible position than simply announcing, to create a stir, that empathy is an unambiguously "bad thing."

Stuurman's *Invention of Humanity* is a vastly different book than the breezy pop psychology and pop philosophy volumes written by Bloom and Bazalgette. Stuurman is a retired Dutch intellectual historian, and he brings to bear a formidable erudition to examine humankind's passage from the earliest recorded history, where strangers were routinely classified as barbarians and inferiors, scarcely human and often treated as less than that, to a world that at least pays lip service to notions of basic equality, a common humanity, and the claim that there exist basic human rights to which all of us are entitled. There is an obvious danger of producing a teleological story here, and inevitably at least some of us living in the twenty-first century prefer the contemporary ideas to the extreme xenophobia and violent hostility so evident in ancient times. We intellectuals, after all, helped invent and propagate these new ideals and often take them to be self-evident, and outside the ranks of the neurological reductionists, we, like Stuurman, believe that "ideas matter and that canonized ideas matter a lot."[28]

Stuurman, however, is mostly alive to the danger of march-of-progress narratives, and he most certainly is aware of the limits and contradictions embodied in successive claims to have embraced unambiguously morally superior ways of being in the world. His is very much an intellectual history, and though he gestures throughout at factors such as travel, cultural contact, and exchange (of both material goods and ideas) as motors of change, his focus is most centrally on the evolution of ideas about equality and cultural difference across the whole arc of human history. The idea of our common humanity is, he insists, an invention, a highly complex cultural construction not somehow given in our genes or mechanically produced by the organization of our brains and nervous systems. To reconstruct its long and tortured history, he turns to a galaxy of major thinkers, seeking to show through a close analysis of their writings how discourses of inequality and inferiority (often extending to enslaving or exterminating the other) were disrupted by different ways of thinking that transformed the ways human relationships were understood and articulated. "How and in what historical circumstances," he asks, "did cross-cultural humanity become thinkable?"[29] His answer relies heavily on an examination of how, why, and to what extent some thinkers found it possible to put themselves in other people's shoes, to begin to comprehend and grant validity to alien cultures, and to develop some degree of critical distance from the culture into which they had been born and in which they lived. As this implies, empathy with the stranger, and what flowed from that empathy, are absolutely central in Stuurman's mind to the halting and uncertain widening of mental horizons and to the emergence of the idea that we share a common humanity, with all that ultimately results from accepting such a proposition.

Careful not to be trapped in an ethnocentric, purely Western mental universe, Stuurman ranges widely across different civilizations. Homer and Confucius, Herodotus and Ibn Khaldun, the Judeo-Christian and Islamic traditions, and the major thinkers of the European Enlightenment are all mustered to the task of unpacking how our common humanity came to be imagined and invented. So too are less obvious figures such as travelers and ethnographers, as well as anthropologists of various stripes. Attention to the language, attitudes, and behaviors of European colonizers is matched by an attempt to recover the sensibilities and reactions of the colonized. The American and French Revolutions sit astride an analysis of the Haitian revolution, and examinations of national liberation movements in the Third World are paired with the African American struggle for equality in the United States.

At times, the exposition can seem a labored and dutiful recital and précis of different strands of social thought. Overall, however, the intelligence and learning of the author shine through, as does his constant attention to the blind spots and limitations of the thinkers whose work he examines. This is not contextual history. Stuurman wants to mine the past, recover what he thinks is valuable in different intellectual traditions, look for commonalities and points of contrast, and search out the problems and persistent inequalities that often lay below the surface of seeming assaults on inequality. Telling here are his critiques, for example, of Enlightenment ideologues and their limitations. "All men"—but what about women? And what about those who lacked the qualities of enlightened gentlemen? "Savages" were fellow human beings who shared the capacity to reason but had developed it in only rudimentary form. Egalitarianism would be realized in the future but only once "advanced" societies had tutored the backward and brought them into the modern world (i.e., remade them in their own image). Here, Stuurman elaborates on how arranging the history of humanity in a temporal sequence engendered a new form of inequality and thus provided a novel way of combining a claim of human equality with continued unequal treatment of some people: temporal inequality meant that one could acknowledge "the equality of non-Europeans as generic human beings but downgrade them as imprisoned in primitive and backward cultures."[30]

In the nineteenth century, such notions justified imperialism by reference to its "civilizing mission," no matter the rapacious realities of colonial rule. In the twentieth century, they were employed to justify authoritarian, dictatorial, and murderous regimes. For their leaders were the enlightened, the vanguard, more advanced than hoi polloi and tasked with overcoming the false consciousness of the masses and leading them to the promised egalitarian paradise. Yet the Enlightenment, Stuurman insists, was Janus faced, and though its ideas were mobilized to underwrite the "scientific racism" of the nineteenth century and the vanguardism of the Leninists and Maoists of the twentieth century, it can be seen as giving a decisive boost to the idea that we possess a common humanity and to efforts to criticize and supersede a whole array of social inequalities. Indeed, it was on the discourses of the Enlightenment that the critics of racism, authoritarianism, and the subordination of women drew to construct their intellectual assaults on these structures, as Stuurman acknowledges others have previously grasped.

The book closes with a discussion of the creation, in the ashes of World War II, of the 1948 Universal Declaration of Human Rights at the newly constituted United Nations, and with the debate over Samuel Huntington's claims about the forthcoming clash of civilizations. Many are inclined to be cynical about the former, and with good reason. All who signed it stand convicted of hypocrisy and worse, and Stuurman concedes as much. Still, he lauds the document's importance, claiming that it "created a powerful global master language of universal equality, which can rightly be counted among the major turning points of the global intellectual history of common humanity and equality."[31] Whether such optimism will prove justified remains to be seen. Huntington's bleak prognosis suggests a much nastier alternative narrative. Where the invention of humanity will lead to next, particularly as we appear to be entering the twilight years of Pax Americana, is anybody's guess. Stuurman's excellent book ought to play an important role in the coming debates—at least for those of us who acknowledge the capacity of humans to reason and to change their minds, and who reject the image of us as machines, automatons ruled by our genes and the mechanical operations of our male and female brains.

15 Mind, Brain, Law, and Culture

Some foolish folks believe that history matters, that human societies and human behaviors have developed over thousands of years largely because of the elaboration of an increasingly complex set of social, cultural, and material phenomena that need to be examined on their own terms. The wiser among us, however, understand that we are only animals and as such are ruled by our biology, just as ineluctably as the ant or the rhesus monkey, and that if we want to understand human action in general, or more specialized realms like the human institution of the law, it is to our biology that we must turn. More specifically, it is mostly our brains that matter, and therefore it is in the elucidation and illumination provided by evolutionary psychobiology and contemporary neuroscience that we need to look for answers. Science, *hard* science, will uncover the secret wellsprings of all our actions, and we can then leave behind once and for all the soft speculations of the social sciences and gratefully set aside the empty verbiage of the philosophers. Or perhaps, if we are a bit more charitable and ecumenical, we can incorporate some bits of the harder social sciences, such as economics, game theory, and cognitive psychology, while abandoning the fuzzy notions foisted on us by soft-hearted and soft-headed anthropologists, sociologists, and historians.

In their book *Law and the Brain* (2006), Semir Zeki, a London-based neuroscientist, and Oliver Goodenough, an American professor of law at the University of Vermont, have assembled a collection of papers embracing this neurobiological perspective and laying out its implications for the law. They, and their contributors, can barely contain their excitement. Technical advances in brain imaging, particularly positron emission tomography (PET) and functional magnetic resonance imaging (fMRI) have allowed us to visualize brain activity with an unprecedented level of precision. Simultaneously, at the conceptual level, we have finally grasped that subjective mental states have direct neural correlates. The implications are profound. Where once "the study of subjective mental states would have been considered by many to be an unscientific pastime, because it was not objectively verifiable," now a whole new vista opens before us, one that will "put a biologically informed psychology front and center in jurisprudential study."[1]

Consider just the implications for criminal law. Here, the editors anticipate, "brain-imaging techniques will replace finger-printing and lie detector tests as reliable indicators of identity and of the truthfulness of a witness's statement."[2] Even more significantly for a common-law system that relies on the notion of mens rea as a key ingredient in the assessment of a defendant's culpability, the fallible assessments of a lay jury can be replaced by hard scientific fact. "In the very near future," we can eschew error-prone human justice in favor of a legal system grounded in "biological justice."[3]

But all aspects of the law will benefit from the new brain science. As we understand that human emotions and cognition are simply the product of the material operations of our brains and are able to provide clear pictorial evidence of how human beings make decisions and determine their preferences, all sorts of subbranches of the legal enterprise, from contracts to marriage law, from property to estate and inheritance law, will fall under the sway of "objective neurobiological evidence."[4] Once we grasp how our brains work, nothing else is material—for all human action, all human thought, all of society and social institutions issue from those billions of cells and their interactions. And the scientific truth of the matter, as Princeton psychologists Joshua Greene and Jonathan Cohen inform us, is that "in a very real sense we are all puppets. The combined effects of gene and environment determine all of our actions."[5]

For too long we have clung to magical fables about free will and human autonomy. At last, with the aid of modern neuroscience, we can appreciate "the mechanical nature of human action in a way that bypasses complicated arguments."[6] Who needs those? As we improve current technology, we can expect the arrival of "extremely high-resolution scanners that can simultaneously track the neural activity and connectivity of every neuron in the human brain, along with computers and software that can analyze and organize these data."[7] And down the road a little further, "this sort of brainware may be very widespread, with a high-resolution scanner in every classroom. People may grow up used to the idea that every decision is a thoroughly mechanical process, the outcome of which is completely determined by the results of prior mechanical processes."[8]

Utopia looms, thanks to the breakthroughs brought forth by the decade of the brain. For it is not just our petty or consequential legal squabbles that will fall by the wayside once we abandon an earlier metaphysics: "In a 'millennial' future, perhaps only decades away, a good knowledge of the brain's system of justice and of how the brain reacts to conflicts may provide critical tools in resolving international political and economic conflicts."[9] Harmony will rule and democracy will triumph when neuroscience at last fulfills its destiny as the queen of all the sciences.

It will do so in part because "democratic institutions are not artificial constructs, but rather are expressions of our own evolved, and complimentary [sic], desires for freedom and social stability."[10] Likewise, "there is an inextricable evolutionary link between justice and democracy."[11] On the mundane, daily level, even the decisions of judges, juries, and legislatures depend on preferences "that reflect the interaction between the case at hand and the neuroeconomically evolved, probabilistic, norms that all judges, jurors, and legislators carry inside their brains."[12] As for the market economy, that too derives from our biology. It is not just that "fundamental principles of property are encoded in the human brain."[13] Even more complex aspects of our economic behavior may be built into us. For example, "we may have an innate sense of alienability"; "instincts may tell us not only how to transfer property, but also to whom"; and "the property instinct connects with an instinct for equity in reciprocal exchanges."[14]

Thus, we can bask in the scientific certainty that "a democratic nation with a free market economy is the highest expression of the human spirit."[15] Truth, justice, and the American way, it turns out, need no Superman to defend them because they are hardwired into our biology. Their triumph in the not-so-long run is inevitable, supported as they are "by psychological characteristics that are probably pancultural and likely to have been the product of natural selection"[16]

"Knowing more about the ultimate evolutionary causes of human brain design"[17] allows us to understand all manner of other social institutions and phenomena. The roles, behaviors, and social situation of the sexes, for example, are heavily influenced by evolutionary biology. After all, "natural selection acts through reproductive success, and the reproductive requirements of the sexes differ. . . . Men must compete for sexual partners, and protect those they have acquired. Male aggressiveness and assertiveness, machismo traditions and protective chivalry towards women are in harmony with this. . . . In most societies men hold the power in the social and political spheres." In contrast, "feminine dispositions" are, because of the same biological mechanisms, more focused on children, and on home and hearth. And "in harmony" once more with built-in biological imperatives, "in probably all societies men are allowed more sexual license than women, . . . [who] are expected to be chaste, modest, and faithful." All these features and more are part of the natural order of things, and "in keeping with evolutionary theory."[18]

From this dream of certitude, however, we may happen to awake. If we do so, we may recall that we have been here more than once before. Many prominent Enlightenment philosophers advanced views of this sort. In 1802, Cabanis famously claimed that the brain secretes thought just as the liver secretes bile, and he neatly anticipated Hinde's claims about the male-female divide: "Men must be strong, audacious, enterprising; and women weak, timorous, hidden away. That is Nature's law." (Il faut que l'homme soit fort, audacieux, entreprenant; que la femme soit faible, timide, dissimulée. Telle est la loi de la nature.)[19] As much as a half century earlier, in 1748, Julien La Mettrie had announced that man was merely a machine.[20] And such views were not the peculiar province of the godless French: Sir William Lawrence, one of the most prominent early nineteenth-century British surgeons, was equally insistent that "physiologically speaking . . . the mind is the grand prerogative of the brain," and he announced that deranged thoughts "have the same relation to the brain as vomiting, indigestion, heartburn, to the stomach, cough, asthma to the lungs, or any other deranged functions to their corresponding organs."[21]

If this crude materialism might be seen as a passing phase, nothing more than a manifestation of Enlightenment enthusiasm, subsequent attempts to reduce human nature to biology have often had more sinister overtones. For nineteenth-century physicians, few facts were more incontestably established than that the female of the species was "the product and prisoner of her reproductive system."[22] A woman's place in society—her capacities, her roles, her behavior—was ineluctably linked to and controlled by the existence and functions of her uterus and ovaries. To the crises and periodicities of her reproductive organs could be traced all the peculiarities of her nature: the predominance in her of the emotional over the rational; her capacity for affection and aptitude for child-rearing; her preference for the domestic sphere; and her "natural" purity and moral sensibility. Her status as "a moral, a sexual, a germiferous, gestative, and parturient creature"[23] thus rested firmly on the findings of science, which repeatedly demonstrated that "the functions of the brain are so intimately connected with the uterine system, that the interruption of any one process which the latter has to perform in the human economy may implicate the former."[24] Such "interruptions," of course, profoundly threatened women's health and formed the physiological foundation of her greater delicacy and fragility. And given that the central mediating role between brain and generative organs was played by the nervous system, it was no wonder that perhaps the most fearsome threats that were thus presented were to the feminine hold on sanity.

Henry Maudsley, who in the late nineteenth century was the leading anglophone student of what he termed the physiology and pathology of the mind,[25] uncompromisingly made clear the implications of the scientific consensus: notwithstanding the selfish protests of the few, there remained the "inescapable fact that the male organization is one, and the female organization another, and that, let come what may in the way of assimilation of female and male education and labor, it will not be possible to transform a woman into a man."[26] The destiny of the overwhelming majority of women remained marriage and childbearing, and their education and upbringing should reflect that fact. With an "enthusiasm which borders on or reaches fanaticism," the advocates of higher education for women overlooked the fact that "the energy of the human body [was] a

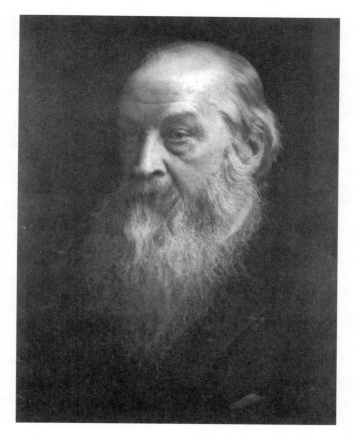

Figure 10. Henry Maudsley as a misanthropic old man. (*Journal of Nervous and Mental Disease* 1, [1874]: 103.)

definite and not inexhaustible quantity,"[27] and women who overexercised their brains risked deadly medical consequences. When all was said and done, "they . . . cannot escape the fact that a woman labours under an inferiority of constitution which there is no gain-saying. . . . This is not the expression of a prejudice nor of false sentiment; it is a plain statement of a physiological fact."[28] Race suicide loomed for societies that permitted women to substitute (indubitably second-rate) intellectual endeavors for their real task: focusing their physical and mental energies on reproduction and on the care of the male of the species.

For Victorian brain scientists, the facts of physiology thus definitively proved that the existing gendered social and moral order was rooted in the stern realities of the natural world. But, it emerged, the findings of biological science had a still broader social relevance. In fin-de-siècle Western society—in France, in Germany, in Britain, and in the United States—the new evolutionary biology was invoked to explain a whole host of social ills: crime, mental illness, alcoholism, epilepsy, feeble-mindedness, poverty— all were a product of inherited inferiority and physical defect. Degenerate specimens, kept alive by the misplaced kindness of civilized societies, repaid that kindness by reproducing at a fearsome rate, for as unreasoning beasts they lacked the moral restraints built into their more intelligent fellow citizens. The upshot was that "every year thousands of children [were] born with pedigrees that would condemn puppies to the horse pond."[29]

Physical isolation of the unfit in state-funded institutions was one scientific solution, but the very size of the problem population made it an extraordinarily expensive one. The United States pioneered an alternative approach: compulsory sterilization. State after state passed such laws, and the policy survived a constitutional challenge before the Supreme Court. The state of Virginia had involuntarily sterilized Carrie Buck, a young woman confined to a mental hospital whose mother had also been institutionalized as mentally defective. (Carrie had been raped by her cousin, and the birth of her child had served as the pretext for her commitment as insane.) When the lawsuit about her case reached the Supreme Court, Chief Justice Oliver Wendell Holmes, claiming science was on his side, wrote for the eight justices who formed the majority: "It is better for all the world if instead of waiting to execute degenerate offspring for crime, or to let them starve for their imbecility, society can prevent those who are manifestly unfit from continuing their kind. The principle that sustains compulsory vaccination is broad enough to cover cutting the Fallopian tubes. Three generations of idiots are enough."[30]

Of course, some might question the wisdom of allowing those cursed with a hopelessly inferior genetic endowment to continue to exist, even as eunuchs or sterilized women. If one set aside sentiment, surely a more efficient solution could be found. Would it not be better "to weed out and exterminate the diseased and otherwise unfit in every grade of natural life"?[31] Regrettably, though, physical elimination seemed to have its

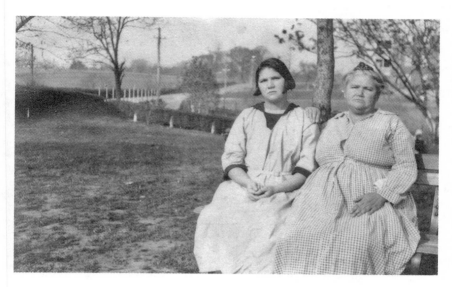

Figure 11. Carrie Buck and her mother, Emma, 1924. (Reproduced by courtesy of the M. E. Grenander Department of Special Collections and Archives, State University of New York at Albany.)

detractors. The American scientist Charles Davenport lamented, "It seems to be against the mores to burn [to death] any considerable part of our population"; and those who sought to popularize the new science of eugenics, like Madison Grant, the president of the Immigration Restriction League, sold lots of books, but they found their insistence that "the laws of nature require the obliteration of the unfit" difficult to translate into the final solution they sought.[32] Except, of course, in Nazi Germany, where the proponents of racial hygiene openly acknowledged their debt to the pioneering work of American science and American legislation when implementing their own program of mass castration, which was soon replaced by the expeditious consignment of the mentally unfit to the gas chambers. The mores might yet prove malleable.

Not sufficiently, it would seem, if they were the product of democratic brains. The "evolutionary" difference between German brains and English and American brains must have been insignificant, and there were surely many Anglo-American brains that were somehow not fully evolved in a democratic direction. Yet the reaction among the victors in the war against Hitler was to recoil from what had been done in the name of science. The Zeki and Goodenough volume contains some wry but circumspect acknowledgments of the cautions this history has thrown up. Owen Jones accepts that "those who voice skepticism about biological perspectives on the brain are sometimes right—because biology has been misused in the past."[33] And the editors themselves acknowledge that "there are particular inhibitions and taboos about the biology of moral judgement that grow from the deployment, in past years, of cartoons of this kind of science as window dressing for ideas, some of them quite hideous, that had their sources in other passions."[34] But our science is a dispassionate science. And recognition of a dreadful past, "properly understood," calls "more for caution than for exclusion."[35] This time around, we can rest assured that things are different.

But it is time to fess up. This time around, things are not different. The "findings" reported in Zeki and Goodenough are for the most part a far-rago of nonsense, unsupported speculation, breathtaking chutzpah, and massive exaggeration. After having been entertained by speculative evolutionary genealogies, we are treated to a host of bathetic insights: "children have propensities for both prosocial and selfishly assertive behaviour"; "the ownership convention is more complicated for humans than for butterflies"; "in practice rights are not quite 'inalienable,' and differ to some extent between cultures"; in potentially cooperative situations, "the decision of whether to take action involves apparently both cognitive mechanisms and trust and reciprocity and social mechanisms"; "because law is generally generated by a subgroup, it most probably will operate to promote that subgroup's welfare."[36] No kidding! I thought sociologists were the ones who recycled the trite and the obvious and called it an addition to knowledge.

Elsewhere, evolutionary biology, psychology, and economics are invoked to support democratic "instincts," property "instincts," and justice "instincts'" that are invented whole cloth in the crudest of fashions and used to provide a naturalistic justification for the particular social arrangements this group of scholars happens to prefer (and that, as it happens, I tend to prefer too). Over and over again in the discussions of the origins and existence of supposed instincts, we encounter weasel words and phrases: "perhaps"; "could have been"; "must have"; "may"; "probably"; "it is not surprising that"; "the evidence [*sic*] favours the view that"; "likely to have been"; "in keeping with the view that"; "it is reasonable to assume that"; "presumably." Instincts are postulated, in a frivolous fashion, to provide support for whatever social arrangement is either observed or desired, and where reality diverges from what the proposed instinct dictates, the authors simply invent another ad hoc explanation of why this might be: "Our operative legal principles exist because they more or less capture an intuitive sense of justice."[37] I see. Then how do we account for Mao's China, Hitler's Germany, Castro's Cuba, Verwoerd's South Africa, or a whole host of patently unjust societies to which one could point? Well, those societies somehow temporarily deviated down pathways at odds with our instincts. Too bad that such deviations make up most of recorded human history.

On the basis of no evidence whatsoever, we are informed that "Homeric Greek society and Medieval Icelandic society . . . probably exemplify the environment within which human brains evolved."[38] Assume for a moment that one were to accept this bizarre claim. How then are we possibly to account for the extraordinary diversity of human societies? Or for the existence of Homeric or Icelandic societies themselves, both of them complex and "advanced" beyond anything our authors appear to dream. So far as I am aware, no respectable scientist argues that the human genome has evolved to any significant degree since the Stone Age. Yet human culture and human society have transformed themselves in a quite extraordinarily diverse array of ways in that period precisely because of the plasticity of human beings, their capacity to learn, and innovate and to transmit what they have learned and invented across generations.

Perhaps the neuroscience in Zeki and Goodenough's volume fares better than the evolutionary psychology? On the whole, I think not. Only to a quite limited degree and in very restricted circumstances are neuroscientific advances likely to have relevance for such things as the current legal system. Much is made of the fact that particular regions of the brain show heightened levels of activity on fMRIs when people, for example, are making choices or telling lies. Even Bishop Berkeley would not be surprised by that. When I move, speak, think, or experience an emotion, one may presume this is correlated with physical changes in my brain, but such correlations prove nothing about the causal processes involved any more than—note well—the existence of a particular sequence of events demonstrates that some early event in the sequence ineluctably caused a later event. Post hoc, ergo propter hoc is an elementary logical fallacy.

And further problems immediately loom. As Paul Zak wistfully but honestly acknowledges, different observers report different results—different locations for the thoughts in question: "There is," for example, "no consistency between the findings of Rustichini et al. and Smith et al. about the neural substrates associated with ambiguity during choice."[39] Likewise, we have no way to translate "heightened activity" into the contents of people's thoughts, and there is no prospect of making such translations. Nor, as Spence and his colleagues acknowledge, in one of the few careful and balanced papers in *Law and the Brain,* do we possess any way of moving from weak inferences based on statistical averages of the gross changes in brain function in large experimental groups to the level of the individual subject.[40] Moreover, just as economists traditionally rely on absurdly oversimplified portraits of human motivation to construct their models, so all the neuroscientific findings that are so proudly proffered reflect simple simulated experiments that in no way capture the intricacies of everyday social situations, let alone the complex interactions over time that make up human history.

One can grant that people who have suffered massive damage to their prefrontal cortex may reason differently from the rest of us, and perhaps be so lacking in inhibition as to find it difficult to exercise the forward planning, emotional self-control, and tact that is required to be a fully functioning member of society. (One can grant, indeed, that dead people do not seem to think at all.) We had a naturalistic experiment of just this sort back in the 1940s, when neurosurgeons and psychiatrists used their primitive understanding of human brains to justify damaging the frontal lobes of the mentally ill to "cure" them—and these lobotomized patients did indeed exhibit such symptoms and deficits. Were contemporary neuroscience to demonstrate the existence of similar physical malfunction in some people who have not had lobotomies, that might very well bear on the issue of holding such people legally responsible. But knowledge of this sort would require no more than a marginal adjustment of existing legal practice, not a wholesale rethinking of our entire judicial system.

One final point: many of the contributors to *Law and the Brain* seem to subscribe (if readers will forgive the awful pun) to a sort of mindless biological determinism. For them, what occurs in the world is simply the predetermined product of our evolutionary psychology and the physical construction of our brains, which respond as they must to the environment that contains them. We are, as Greene and Cohen would have it, mere puppets, helplessly following our preprogramed pathways in a purely mechanical way. If so, I am at a loss to understand what these folks are doing when they publish books like this one. They seem to be trying to persuade us of something, to convince us to amend our ways and acknowledge their superior wisdom. But that would necessitate our ability to assess arguments, to reason, to choose. And those, of course, are capacities for which their world has no place. Too bad. And not good (enough).

Much better is Bruce Wexler's extended essay on the links between *Brain and Culture* (2006). Rather than positing a rigid separation between the biological and the social, Wexler insists that the two interact and mutually influence each other in powerful ways. It makes no sense, in his view, to regard the brain as an asocial or a presocial organ, because in important respects its very structure and functioning is a product of the social environment. For the most remarkable feature of the human brain is "its deep and extended sensitivity . . . to shaping by psychosocial and other sensory inputs."[41] What this means, he contends, is that "our biology is social in such a fundamental and thorough manner that to speak of a relation between the two suggests an unwarranted distinction."[42]

To an extent unprecedented in any other part of the animal kingdom, humans' brains continue to develop postnatally, and the environmental elements that most powerfully affect the structure and functioning of these maturing brains are themselves human creations. As one would expect of a psychiatrist and neuroscientist, Wexler's "conceptual starting point and foundation are . . . biological."[43] What he emphasizes, however, is the remarkable neuroplasticity of human beings, at least through adolescence, and the critical importance of nonbiological factors in transforming the neural structures we are born with, thereby creating the mature brain. The very shape of the brain, the neural connections that develop and that constitute the physical underpinnings of our emotions and cognition, are profoundly influenced by social stimulation and by the cultural and especially the familial environment within which these developments take place. It is in these settings that "the fine-grained shaping of the structural and functional organization of the human brain takes place."[44] Quite simply, "human nature . . . allows and requires environmental input for normal development."[45] And that development continues for a very long time, with increases in connectivity and changes in brain organization, especially in the parietal and frontal lobes, taking place well into the third decade of life, whereas "corresponding changes in the brains of chimpanzees and other higher primates reach comparable levels of maturity during the second and third years of life."[46]

Wexler stresses that rather than being localized in particular regions of the brain or being the properties of individual neurons, thinking, feeling, and remembering are the product of complex networks and interconnections that form as we mature. These in turn derive from the selective survival and growth of cells and the pruning of connections among cells—processes that are heavily dependent on the interactional environment in which the human infant is raised and that are particularly important for the development of the cerebral cortex, whose size "relative to the rest of the brain is greater in humans than in any other species."[47] That environment, of course, is to an unprecedented extent a human-made environment, much of it taking effect through the medium of language. And crucially, "it is this ability to shape the environment that in turn shapes our brains that has allowed human adaptability and capability to develop at a much faster rate than is possible through alterations of the genetic code itself."[48]

In support of these propositions, Wexler deploys evidence from a wide variety of human and animal studies on the effects of the social environment and sensory deprivation on mental functioning and neural development, attempting to bolster his arguments by drawing on a variety of disciplines, ranging from neuroscience to linguistics to academic psychology to psychoanalysis. He argues that, though these bodies of knowledge have developed independently and separately, their findings on these fronts largely complement one another, a convergence reflecting the fact that "neurological and psychological function are two sides of a coin, and different aspects of each are joined in the organic wholeness of the individual."[49]

Wexler writes gracefully and clearly, and in the first two-thirds of his book makes a powerful case for his point of view. Some might argue that he underestimates the degree to which intelligence, temperament, and individuality are dependent on inherited, presocial characteristics of a person, and there is weight to this criticism. And yet to acknowledge that he may on occasion slight nature in favor of nurture does not, in my view, invalidate the fundamental thrust of Wexler's argument.

That said, the final portions of *Brain and Culture* struck me as far more speculative and vulnerable to criticism than the earlier chapters. Wexler's claim that the neuroplasticity of humans has sharply declined by early adulthood seems consonant with much of the available evidence. This remains true whether one focuses on such things as the increased difficulty of learning new languages or on the evidence about the growing stability of brain structure. But the extrapolations that Wexler makes in the last chapters from this state of affairs struck me as strained and selective. The greater rigidity of adult brains leads, he suggests, to such phenomena as a "neurobiological antagonism to difference,"[50] a resistance to novelty and change, a state of misery and illness in the face of altered worlds, and even a propensity "to eliminate strange and foreign people."[51] Whereas earlier in life we change our brains to match our circumstances, later on we try to change the world to match our newly static internal dispositions.

Significantly, these generalizations are supported not by the sorts of evidence that are invoked earlier in the book but by selective snippets from history and anthropology, allied to anecdotes about the effects of losing a spouse, the dread of seeing one's child marrying someone from another ethnic group or culture, and the dislocations attendant on immigration to another country as an adult. We are invited to view the genocide in Rwanda, the Crusades against the Muslims and against the Albigensian heretics in Languedoc, the Inquisition, and a variety of other lethal encounters between disparate people and cultures as, in substantial part, the product of a biologically rooted conservatism and ethnocentrism. To be sure, Wexler acknowledges that "data to support [these] assertion[s] are not as clear-cut as the data . . . that support the arguments for environmental shaping of brain development."[52] But it does not stop him speculating along these lines, ignoring all the counterexamples that history and our own daily experience can just as easily offer: of adults embracing and seeking out novelty; of cultures comfortably coexisting; of delight in difference. The fact that even someone with generally so subtle a perspective on the interactions between brain and culture feels impelled to advance simplistic notions of this sort is a pity. It would seem that the siren song of biological reductionism is not easily resisted, even by those who ordinarily know better.

16 Left Brain, Right Brain, One Brain, Two Brains

It struck me as odd that I was invited to write an essay review of Iain McGilchrist's new magnum opus. It was not all that strange to receive a request as a non-neuroscientist to write a review of a book on the structure and functioning of the left and right hemispheres of the brain, for *The Master and His Emissary* is after all aimed at the intelligent general reader, and in this context I can at least lay claim to being a general reader. What was peculiar was that the invitation came from the editor of the oldest neurological journal in the world, *Brain*—the readership of which is largely confined to neurologists and neuroscientists, an audience whose expertise on the underlying brain science is orders of magnitude greater and more sophisticated than mine. How to tackle such a task? It makes no sense for me to devote much space to a critique of McGilchrist's mastery of the research literature on which he draws to make his case, for there are literally thousands of reviewers more competent than I to undertake such an assessment. Instead, like other nonspecialist readers, I must perforce take largely on trust his claims to represent the current state of neuroscientific knowledge and turn most of my attention elsewhere: to where his analysis sits in a long-running historical debate on the duality of the brain; and to an examination of his attempt to move from the narrow findings of neuroscience to a remarkably bold and ambitious attempt to understand their implications for, as he puts it in his subtitle, "the making of the Western world."

That human and mammalian brains are composed of two hemispheres has long been known. Greek physicians from the third century BCE knew of and speculated about the divided brain, and McGilchrist mentions, largely in passing, that Galen's anatomical researches, mostly conducted on animals, made the basic duality of the brain known to all interested parties in the second century CE. Other organs are also doubled, of course: ears, eyes, lungs, kidneys, testicles, and ovaries, to point to just a few important examples. Until relatively late in the nineteenth century, most observers seem to have believed or assumed not only that the brain was composed of two hemispheres but that these hemispheres were essentially bilaterally symmetrical and simply duplicated one another's functions. Such was emphatically the view of the British physician Arthur Wigan, whose *New View of Insanity: The Duality of Mind* (1844) gave new prominence to the phenomenon and propounded the view that "each cerebrum is a distinct and perfect whole, as an organ of thought."[1] When the action of these two halves failed to parallel one another, through disease or faulty education, mental incoherence and insanity were too often the result.

Two centuries earlier, René Descartes had advanced a different sort of dualism, one that distinguished sharply between the mind (immaterial, immortal, and identical to the soul) and the body. But Descartes, too, was aware of the doubling of the brain and turned this knowledge to account when he grappled with the puzzle of how mind and brain interacted. If the brain itself was double, allowing our twinned eyes, ears, hands, and nostrils to feed sensory data into the system, there was an organ deep within its structure, the pineal gland, that was not. Here, Descartes hypothesized, the two sets of sensory impressions came together, uniting before passing their input to the unitary soul. It was a theologically satisfying solution whose attractions for Descartes were amplified by his (false) belief that animals do not possess a pineal gland, for only humans, of course, were supposed to possess a soul. (Descartes notoriously claimed that animals were simply machines.)

There were thus good extrascientific reasons to believe that the two halves of the brain were precise mirror images of each other, an integrated

brain sustaining an indivisible soul. Xavier Bichat, one of the central figures in the rise of Paris hospital medicine in the early nineteenth century,
added his prestige to the doctrine of anatomical symmetry, arguing that
"harmony is to the functions of the organs what symmetry is to their con-
formation. . . . Symmetry indicates an exact analogy in the external forms
and internal structure."[2] To be sure, at almost the same time, the founders
of phrenology, Franz Gall and Johann Spurzheim, asserted that the brain
was nothing but a congeries of organs and claimed that they had localized
psychological functions in these different organs or regions of the brain.
But theirs was a doctrine that (rightly) led to accusations of materialism,
and soon enough phrenology was condemned as a pseudoscience, its practitioners relegated to the fairground and its claims of localized function
read out of the mainstream.

The revival of the notion of localized function is generally attributed to
Pierre Broca's discovery of a lesion in the third convolution of the left frontal cortex that produced aphasia. Broca's discovery of this region is held to
have led to a general reinterpretation of the functioning of the two halves
of the brain and to have launched a more systematic study of the differences between the two hemispheres. And so, in a sense, it did, though the
story is considerably more complicated than it appears at first sight. In the
first place, as McGilchrist notes, the discovery in question had actually
been made some decades earlier by an obscure provincial French doctor,
Marc Dax, who never received credit for his priority. Secondly, and perhaps more importantly, when Broca made his first examination of the
brain of an aphasic (or, as he preferred, aphemic) patient who had lost
the power to speak, he was as fully committed as most of his generation to
the notion of brain symmetry. Observing a lesion in the left frontal lobe,
he assumed that in other similar cases, he would be just as likely to find a
lesion on the right frontal lobe, but not necessarily in its third convolution.
Only when an accumulation of cases disappointed his initial expectation
was he led to revise his view and identify what we now call Broca's area. In
the process, the attention of other researchers finally began to shift, and
the doctrine of cerebral asymmetry started to develop.

In the hands of Broca and his successors, as Anne Harrington has
shown,[3] the left hemisphere increasingly came to be regarded as the dominant hemisphere, one that essentially held a monopoly on the most central

social and scientific virtues. The left hemisphere was the seat of reason, logic, language, balance, and willpower. Its thankfully largely silent counterpart on the right of the brain was where one encountered animality, instinctual action, impulsiveness, and intuition (as contrasted, unfavorably, with rationality). Many found it irresistible to incorporate their own prejudices into their science, and they labeled the left hemisphere the "male" half of the brain and the right hemisphere the "female" half. Women's inferiority, and their incapacity for higher education, was, they "discovered," built into the organization of their brains.

Curiously, McGilchrist has little to say about the differences between male and female brains. Perhaps he remembers the fate of a certain Harvard president who trespassed not so long ago on to this contested terrain,[4] or perhaps he feels he already gives enough hostages to fortune. McGilchrist's book, after all, is likely to stir up enough of a hornet's nest without venturing to address questions of gender. Still, the issue lingers, and the failure to address it—remarkable given his unapologetic embrace of the superiority of the right brain, with its connections to the world of the social, the emotional, the contextual, and the intuitive—seems egregious and unfortunate.

Once neurologists' attention began to be focused on brain asymmetry, the structural dissimilarities of the two hemispheres swiftly surfaced. Hitherto overlooked, the differences were now laid bare: typically, the left hemisphere is larger, wider toward the back, and extends further toward the rear than its counterpart; while the right hemisphere is wider toward the front of the brain and even overlaps a bit there with the left. But were these anatomical asymmetries related to functional ones? The answer for most neuroscientists was increasingly yes. Size matters, it appears (at least for brains), and over the ensuing century and more, the left hemisphere was increasingly spoken of as the "dominant" hemisphere. In the words of Salomon Henschen, the Swedish neuropathologist writing in the pages of the journal *Brain* in 1926, the right hemisphere displayed "a manifest inferiority when compared with the left, and plays an automatic role only. . . . The right temporal lobe is, of course, sufficient for the more primitive psychical life; only by using the left temporal lobe can man reach a higher level of psychical life."[5] Later generations of experts have largely agreed. McGilchrist quotes Michael Gazzaniga, for example, speaking of "the shocking differences between the two hemispheres," differences he summed up on another occasion with the tart remark, "It could well be argued that the cognitive skills of a normal disconnected right hemisphere without language are vastly inferior to the cognitive skills of a chimpanzee."6

The past half-century has witnessed an ongoing effort to unravel the mystery of the two hemispheres and how exactly they function. Total war helped the process along, the traumatic brain injuries it brought in its train creating a series of naturalistic experiments that helped to unravel the effects of particular sorts of brain injuries. Tumors, strokes, and other sorts of insults to the integrity of the brain provided another avenue to knowledge, as for a time did neurosurgical interventions in some serious cases of epilepsy where the corpus callosum—the bundle of fibers linking the two hemispheres—was often severed in a desperate and sometimes successful attempt to control seizures. More recently, imaging technologies have been recruited to the task, as have experiments where one half of the brain is anesthetized while the other remains active. None of these sources of information is without its problems, but collectively they have contributed to considerable advances in our knowledge of brain function.

For many neuroscientists, this accumulating volume of evidence has served, in McGilchrist's words, to reinforce "the entrenched prejudice that, while the right hemisphere may add a bit of color to life, it is the left hemisphere that does the serious business."7 As his use of the term "prejudice" signals, this is the very opposite of the conclusion McGilchrist draws, and he devotes a great deal of his attention to arguing forcibly (and largely persuasively, in my view) that on the contrary, the right hemisphere is the more important of the two. The point is hammered home repetitively (some might say obsessively), but among McGilchrist's central aims in *The Master and His Emissary* are to convince his neuroscientific colleagues of the error of their ways, and to rescue the right hemisphere from undeserved opprobrium and neglect. Far from being of marginal importance, our right hemisphere, he claims, gives us our most central and human qualities. The left hemisphere, by contrast, is a dry, desiccated sort of fellow, given to arid abstractions that denature our existence and leave us to contemplate a mechanical, lifeless universe. The two halves of our brain, it would appear, have radically different agendas, something many of

McGilchrist's neuroscientific colleagues have missed, captured as they have been by the left sides of their own brains. After all, most conventional neuroscience is committed to breaking down and analyzing how brains are put together, on the analogy of machines—by McGilchrist's account, a classically left-hemispheric approach. In the process, neuroscience has lost sight of the forest by focusing too much on the trees or, to put it another way, "has largely given up on the attempt to make sense of the findings, once amassed, in any larger context."[8]

If all this sounds as though there is a tendency in *The Emissary and His Master* to reify and anthropomorphize the two halves of the brain, this is indeed a feature of McGilchrist's account. His version of our mental life often reads like a drawn-out battle between two homunculi rattling around inside our skulls, each bent on the subjugation of the other, engaged in an unequal contest, with the corpus callosum acting the part of some feeble referee, mediating between the contenders and fruitlessly attempting to inhibit their excesses. Hence the book's very title, which derives from a Nietzschean fable: There was once a sage philosopher king, whose rule over a small but prosperous domain was selfless and benign. The kingdom flourished and its borders grew. The king trained advisors to administer his growing territories. Eventually, the cleverest and most ambitious vizier began to see himself as wiser than his master, and he used his position to advance his own wealth and influence. He grew contemptuous of the king and ended by usurping his authority. The upshot was a tyranny, before the vizier's rule collapsed in ruins. It is, McGilchrist suggests, a parable for our times, and for our brains: "At present the domain—our civilization—finds itself in the hands of the vizier [the left side of our brains], who, however gifted, is effectively a regional bureaucrat with his own interests at heart. Meanwhile the Master, the one whose wisdom gave the people peace and security, is led away in chains."[9]

McGilchrist recognizes that both hemispheres are vital to humans and acknowledges that many of the achievements of civilization would have been quite impossible without the influence of those features of our mental life he believes can be attributed to our left hemispheres. Left hemispheres abstract, they bring to bear focused attention, they isolate, fix, and make explicit certain features of the world, giving us the power to learn and to make things. But these are, on McGilchrist's account, lesser if still important attributes. And it is a measure of how powerfully his account favors the characteristics he ascribes to the right side of our brains that at one point he is driven to insist, "I do not wish to leave the impression that it might be a good thing [disregarding the fact that the right side of everyone's body would be paralyzed!!] if the entire population suffered a left hemisphere stroke."[10]

It is the right hemisphere, he insists, that is linked to the highest achievements of the human mind. Where its opponent is literal-minded, narrow, inflexible, given to perseveration, incapable of creativity, and lacking any capacity for empathy with others, the right side of the brain embraces irony and metaphor. It grasps things as wholes, exhibits a broad perspective on the world, is capable of taking the perspective of the other, and thus allows empathy and the social side of human beings to flourish. The right hemisphere is open to ambiguity and novelty. It is the source of creativity and imagination, poetry and music, humor and our moral sense. Quite a list. "Until recently," McGilchrist claims, "everything about the right hemisphere has been shrouded in darkness. It was, after all, considered to be silent; and to the verbal left-hemisphere way of thinking, that means dumb."[11] From this misplaced condescension, our knight errant rides to rescue the poor right side of the brain.

One is tempted at times to view Iain McGilchrist as a sort of neuroscientific Quixote, a tilter at windmills who has lost his sense of perspective, if not quite his mind. But in fact, he cleverly marshals his forces and attempts with no inconsiderable success to tie the broad claims he is making back into the details of left-brain neuroscientific research. It is no exaggeration to say that part 1 of the book is a tour de force. Yet it is also the case that McGilchrist's task is not as lonely as it might seem, for it turns out that he is not bereft of allies among his fellow scientists, others of whom have also broken with prior orthodoxy.

Having thus established which is master, at least to his own satisfaction, and in the process provided a quirky but fascinating synthesis of how brains work, he turns in part 2 of his book to an even more ambitious task, an attempt to connect his model of how the brain functions to an account of the path taken by Western civilization and the crisis that he believes it currently confronts. It is an endeavor that once more has Quixotic overtones, and at the very least, one has to admire his chutzpah.

And not just that. McGilchrist puts on display a remarkable erudition, an ability to discuss with intelligence and insight the history of Western art and literature, philosophy of a whole range of stripes, musicology (and the relationships between music and the brain), and the varieties of religious experience, to mention just a few of the topics he touches on. In a prior life, McGilchrist was an English don at Oxford, and he has some of the qualities of a Renaissance man—an epithet he would surely embrace. One suspects that not many psychiatrists or neuroscientists could demonstrate such a broad acquaintance with humanistic learning (and conversely, the list of literature professors who could deal fluently and convincingly with contemporary neuroscience must be shorter yet, perhaps even an empty set).

Even in a book as long as *The Master and His Emissary*, and even with a relentless Western and elitist focus, there is space for only what McGilchrist acknowledges is a "hugely selective" gallop through the historical cosmos. Somewhat breathlessly, we are ushered through the rise of the written word (a splendid aside here on the differences between and cognitive implications of pictograms, ideograms, and phonograms) and the origins of classical drama into a discussion of thought and experience in classical Greece and Rome. Then we fast-forward to the Renaissance and the Reformation, the Enlightenment and Romanticism, and the world of the modern and the postmodern, an era McGilchrist seems to approach with some distaste. Our neuroscientific Quixote sees history as oscillating between periods of right- and left-brain dominance (though his attempts to explain how this sort of alternation has come about are uncharacteristically feeble and in my judgment not up to the task). Greece has its right-brain thinkers (Homer and the great dramatists, as well as pre-Socratic philosophers like Thales and Anaximander), but later the quintessential left-brain philosopher Plato comes to the fore, and with him "the (left-hemisphere-congruent) beliefs that truth is in principle knowable, that it is knowable through reason alone, and that all truths are consistent with one another."[12]

If Plato is pernicious, so too are Enlightenment thinkers and their present-day successors. It is to the achievements made during the Renaissance and the Romantic era that McGilchrist likes to point. Here, in his perspective, are periods of right-brain dominance, marked by an unprecedented flowering of human creativity, artistic accomplishment, and balance in people's lives. Contrast that with the empty material progress of the Industrial Revolution and capitalism and the period of left-brain dominance that has persisted all the way up to our own era, with its greed, ruthlessness, exploitation, Gradgrindian philistinism, and sheer bureaucratic soullessness. Even the art of the current era reveals its one-sided emptiness: a caption beneath a reproduction of Matisse's *Large Reclining Nude* invites us to contemplate how the "loss of proportion and perspective in modernism emphasizes emotional detachment. Like harmony [in music], perspective arrived with the Renaissance, and left with modernism."[13] "Down with the left" would seem to be McGilchrist's motto, and not just when it comes to the brain.

17 Delusions of Progress

How should we decide who is mad and who is sane? It is a question psychiatrists and society as a whole still wrestle with—largely fruitlessly, as the endless iterations of the APA's *Diagnostic and Statistical Manual* vividly illustrate. X-rays, MRIs, blood tests, and laboratory findings don't provide any help to those who must make this most basic of distinctions.

The followers of Thomas Szasz dismiss the whole business as a massive fraud on the public, insisting that "mental illness" is nothing more than a myth. But all competent members of a culture know better: some of our fellow creatures—deluded, distracted, depressed, or demented—are so alienated from the reality the rest of us seem to share that we routinely label them mad (or, more politely, mentally ill). With respect to the most serious cases of alienation, we would likely be tempted to question the sanity of someone who dissented from the consensus. Where do we draw the line, though, in less obvious cases? We laugh when we read the courtroom testimony of John Haslam, one of the most famous (or infamous) mad-doctors practicing in the early nineteenth century: "I never saw any human being who was of sound mind."[1] But in truth, beyond the hard core of easily recognizable behavioral or mental disturbance, the boundary between the normal and the pathological remains extraordinarily vague and indeterminate. And yet lines are drawn, and lives lie in the balance. Crazy or merely eccentric? It matters greatly.

In the past, in the era of the madhouse and the asylum, how we drew the line between sanity and madness mattered perhaps even more than it does now. For to be certified as mad was to lose one's civil rights and one's liberty—to be shut up, in multiple senses of that term. It was a social space, however, that shielded families from the scandal and turmoil that madness brought in its train. So it was that England's growing affluence in the eighteenth century gave birth to such establishments. Here were places that allowed families to rid themselves of the insufferable and impossible people who put their lives, their property, their peace of mind, and their reputations at risk. The calculus for those who were locked up was very different, though. Many patients likened the experience to being confined in a living tomb, a cemetery for the still breathing.

The mass incarceration of the seriously mad that was adopted all across Europe and North America in the nineteenth century meant that many more people found themselves inside the walls of reformed asylums. The cure rates that had been promised when advocates of the new moral treatment persuaded societies to adopt an institutional approach to the management of mental illness largely failed to materialize. Yet for over a century, these total institutions continued to absorb an ever-larger number of people. The periodic scandals that engulfed individual asylums seemed to have very little effect on the remorseless rise in the number of institutionalized patients, most of whom were committed involuntarily. Isolated and vulnerable, the lot of the mental patient was an unenviable one in many respects, especially when their stigmatization and isolation led to the orgy of experimental treatments that marked the years between 1910 and 1950. The periodic spasms of anxiety about the improper confinement of the sane and the rough treatment psychiatrists often received in the courtroom when they laid claim to expertise in the identification of mental illness in criminal defendants demonstrate that doubts about the profession's capacities were never far from the surface. But ironically, it was only as asylum populations began to collapse in the 1960s that concerns about the profession's capacity to diagnose mental illness accurately and reliably became a central and ongoing object of concern—not just outside the profession but within it as well.

The crisis of legitimacy that erupted during the 1960s has produced a series of novel attempts by the psychiatric profession to solve the problem of separating the mentally ill from the rest of us. Those responses have a common framework and have formed part of a dramatically changed psychiatric landscape—a transformation to which these concerns with diagnosis and nosology have contributed a great deal. But the very fact that the underlying issues need to be revisited every few years suggests all is not well in the state of Denmark. Though the initial major shift in diagnostic practices that was ratified in 1980 was managed with consummate political skill by its principal architect, the Columbia University psychiatrist Robert Spitzer, later revisions of the edifice he created have engendered more and more controversy. Indeed, as we will see, the adoption of the most recent "solution" to the conundrum was marked by massive professional infighting before it saw the light of day, and by devastating criticism from some of the most powerful figures in the profession when it was finally, belatedly, published.

The world before the publication in 1980 of the third edition of the APA's *Diagnostic and Statistical Manual* was not without its charms and complications. When the modern profession of psychiatry began to emerge in the nineteenth century, one of the preoccupations of many in its founding generation was the construction of new maps of the universe they sought to rule. Complicated nosologies were the order of the day. They proliferated endlessly and seemed to be of little clinical use, not least because they were so hard to operationalize. The first generally accepted subdivision of the psychoses was established in Germany in the late nineteenth century by Emil Kraepelin, who claimed to have inductively developed a distinction between two basic subtypes of serious mental disorder: dementia praecox (later relabeled schizophrenia) and manic depressive psychosis. For Kraepelin, the latter was a sort of residual category for psychotics who didn't manifest the symptoms or have the hopeless prognosis of dementia praecox, and it was generally regarded at the time as a more hopeful diagnosis. It was a testament to the wide and continuing influence of Kraepelin's endeavors that the revolution in psychiatric nomenclature launched by *DSM III* in 1980 is commonly referred to as the neo-Kraepelinian revolution in psychiatry. Both sought to transform a disorderly chaos of symptoms into an orderly list of illnesses. Kraepelin's broad-brush distinctions between major psychiatric disorders enjoyed a very long half life, and indeed it is fair to say that these distinctions still exercise a profound influence on contemporary psychiatry.

Still, the APA's diagnostic manual, in all its incarnations, introduces many more psychiatric symptoms and syndromes, and it claims to be a more comprehensive guide to the psychiatric universe. As its title indicates, *DSM III*, the third edition of the manual, had some predecessors. American psychiatrists had constructed two previous official diagnostic systems, small pamphlets that appeared in 1952 and 1968. Both set up a broad distinction between psychoses and neuroses (roughly speaking, between mental disorders that involved a break with reality and those that, less seriously, involved a distorted view of reality), and they divided up many of a hundred or so varieties of mental illnesses that were recognized in accordance with their alleged psychodynamic etiologies. In that respect, they reflected the dominance of psychoanalytic perspectives in post–World War II American psychiatry. Of marginal use bureaucratically in the large state hospitals that still housed hundreds of thousands of inmates, the first two editions of the manual had even less appeal to the psychiatrists who practiced outpatient psychiatry, who by now made up the majority of the profession. Diagnostic distinctions of the broad, general sort these first two editions set forth were irrelevant for most analysts, focused as they were on the individual dynamics of the particular patient they were treating. The first two editions of the *DSM* were therefore seldom consulted and were seen as little more than paperweights—and rather insubstantial paperweights at that. *DSM II* was a small, spiral-bound pamphlet running to no more than 134 pages and encompassing barely a hundred different diagnoses accompanied by the most cursory of descriptions. It sold for a mere $3.50, which was more than most professional psychiatrists thought it was worth.

By contrast, the current version of the manual, *DSM 5*, sells for $199, and over its expected lifetime, it will realize profits running into the tens of millions of dollars for the APA, which owns (and jealously defends) its copyright. Its immediate predecessor, the *DSM IV TR* (the "TR" stands for "text revision"), was still contributing $5 million a year to the APA's coffers as it stood on the brink of being discarded. Any mental health professional who expects to be reimbursed by an insurance company for his or her services—even clinical psychologists who reject the model of mental illness it is built on—must use the manual's categories. All patients must somehow be fitted into its preordained patterns. Choose the wrong category, and payment will be denied or reimbursement levels curtailed. But since the verbiage is vague and the categories broad and overlapping, it doesn't take much effort to find something to suit any patient. The reach of the *DSM* now extends far beyond the US borders, for drug trials and drug treatments have come to be tied to its diagnostic categories, and so non-Americans increasingly rely on it too.

This shift to a psychiatric world dominated by a book, or rather an anti-intellectual collection of categories jammed between two covers, can be dated quite precisely. The publication of *DSM III* in 1980 ushered in this so-called neo-Kraepelinian world. Each of the successive revisions of psychiatry's manual since that time has embodied its fundamental approach to the universe of mental disorder, and that view has come to completely dominate our society's approach to mental illness. Not entirely coincidentally, the appearance of *DSM III* was followed, within a few years, by the collapse of psychoanalytic hegemony in American psychiatry and its replacement by an emphasis on biology, neuroscience, and drugs.[2]

By the 1970s, psychoanalysts were bored by the whole question of how to classify mental illness, and when the APA set up the *DSM* Task Force in 1974, they treated the enterprise with disdain. In their eyes, diagnostic categories and questions of nomenclature were supremely unimportant. Their complacency would prove to be a stunning political misjudgment.

The task force quickly came to be dominated by its chairman, Robert Spitzer, and by a group of biologically oriented psychiatrists who liked to refer to themselves as DOPs (data-oriented persons), which was an interesting conceit, since data and scientific evidence had remarkably little to do with what emerged from the committee's deliberations. Instead, the work produced by the task force had much to do with the preferences and prejudices the self-anointed DOPs shared. These were psychiatrists (many of them hand-picked by Spitzer) who preferred pills to talk, and for whom creating a wholly distinctive new approach to the diagnostic process became a decisive weapon in their battle to reorient the profession. Psychoanalysts had placed but a single member of their fraternity on the major committee, and he was so swiftly marginalized that he ceased attending the sessions at which the proposed changes were discussed and finalized.

Having stacked the task force with allies who shared his desire to relink psychiatry to biology and to mainstream medicine, Spitzer was determined to eliminate the gestures toward the purported psychodynamic etiology of mental disorders that had marked the first two editions of the manual, and, indeed, to do away with the very categories of mental disorder that the psychoanalysts most depended on in their everyday practice: hysteria and the psychoneuroses and depressive neuroses. And in this he largely succeeded. Too late, the analysts realized the devastation the new manual could potentially wreak on their practice. They fought back, and as a sop, Spitzer placed some psychoanalytic terms in parentheses after the diagnoses his team had created. *DSM III* was adopted by the APA, and seven years later, when Spitzer presided over the next revision, the parenthetical diagnoses were eliminated. Psychoanalysis by then was in such sharp decline that it was incapable of resisting what had become inevitable.

Over the nearly four decades since Spitzer loosed his revolutionary text on the world, the manual has gone through a number of further revisions. The revised third edition, published in 1987, was still entrusted to him. Subsequently, Allen Frances, then chair of the Department of Psychiatry at Duke University, took over the task of creating a new version. With each edition, the size of the manual grew, and each time new disorders entered the psychiatric lexicon. Spitzer had introduced such novel diagnoses as PTSD and ADD (later renamed ADHD) and had radically reconceptualized other areas of mental disturbance, especially depression, bipolar disorder, and a whole spectrum of anxiety disorders, and his successor was similarly receptive to adding new "diseases" to the panoply. The process seems to feed on itself, even as the proliferation of diagnostic categories has encountered skepticism and ridicule in some quarters.

Post Spitzer, biology took center stage in American psychiatry. Nearly a quarter-century ago, in a decision symptomatic of this major shift in the field's orientation, President George H. W. Bush proclaimed the 1990s "the decade of the brain," and the federal government launched a campaign to unlock the organ's secrets. Neuroscience would surely at long last reveal the origins of mental illness. As that decade drew to a close, the APA began to assemble a new task force of experts to begin the long process of completely revising the criteria it uses to diagnose mental disorders. Its charge was to develop a new version of the *DSM*—one that, it was assumed, would bring our understanding of mental illness into conformity with the most recent and remarkable advances in brain science. Nearly a decade and a half later, that enormous cooperative effort, which enlisted the assistance of thousands of skilled mental health professionals, reached fruition with the publication of *DSM 5*. The partial and flawed manuals of the past were replaced by this shiny new version, running to more than a thousand pages. The revision promised to transport us into a brave new psychiatric world—one that took account of all the enormous progress that had been made in recent decades in neuroscience and psychopharmacology. Its cheerleaders expected it to mark a major step forward for the profession of psychiatry and those who need its services. So we should mark down May 22, 2013, the day the new edition was released, as a remarkable date in medical history.

Or so *DSM 5*'s architects—and the APA, which employed them and makes millions of dollars a year from peddling the enormous tome—would have you believe. But perhaps all is not quite so rosy. The objections some had raised to the manual's earlier versions have multiplied rather than diminished during the creation of this new revision and have shown no signs of abating after its publication. A long list of well-known British psychiatrists wrote an article in the *British Journal of Psychiatry* objecting vociferously to its use.[3] The leadership of the National Institute of Mental Health reacted with disdain to the new edition and announced that the agency would no longer rely on *DSM* categories when it decides where to direct its research funding. And within a few months of *DSM 5*'s publication, two books had already appeared denouncing it and attempting to undermine its credibility.

Gary Greenberg (a PhD psychotherapist) and Michael Taylor (who prefers to call himself a neuropsychiatrist) present equally scathing assaults on the new manual's value and scientific credentials, though they approach the problem of mental illness from completely opposing points of view. In *The Book of Woe: The* DSM *and the Unmaking of Psychiatry*, Greenberg is clearly deeply skeptical of psychiatry's claim "that psychological suffering is best understood as medical illness." Taylor, on the other hand, in *Hippocrates Cried: The Decline of American Psychiatry*, regards Freud as a fraud, disdains the notion that mental illness has any meaning or has its roots in meaning, and rejects the idea that mental illness can possibly by treated by addressing psychological issues. For him, mental symptoms are so much epiphenomenal noise, the surface manifestations of disorderly functioning brains that are the sole and singular source of mental troubles. Greenberg sees the attempt to reduce human woes to defective brains as a sort of category mistake (though he seems willing to cede a place for biology in the genesis of some kinds of mental disturbance). Taylor minces no words when expressing his disdain for psychotherapeutics, and psychoanalysis in particular. He uses such adjectives as "baseless," "silly," "useless," and "destructive," and he truculently asserts that "if psychodynamic therapies were medications, their support by the U.S. psychiatric establishment would be a scandal."[4] Both men, though, as I have indicated, see the *DSM* as a disaster and a psychiatry built on such foundations as a rickety, unsafe, unscientific enterprise that faces looming catastrophe. And as disorienting as some may find it to see these two agreeing on anything in view of their completely divergent starting points, they may well be right.

The new *DSM* is by its own count the fifth iteration of American psychiatry's attempt to create some order out of the chaos that mental illness is and causes. Some might quibble and call it the seventh version (a revised version of the third edition, *DSM III R*, was published in 1987; and *DSM IV TR*, which I referred to earlier, came out in 2000). But let us keep the count at five for simplicity's sake, and note only that in its most recent incarnation, the manual has moved from Roman numerals to the Arabic numbering system the rest of us use, except when trying pretentiously to elevate the importance of Super Bowls. This is not because its architects wanted to avoid pretension, though that would have been a laudable goal, but because they wanted to borrow from the conventions of the software industry and pave the way for interim revisions: no more III Rs or IV TRs; now we can switch to *DSM 5.1, DSM 5.2,* and so on.

The advent of the *DSM III* world was a response to a political and epistemological crisis in American psychiatry. In a Cold War context, much was being made of the way the Soviets were stretching the boundaries of mental illness to label dissidents as mad, thus licensing their incarceration and forcible medication.[5] But Western voices also began to look askance at their own profession and to allege that the psychiatric emperor had no clothes. In 1961, a renegade psychiatrist, Thomas Szasz, published a best-selling broadside called *The Myth of Mental Illness*,[6] in which he suggested that psychiatrists were pernicious agents of social control who locked up inconvenient people on behalf of a society that was eager to be rid of them. "Mental illness," he alleged, had the same ontological status as the label "witch" that had been employed in prior centuries. Illness, on his account, was a purely biological phenomenon, a demonstrable part of the natural world. Mental illness, by contrast, was a misplaced metaphor, a socially constructed way of permitting an ever-wider selection of behaviors to be forcibly controlled, all under the guise of helping people.

The problem was exacerbated when some psychiatrists sought to examine the diagnostic process. The data that these people produced were disturbing and dramatically reinforced the growing suspicion that their profession's claims to expertise were spurious. Prominent figures such as Aaron Beck, Robert Spitzer, M. G. Sandifer, and Benjamin Pasaminick published systematic findings that dramatized just how tenuous agreement was among psychiatrists about the nature of psychiatric pathology.[7] Whether the subjects were patients in state hospitals or people being treated in outpatient settings, agreement between two psychiatrists rarely reached 50 percent. The profession was soon deeply embarrassed again when a careful study of comparative diagnostic practices of psychiatrists in London and New York showed a stunningly wide discrepancy between the two groups: New York psychiatrists diagnosed nearly 62 percent of their patients as schizophrenic, while in London only 34 percent received this diagnosis. And while less than 5 percent of the New York patients were diagnosed with depressive psychoses, the corresponding figure in London was 24 percent. Further examination of the patients suggested that these differences were byproducts of the preferences and prejudices of each group of psychiatrists, and yet the diagnoses resulted in consequential differences in treatment.[8] Science in the modern world is supposed to travel. Here it clearly did not.

And this chaotic situation was not hidden from a larger public. In the legal profession, the civil rights movement of the 1960s led to the emergence of public interest law. A number of these attorneys broadened their focus from race to include other stigmatized and disadvantaged populations. In the early 1970s, a mental health bar was created, two of whose prominent practitioners, Bruce Ennis and Thomas Litwack, seized on the results reported in the aforementioned studies. They intimated that psychiatrists should no longer be credited with the status of "expert witnesses" since their judgments amounted to little more than "flipping coins in the courtroom."[9]

Drug companies, who were by now making huge profits from drugs designed to treat mental illness (the first so-called antipsychotic, Thorazine, had been marketed in 1954 and had catapulted its owner, Smith, Kline and French, into the first rank of pharmaceutical houses),[10] were increasingly disturbed by this state of affairs: How could they develop profitable new compounds, and persuade the FDA to allow them to come to market, if they could not find homogeneous (or apparently homogeneous) groups of patients to assign to placebo groups and active treatment groups? This problem grew more urgent as the years passed and larger and larger numbers of patients were needed across a multitude of cross-national sites to generate the slight differences in statistical (not clinical) significance that were needed to secure regulatory approval. When drug effects are large and unambiguous, small groups suffice to generate statistically significant results. When effects are comparatively tiny, as is generally the case in the psychiatric realm, larger and larger samples are needed. The more trials that are conducted, the higher the probability that a couple of them, by chance, will be positive, which is all that is needed to secure FDA approval. Meanwhile, the data on failed trials can be buried—though not always securely, as we will see.[11]

Worse was ahead. In 1973, as mentioned in chapter 12, a Stanford social psychologist, David Rosenhan, published a paper that purported to put psychiatry's diagnostic acumen to the test. He claimed to have recruited a number of pseudopatients, screened them to exclude anyone with a prior history of psychiatric disorder, and instructed them to show up at a local mental health facility complaining they were hearing voices that were saying things like "empty" and "thud." Otherwise, they were to behave completely normally and await developments. All of them, on his account, were admitted as inpatients and diagnosed as psychotic, most as schizophrenic, an extremely grave diagnosis implying an unfavorable prognosis. The other patients, the paper reported, recognized that the pseudo patients were faking their illness. Doctors did not. Many were eventually discharged as having "schizophrenia in remission," but one patient had to be rescued after several weeks as confinement dragged on, seemingly without end.

Reported in the august pages of *Science*, the most important general circulation science journal published in North America, under the title "On Being Sane in Insane Places," Rosenhan's study caused a furor.[12] In vain, psychiatrists complained that the study was unfair and methodologically flawed. They were flayed in the court of public opinion as charlatans who were incapable of making even basic judgments about health and illness. Psychiatric diagnosis seemed a joke, an arbitrary business with horrendous potential consequences for those given a psychiatric label. And if psychiatrists were incapable of judging who was mad and who was sane, why should anyone think they were any better at treating patients? The legitimacy of the entire profession hung in the balance.

Recent work by a determined and highly talented New York investigative journalist, Susannah Cahalan, suggests that the critics of Rosenhan's study were insufficiently critical.[13] For example, Rosenhan's own clinical records, which Cahalan obtained from his files, show that his published account of his own pseudopatient experience (he was a participant in his own experiment) is falsified in many crucial respects, including very significant discrepancies from his published account of his presenting symptoms.

Cahalan's own attempts to secure documents related to the peer review of Rosenhan's paper were ignored by *Science*. I offered to help. We both hoped that my position as a scholar might produce a different result. With Cahalan's permission, I wrote to *Science* requesting copies of the peer review of Rosenhan's paper, noting that the names of the referees could be redacted if the journal felt impelled to do that. We were seeking answers to a number of specific questions about the vetting of the paper. My inquiry to Monica Bradford, the current editor of *Science*, was designed to secure the basic information Cahalan sought, and it read in part:

> There is much to worry about in reading [Rosenhan's] paper 40 odd years on. The pseudo-patients who are the key to the paper's explosive findings are anonymized, as are the institutions where they apparently sought admission. While understandable on some levels, this means that the author's fundamental honesty has to be taken on trust—a trust that was greatly bolstered by the prestige of the journal where these results were published—

yours. As someone deeply committed to the peer review process, I both understand its limits and also the need for anonymity to protect referees. But in this instance in particular, it seems to me to be of great importance to understand the basis on which *Science* accepted the paper for publication, and what the peer reviewers saw and requested to see. Did the journal check on the identity, even the very existence of the pseudo-patients? Were they made aware of which mental hospitals had supposedly admitted them? Did they verify the account Professor Rosenhan provided of how long they remained patients or what the attending psychiatrists had to say in their case notes? These are all matters of great moment, and at present all one has to go on are the apparently uncorroborated statements of an academic whose entire career was built on this single foundation.

Would it be possible for you to share redacted versions of the referees' reports with me, removing anything that might identify them? Could you or someone else on your staff also enlighten me on what steps, if any, *Science* took to ensure the validity of Dr. Rosenhan's work? Given the extraordinary real world impact of this paper, these are questions that really need to be answered satisfactorily. Dr. Rosenhan published no other work of comparable importance in his career, and I find what appears in the public record less than fully convincing. Given all the current controversy swirling around the replicability of findings in psychology and economics, these issues have even greater salience, and it seems to me, as one of the leading journals for the sciences, *Science* itself has a vested interest, indeed an obligation, to look closely into the verifiability of these reported findings.[14]

It turns out that the Columbia psychiatrist Robert Spitzer, who engaged in spirited private correspondence with David Rosenhan at around the time the paper was published, sought answers to some of the same questions, only to be rebuffed. As Cahalan's researches showed, Rosenhan wrote back declining to answer: he refused to supply case records or to name the institutions to which the alleged pseudopatients had been admitted. "I am," he contended, "obliged to protect these sources."[15] Two weeks after receiving my inquiry, Monica Bradford wrote to inform me that she could not answer the questions either: "We do not have manuscript/peer review records from that time period."[16]

In my view, that leaves us with serious doubts about the truth of Rosenhan's claims. It would not be the first time *Science* (like other journals) has been deceived.[17] But such queries decades after the fact are irrelevant, of course, to the question of the paper's impact at the time and for many years following its appearance. As I noted in my correspondence with Monica Bradford, "Rosenhan's study played an absolutely critical role in discrediting the ability of psychiatrists to diagnose mental illness reliably. As such, it did much to persuade the American Psychiatric Association to revamp its diagnostic and statistical manual. *DSM III* in turn radically altered the future direction of American and world psychiatry, helping to bring about the virtual collapse of psychoanalytic psychiatry and ushering in the current era where biological psychiatry dominates research and therapeutics for mental illness."

For Spitzer, paradoxically, Rosenhan's study and the extraordinary publicity it received was manna from heaven. It provided the final impetus for a project he had been agitating to conduct for some time. The next year, he was commissioned to set up a task force of the APA charged with overhauling psychiatry's approach to diagnosis. Spitzer and the team he recruited now went to work. In many respects, their efforts must be judged a remarkable success. Early on, they disdained any concern with validity—that is, with making sure that the distinctions they drew up corresponded to real differences out there in the world or, to put it another way, that they were cutting nature at the joints. Few of us doubt that the distinctions between, say, pneumonia and tuberculosis are grounded in real pathological differences between the two diseases and real internal commonalities in the pathology of each. We would be wise not to invest as much confidence in differences between psychiatric labels. But if validity was to be set aside, reliability—the statistically demonstrable ability of any two clinicians confronted with the same patient to assign him or her the same diagnostic category—most certainly was not. This was where Spitzer and his team concentrated their efforts.

Unable to demonstrate convincing chains of causation for any major form of mental disorder, the Spitzer task force abandoned any pretense of doing so. Instead, they concentrated on maximizing inter-rater reliability—that is, the degree of agreement between psychiatrists when diagnosing the same patient. Spitzer's team developed lists of symptoms that allegedly characterized different forms of mental disturbance and used that list to create a tick-the-boxes approach to diagnosis. Faced with a new patient, psychiatrists would record the presence or absence of a given set of symptoms, and once a threshold number of these had been reached, the person they were examining was given a particular diagnostic label, with comorbidity invoked to explain away situations where more than one condition could be diagnosed. Alternatively, one could set up a hierarchy of psychiatric diseases and award the patient the most serious of them. Disputes about what belonged in the manual were resolved by committee vote, as was the arbitrary decision about where to situate cut-off points: that is, how many of the laundry list of symptoms a patient had to exhibit before he or she was declared to be suffering from a particular form of illness. Questions of validity were simply set to one side. If diagnoses could be rendered mechanical and predictable, consistent and replicable, that would suffice.

To accomplish their ends, the *DSM III* Task Force thus adopted a mechanical approach to assigning illness labels. If a patient exhibited any six of a list of ten symptoms—voilà, he or she was a schizophrenic. Why six? Well, as Spitzer later put it, that felt about right. Tick another set of boxes and you had general anxiety disorder, and so on. How many categories of illness to accept, and which ones? Here, there was much politicking at work. And so the number of mental illnesses proliferated, a process that has continued unchecked all the way up to the publication of *DSM 5,* which for the first time contains such new "diseases" as hoarding disorder, disruptive mood dysregulation disorder (proneness to outbreaks of violent, uncontrollable rage), and, listed in an appendix, attenuated psychosis symptom syndrome, a category particularly likely to be applied to young children that supposedly identifies those likely to become full-blown psychotics, though the vast majority of children so labeled do not proceed down that pathway.[18] With each iteration, the manual has grown larger, and the range of human behavior brought within the ambit of the psychiatric profession has grown ever more extensive. The latest version, for example, controversially erases a distinction between bereavement and depression, accentuating the danger, as other critics have commented, that ordinary sadness and other human emotions will be pathologized and then treated with powerful, dangerous (and profitable)—but not necessarily effective—pills.[19] Pills that are certainly not some sort of psychiatric penicillin.

DSM III's triumph marked the advent of a classificatory system that increasingly linked diagnostic categories to specific drug treatments, and of an embrace on the part of both the profession of psychiatry and the public of a conceptualization of mental illnesses as specific, identifiably different diseases, each amenable to treatment with different drugs. In subsequent years, particularly once antidepressant drugs took off in the 1990s, biological language saturated professional and public discussions of mental illness. In 2005, Steven Sharfstein, the president of the APA at the time, referred to the upshot of this process as the transition from "the biopsychosocial model [of mental illness] to . . . the bio-bio-bio model."[20]

That the specificity of the treatments was largely spurious, and that the various editions of the *DSM* from the third edition onward emphasized reliability and essentially ignored the more central issue of the validity of psychiatric diagnoses, proved largely irrelevant to the manual's success in reorienting perceptions, lay and professional alike. Linked to expanded insurance coverage for the treatment of mental disorders, and providing a new grounding for psychiatric authority and a less time-consuming and more lucrative foundation for psychiatric practice, psychopharmacology encouraged a distancing of psychiatrists from the provision of psychotherapy. And because of the seemingly scientific basis of the labels, the consistency with which cases are judged, and the translation of human judgment by means of this verbal alchemy into statistics, the multiplication of the anxious and the nervous, as with other psychiatric casualties, has proceeded in relentless fashion.

In 1994, a task force led by Allen Frances published the fourth edition of the *DSM*. In many respects, it followed dutifully in Spitzer's footsteps, though it included new diagnoses and broadened and weakened the criteria that had to be met for any particular diagnosis to be assigned. Frances would later issue a mea culpa, claiming that the epidemics of autism and depression that followed the issuance of *DSM IV* were largely iatrogenic, the product of a series of well-intentioned mistakes on his part that served to greatly expand the numbers of children diagnosed with autism. It would prove a highly controversial assertion, sparking angry responses not just from fellow psychiatrists but also from the families of patients with children diagnosed with Asperger's syndrome or autism. Parents saw him as belittling or denying the troubles and difficulties they and their offspring faced, and as threatening their access to needed social and educational services, since that access was dependent on their children's diagnosis.[21]

At times, the vituperation that rained down on Frances's head was extraordinary. It is hard not to form a mental image of families all across the country sticking pins into a Frances voodoo doll. Whatever other lessons are derived from this state of affairs, one point is obvious, but it nonetheless deserves emphasis: neither professional imperialism on the part of psychiatrists nor the greedy machinations of Big Pharma can singlehandedly explain the burgeoning problem of mental disorder in early twenty-first-century America. Patients and their families are also deeply implicated in these developments.

DSM 5 was supposed to be different from its predecessors. Those put in charge of producing it announced that the logic that had underpinned the two previous versions was deeply flawed and declared that they would fix things. Drawing on the findings of neuroscience and genetics, they would move away from the symptom-based system that they now acknowledged was inadequate and build a manual that linked mental disorders to brain function. They would also take account of the fact that mental disorder is a dimensional, not categorical, issue; it is a matter of being more or less sane, not a black and white world with sanity in this corner and mental illness in that. It was a grand ambition. The only problem was that these goals were impossible to achieve. All the pretty pictures conjured up by neuroscientists playing with fMRI images could not and did not provide what the architects of the *DSM* needed. Crude measures of blood flow to different regions of the brain (which is what fMRI images display) were a poor substitute for tying together behavioral symptoms and brain defects in a robust causal fashion. And genetics wasn't any better at providing the necessary answers. Having thrashed about at the outset pursuing this chimera, those running the task force were ultimately forced to concede defeat, and by 2009 they were back to tinkering with the descriptive approach.

Then the fun began. The architects of *DSM III* and *DSM IV,* who had built their careers on this very approach, undertook an increasingly fierce attack on the work of their successors. Robert Spitzer began the assault, but he was ailing from a bad case of Parkinson's disease. Soon the cause was taken up by Allen Frances, who had retired to Southern California to take care of his wife, who was sadly stricken by the same disorder as Spitzer. Frances proved a tenacious critic who soon moved beyond purely intraprofessional criticism to launch a sustained campaign of vilification in the mainstream media. Relentlessly, he and Spitzer attacked the science (or lack of science) that lay behind the proposed revisions and raised warnings that these revisions would further encourage psychiatry's tendency to pathologize normal human behaviors.[22] For orthodox psychiatrists, it was a deeply embarrassing spectacle. It is one thing to be attacked by Tom Cruise and the Scientologists, who can be dismissed as a vicious cult, but quite another to come under withering assault from one's own. Wounded, the leaders of American psychiatry struck back with ad hominem attacks, alleging that Spitzer and Frances were clinging to past glories and going so far as to suggest that the latter, by far the more energetic of the two, was motivated by the potential loss of $10,000 a year in royalties he still collected from *DSM IV*.[23] (Left unmentioned was how dependent their professional association had become on the many millions of dollars in royalties a new edition promised to provide.) The prolonged spat forced a delay in the issuance of the new manual, but it seems to have done little to alter *DSM 5*'s basic structure and contents.

All this suggests a profession in crisis. One particular diagnosis of the nature of that crisis, and a suggested way forward for the profession, is offered by Michael Taylor, who suggests the need for a re-engagement with biology, coupled with an insistence on psychiatry's exclusively medical identity. As far as he is concerned, such a reorganization of the profession has not happened to date. Consequently, his book is a lament, as its subtitle indicates, for "the decline of American psychiatry." It is an interesting notion, because to speak of a decline suggests that once upon a time—who knows quite when—the profession was in healthy shape, only to have since fallen victim to bad choices and to have lapsed from its previous state of grace.

True or not, Michael Taylor's cri de cœur is for a world he claims we have lost. His is a very personal story that mixes large quantities of personal experience and partially disguised anecdotes about individual patients with some sweeping characterizations of a whole series of changes in the psychiatric universe. Virtually all of these changes, if he is to be believed, are changes for the worse, betrayals of the one true path that ought to have characterized his profession. But the arduous path of true psychiatric science has been ignored by everyone except Michael Taylor and a handful of other enlightened psychiatrists (or neuropsychiatrists, as he would prefer that we call them). Taylor's first chapter is titled "The Origins of Indignation," and his book is in many ways an unrelieved jeremiad.

But in this case, it is hard to know quite where to locate the missing golden age. Certainly it did not exist when Taylor joined the profession in the 1960s, the last decade of the psychoanalytic dominance he deeply deplores. Nor can it be found, as he is at pains to make clear, in the years since.

At one point in his reflections, he does suggest a time and a place for his psychiatric paradise. Astonishingly (at least so far as this psychiatric historian is concerned) he points to the late nineteenth century as that paradise lost. During this period, he asserts, "U.S. psychiatry, at least in the Northeastern part of the country, was as good as any in the world."[24] The narrow geographical focus is, I think, an attempt to make plausible what otherwise would seem a bizarre claim. After all, as the nineteenth century drew to a close, America's mental hospitals, like their counterparts elsewhere, were widely seen as little more than cemeteries for the still breathing. The alienists who ran them (the term "psychiatrist" had not yet been embraced by the asylum superintendents) explained that mental illness was hereditary and hopeless; their charges were a bunch of degenerates; and the primary justification for vast mental hospitals was that they were a crude way of isolating these defectives and preventing them from reproducing more of their own kind. That sort of late nineteenth-century psychiatry would be an odd sort of Nirvana.

In the northeastern United States, however, a new group of specialists had emerged in the aftermath of the Civil War, and these men appear to be the object of Taylor's veneration. They called themselves neurologists, and, like Taylor and his embattled coterie of the enlightened in the early twenty-first century, they "understood behavioral symptoms to be reflections of brain or nervous disorder. The medical model of diagnosis prevailed," and psychiatric disorders were seen "as reflections of different brain diseases that were only awaiting the detailing of their neuropathology."[25] Here is "the neuropsychiatric alternative" that is the otherwise obscure object of Taylor's desire and the foundation for the prescription he has to offer his profession as it seeks a way forward out of what he regards as its current epistemological and clinical swamp.

This choice is still, I think, a curious one, and not just because we are still waiting—like the poor folks waiting for Godot—for those mysterious and long rumored neuropathological causes of mental illness to surface. After all, Taylor's heroes—he seems particularly enamored of William Hammond and Edward Spitzka—had no scientific warrant for their claims that mental illnesses were brain diseases. Theirs were claims based on faith, wagers on what medical science would discover at some uncertain point in the future. They are wagers that have yet to pay off (save in the important case of the syphilitic origins of what used to be called general paralysis of the insane). The same objection can be raised about Taylor's assertion that he knows the one true way forward for his profession. As for the therapeutics of the golden age—those fin-de-siècle gentlemen's prescriptions for their "brain diseased" patients—they ran the gamut from shiny machines made of polished brass and chrome that delivered jolts of static electricity to stimulate the nerves to periods of enforced bed rest and high-calorie diets that were meant to build up "fat and blood" and restore the elasticity of the nervous system, not to mention the nerve tonics and the extracts from animals' testicles that William Hammond peddled on a large and profitable scale to his many anxious patients.

That would be an odd sort of golden age.

Leaving Taylor's unrequited quest aside, how does he justify the claim that his profession is in decline? As I've suggested, if Taylor loathed the psychoanalytically inclined profession he joined in the 1960s, he is no more enchanted by what has succeeded it. In his eyes, the *DSM* from the third edition forward—and of course the less said about its Freudian predecessors the better—has been "a political rather than a scientific document. . . . The process was and is very much like congress writing legislation. The procedure is messy and the results are wanting. Instead of 'earmarks' we have new never validated labels and distinctions, such as shared psychotic disorder, identity disorder, schizophreniform disorder, bipolar I, II, III as separate diseases, and many other 'bridges to nowhere.'"[26] Diagnoses have proliferated, according to Taylor, but not because of any advances in the profession's scientific understanding of mental illness: "The explosion of diagnoses . . . is a fabrication of the political process. . . . The pharmaceutical industry adores the explosion of conditions, because as 'medical diagnoses' the *DSM* categories provide the rationale for prescribing drugs."[27]

Most outside observers looking at American psychiatry since 1980 see a profession seemingly wedded to biological reductionism, one that insists that all mental illness is rooted in the brain and is thus a disease like any other. But Taylor is convinced that these assertions are no more than ideological window dressing. There is no serious attempt, he asserts, to pay proper attention to brain pathology and to connect it to the diagnostic process and to treatment. Residents are not trained as they should be, and they still get instruction in the ridiculous enterprise that is psychotherapy—which he dismisses as a useless form of treatment that they generally don't use much when they become professional adults. In day-to-day practice, his colleagues have become wedded to a descriptive manual that is founded on pseudoscience and have sold out to the blandishments of the drug companies, becoming little more than glorified pill pushers.

One dimension of the penetration of psychiatry by Big Pharma is the sheer number of practitioners who depend on industry funding for their research. One questions the independence of the judgments brought to bear by the *DSM* Task Force when one learns that of those in the group working on mood disorders, 100 percent had financial ties to the drug industry, while in the groups working on anxiety disorders, it was "only" 80 percent. Close relationships between clinicians and industry remain the norm, and even the top medical journals make no serious effort to police rampant failures to disclose these potential conflicts of interest.[28] The incestuous relationship between academic psychiatry and the pharmaceutical companies has intensified, in fact, in recent years: while 57 percent of the *DSM IV* Task Force had connections to the drug industry, 80 percent of the *DSM 5* Task Force had ties to it. And although this pattern is not unique to psychiatry, it is particularly pernicious here because of the subjectivity that surrounds the very definition of what constitutes psychiatric illnesses. Just how troubled we should be by the extent of these relationships and the conscious and unconscious bias they may introduce into the reported outcomes of drug trials is suggested by the systematic research on the connections between the published results of supposedly double-blind clinical trials of new drugs and the sources of the funds underpinning the research.[29]

Unsurprisingly, as Taylor reports, in the latest iteration of the *DSM*, "Guidelines were weakened for identifying several conditions, raising concerns that the mental health system would be overwhelmed by persons meeting the new diagnostic criteria but who would not be ill. Standards for acceptable reliability were also watered down so that the present field trials of the proposed system yielded results that were worse than what was experienced in previous versions, including *DSM III*. The watering down will help the pharmaceutical industry because as more persons are identified as ill, the justification grows for increased numbers of prescriptions."[30]

The problem runs deeper than professional corruption, however. In at least one highly publicized instance, a preliminary draft of *DSM 5* proposed to tighten a set of definitions. The label of autism, along with a number of related "illnesses," was to be replaced by the global category of "autism spectrum disorders," and in the process, Asperger's syndrome, a widely used diagnosis, was slated to disappear, meaning that many people presently with such a diagnosis would have found themselves cast adrift. For these patients and their families, the loss of the label threatened what they viewed as catastrophic consequences, since access to an array of publicly funded social and educational services is conditional on having the requisite medical diagnosis. The backlash was predictable and fierce. It turns out that it is easy to broaden the criteria of psychiatric disability. Reversing the process, however, is extraordinarily hard.

In fact, as some troubling passages in Gary Greenberg's book make clear, the insidious and corrupting influence of Big Pharma and its allies on the practice of psychiatry runs much deeper than its influence on the manuals themselves. Not content with the vast array of "diseases" they were already licensed to identify, "opinion leaders"—prominent academic physicians—have constructed still more disorders from which to profit. A particular target of Greenberg's ire is Joseph Biederman, a leading child psychiatrist at Harvard, who, together with his associates, masterminded the construction of childhood bipolar disorder and then began to prescribe particularly dangerous and often life-threatening drugs to children off-label—that is, without even a modicum of testing for safety and efficacy in such patients.[31]

It is one of the peculiarities of American medicine that once drugs have undergone the long and expensive process of being licensed for one purpose, clinicians may prescribe them casually for others, despite the lack of scientific data to warrant such practices. Drug companies themselves are forbidden to overtly endorse this practice—more on that anon—so the workaround has been to get opinion leaders to tout the off-label uses and encourage their sheep-like followers (and desperate consumers who are eager to find new remedies for the troubles they are grappling with) to embrace the new magic bullet. Biederman, Charles Nemeroff (who was a member of the psychiatry department at Emory University from 1991 to 2009), and Alan Schatzberg (a professor at Stanford and the 116th president of the APA) exemplify the ways this sort of behavior has become the norm, even among the most prominent members of the profession. Grant moneys and long lists of publications in prominent journals are the currency of the realm in our modern knowledge factories, and universities have come to reward rather than sanction activities that may prompt ethical qualms in other quarters.

Ironically, it was Schatzberg, during his year as APA president in 2009, who responded vehemently to Allen Frances's criticisms of the work of the *DSM 5* task force by pointing to the $10,000 in royalties Frances was still receiving from *DSM IV* and claiming that this was a major reason for his complaints. Apparently, the $4.8 million in stock options Schatzberg had in a drug development company and the large fees he received from such companies as Pfizer had no similar distorting effect on his judgment. Likewise, we are supposed to believe that the $960,000 Charles Nemeroff received to support his research from GlaxoSmithKline (although he reported only $35,000 to his university) had no influence on him whatsoever; and that the millions of dollars that Biederman and his associates at Harvard received for creating a new diagnosis and a massive new market for antidepressants and second-generation antipsychotics (drugs associated with massive weight gain, metabolic disorders, diabetes, and premature death) among young children had no impact on their behavior.[32] Greenberg quotes the Columbia child psychiatrist David Shaffer of Columbia on the epidemic Biederman helped to create: "Biederman was a crook. He borrowed a disease and applied it in a chaotic fashion. He came up with ridiculous data that none of us believed"—but that was swallowed wholesale by many in the media and by desperate parents. "It brought child psychiatry into disrepute and was a terrible burden on the families of the children who got that label."[33]

It is interesting to observe how the elite universities on whose faculty these individuals served responded to these revelations. Harvard launched an internal inquiry into Biederman's ties to the drug industry that funded him. University regulations prohibited researchers running drug trials from accepting more than $10,000 a year from the companies whose products were being assessed. It turned out that Biederman and his team, while claiming to have abided by this regulation, had received a total of $4.2 million. Harvard and the Massachusetts General Hospital announced that these violations were to result in "appropriate remedial actions." The academics involved, they decided, should be banned from participating in "industry-sponsored outside activities" for a year, and there would be an unspecified delay in considering them for promotion. A decade later, Biederman remains at his post at Harvard, as influential as ever.[34]

Stanford launched its own in-house investigation, under pressure from Charles Grassley, the United States senator from Iowa, whose subcommittee had brought these drug company connections to light. It absolved Schatzberg of violating university policy, and he is still at Stanford (though, perhaps coincidentally, perhaps not, he ceased chairing its department of psychiatry in 2010).

Charles Nemeroff had faced ethical complaints on two other occasions before the Grassley hearings. Emory University had launched an investigation of his outside consulting arrangements in 2004 and had found "multiple 'serious' and 'significant' violations of regulations intended to protect patients." He had, for instance, failed to disclose conflicts of interest in trials of drugs from Merck, Eli Lilly, and Johnson & Johnson. Nothing came of this internal university report. In 2006, Nemeroff favorably reviewed a controversial medical device in a medical journal he edited, neglecting to mention that he had financial ties to Cyberonics, the company that made it. When a university dean called him to account for producing a "piece of paid marketing" that purported to be an academic paper, Nemeroff blamed the episode on a "clerical error." No action appears to have been taken. Earlier, when concerns had arisen about Nemeroff's membership on a dozen corporate advisory boards, he had responded by reminding the university of the benefits *it* derived from the arrangement: "Surely you remember that Smith-Kline Beecham Pharmaceuticals donated an endowed chair to the department and that there is some reasonable likelihood that Janssen Pharmaceuticals will do so as well. In addition, Wyeth-Ayerst Pharmaceuticals has funded a Research Career Development Award program in the department, and I have asked both AstraZeneca Pharmaceuticals and Bristol-Meyers [*sic*] Squibb to do the same."[35]

Emory adopted a different response to Nemeroff's actions only in the aftermath of intense political pressure from the United States Senate, and from Senator Chuck Grassley in particular. Grassley's staff had discovered that, while overseeing a federal grant designed to evaluate a GlaxoSmithKline drug, Nemeroff had received more than $960,000 from the company. Of this, he had disclosed only $35,000 to Emory. The public relations damage to the university was something that might have been manageable. More serious was the threat that its access to federal grant money might be curtailed or eliminated. Action was finally forthcoming: Nemeroff was stripped of his department chairmanship (a highly unusual step in academic medicine) and forbidden to accept more drug company largesse. Not long afterward, he left the university. He promptly resurfaced, however, as chair of psychiatry at the University of Miami.

Research universities depend for their very existence on the constant flow of research dollars into the institution. Their levels of funding from other sources are grossly inadequate to sustain their operations. The Nemeroffs, the Biedermans, and the Schatzbergs of the academic world are experts at securing millions of dollars to fund their research, and those grants come with 50 to 60 percent overhead charges that accrue to the university budgets. It is no wonder that America's research universities have learned to turn a blind eye to ethical failings if the money on offer is sufficiently tempting. As these scandals proliferate, however, they threaten to inflict major damage on the legitimacy of psychiatry and on the medical-industrial complex more generally. University research and the endorsement of particular therapeutic interventions by leading academics are valuable because they reflect disinterested, "pure" science. If this isn't the case, they lose that value.

If this pattern of behavior provides ample support for Taylor's claim that his is a profession in crisis, the problems facing contemporary psychiatry do not stop there. Antipsychotic and antidepressant drugs routinely rank among the top five most profitable classes of prescription drugs on the planet, and, as always, the great bulk of those profits are earned in the United States. In pursuit of them, the multinational drug industry has been both ruthless and unscrupulous. There has been much talk in recent years about evidence-based medicine, but for such an approach to work, the evidence has to be what it seems. And it is not.

The double-blind controlled trials we rely on to assess the worth of new medications are increasingly funded exclusively by major drug companies. The plaintiffs' bar in America's unusual legal system has periodically exposed the consequences that flow from this situation. The corporations own the data. They manipulate the data. They conceal the data they don't like and that are at odds with their interests. Their public relations staffs ghostwrite scientific papers that then appear in the most prestigious medical journals—*Journal of the American Medical Association, New England Journal of Medicine, The Lancet*—with the names of the most prominent academic researchers appended.[36] Data about side effects, even fatal side effects, are suppressed and hidden and have seen the light of day only occasionally through the discovery process provided by class action lawsuits.[37] Meanwhile, direct-to-consumer advertising increasingly drives drug sales, and neither physicians nor their patients seem to grasp or act on the difference between statistical significance and clinical significance. This whole sorry aspect of the mess that is contemporary psychiatry is at best mentioned in passing by Greenberg and Taylor, but it has recently been dissected at length by David Healy, an Anglo-Irish psychiatrist who ranks high on Big Pharma's most-hated list. His *Pharmagedon* deserves much more attention than it has received to date.[38]

Problems of this sort are most certainly not unique to psychiatry, as anyone who recalls the scandals over the Vioxx painkiller or the more recent revelations about the chief medical officer at Memorial Sloan Kettering Cancer Center, will know.[39] But they have been a notable feature of the psychiatric landscape over the past decade, creating an avalanche of bad publicity and leading on occasion to the award of huge damages. GlaxoSmithKline, for example, pled guilty to criminal charges and paid $3 billion to settle charges of consumer fraud in the marketing of its antidepressant Paxil, whose annual sales, it should be noted, were $2.7 billion.[40] Pfizer paid $430,000 in damages in a single lawsuit over its illegal promotion of off-label use of Neurontin, an anti-seizure drug, for psychiatric disorders—a campaign that had propelled the drug to $2.7 billion in sales in 2003—and subsequent lawsuits brought the total paid out to $945 million.[41] Bristol-Myers Squibb settled similar claims in 2007 about its marketing of its drug Abilify, a so-called atypical antipsychotic, for $519 million.[42] Johnson & Johnson was fined $2.2 billion for concealing the risks of weight gain, diabetes, and stroke associated with its antipsychotic drug Rispidal.[43] And these are not isolated instances. Other lawsuits, for example, have brought to light the deliberate suppression of data pointing to a higher risk of suicide among children and adolescents taking selective serotonin reuptake inhibitors (SSRIs), the most widely prescribed group of antidepressants, despite years of denials by Big Pharma that such data or risks existed.[44]

Perhaps these awards, and the associated unfavorable publicity, help to explain why Big Pharma now seems reluctant to fund much further research in psychopharmacology and has sharply cut the financial subventions it used to provide to the APA. Greenberg reports that the APA's "income from the drug industry, which amounted to more than $19 million in 2006, had shrunk to $11 million by 2009, and was projected to fall even more. . . . [In addition,] journal advertising by the drug companies was off by 50 percent from its 2006 high."[45]

From a variety of perspectives, the APA's decision to issue yet another flawed version of its *DSM* constituted a huge gamble. The organization had built a vast and ramshackle superstructure on impossibly frail foundations, and it had to be praying that the whole Rube Goldberg contraption didn't come tumbling down. Like most prayers, this one went unanswered—or perhaps it has received an answer that the organization's sins deserve: prominently reported statements from Thomas Insel, the then director of the profession's academic paymaster, the NIMH, and from his immediate predecessor, Steven Hyman, publicly denouncing the new manual as an unmitigated unscientific disaster; calling its most basic diagnostic categories illusions and artificial constructs that need to be abandoned; and urging psychiatry to reject the whole approach *DSM 5* embodied.[46]

Robert Spitzer and Allen Francis, not to mention Michael Taylor and Gary Greenberg, appear to have found sympathetic ears for their criticisms, although it is a bit more complicated than that. Insel, I think, would have no truck with the approaches to mental disorders that underlie Gary Greenberg's critique. His sympathies lie firmly with the brand of neuropsychiatry that Michael Taylor argues is the way forward for the profession: one that places an emphasis on the putative biological bases of mental disorder, to the exclusion of any other approach. It is a pretty fantasy, one that aligns nicely with President Obama's announcement on April 2, 2013, that he planned to fund a $100 million initiative—BRAIN, or Brain Research through Advancing Innovative Neurotechnologies—to unlock the "enormous mystery" of the human brain. There's only one problem: as yet we lack even the rudiments of the knowledge we would need to reconstruct psychiatry on such a biological foundation. We don't even possess enough knowledge to allow us to put all our eggs safely in this basket. Indeed, many of us would agree with Gary Greenberg that it is highly unlikely that the complexities of mental illness can be reduced to such crude oversimplifications.

Where should the profession turn? Descriptive psychiatry is in shambles, as both Taylor's and Greenberg's books help to show, and as the events of May 2013 have made even more dramatically obvious. But it has, at present, no plausible rival. Psychiatry confronts an impossible bind.

Speaking to Greenberg some months before the new edition of the manual finally appeared, Insel—the selfsame person who had given his official thumbs down to *DSM 5*—commented casually that most of his psychiatric colleagues "actually believe [that the diseases they diagnose using the *DSM*] are real. But there's no reality. These are just constructs. There is no reality to schizophrenia or depression. . . . We might have to stop using terms like depression and schizophrenia, because they are getting in our way, confusing things."[47] Remarks like these seem to suggest the diagnosis of mental disorders is bereft of all scientific validity, nothing more than a con game. Scientologists and their ilk must be rubbing their hands with glee.

Imagine a world like the one Insel seems to invite, in which psychiatrists actually leveled with us about the limits of their knowledge. Greenberg has outlined such a thought experiment: "What would happen," he asks, "if [psychiatrists] told you that they don't know what illness (if any) is causing your anxiety or depression, or agitation, and then, if they thought it was warranted, told you that there are drugs that might help (although they don't really know why or at what cost to your brain, or whether you will be able to stop taking them if you want to; nor can they guarantee that you (or your child) won't become obese or diabetic, or die early), and offer you a prescription [for these substances]."[48] Psychiatry's status is precarious enough as it is. One can only guess to what depths it might sink in a world like that one.

Perhaps on reflection both doctors and patients would prefer to cling to their illusions. But it seems they may not be able to do so for much longer. And when they can't, then what? The classificatory mania embodied in the *DSM* from the third edition onward arose from an attempt to lend an aura of "facticity" to psychiatric diagnoses and to stave off the ridicule that threatened the profession's legitimacy when its practitioners were shown to be unable to agree about the nature of the illness that confronted them (or even about whether the patient was sick at all). But as "illnesses" proliferated in each revision and the criteria for assigning diagnoses were loosened (as they were again in *DSM 5*), the very problem that had created a need for a new version of the *DSM* in the 1970s recurred, and major new threats to psychiatric legitimacy surfaced.

Relaxed diagnostic criteria led to an extraordinary expansion of the number of mentally sick individuals. This has been particularly evident among, but by no means confined to, the ranks of the young. Juvenile bipolar disorder, for example, increased fortyfold in just a decade between 1994 and 2004. An autism epidemic broke out as this formerly rare condition, seen in less than one in five hundred children at the outset of the 1990s, was found in one in every ninety children only ten years later. The story for hyperactivity, subsequently relabeled ADHD, is similar, with 10 percent of male American children now taking pills daily to treat their "disease."

We are almost as far removed as ever from understanding the etiological roots of major psychiatric disorders, let alone the profession's more controversial diagnoses (which many people would argue do not belong in the medical arena in the first place). Psychoactive drugs are associated with rising concerns about major side effects (ranging from iatrogenic and permanent neurological damage to increased risk of child and adolescent suicides, massive weight gain, metabolic disorders, diabetes, and premature death)—a situation that only compounds the problems psychiatry faces in the twenty-first century. Weighing risks and benefits in the psychiatric arena seems to be an increasingly fraught business.

Relying solely on symptoms and behavior to construct its illnesses, and on organizational fiat to impose its negotiated categories on both the profession and the public, psychiatry is now facing a revolt from within its own ranks. Descriptive psychiatry seems to survive only because it lacks a plausible rival. It is, however, an increasingly tenuous basis on which to rest claims to professional legitimacy. Words like "schizophrenia" and "depression" are engraved on our collective consciousness, and the misery and suffering these terms encapsulate are real and terrifying. Yet some of the most prominent voices within the academy denounce them as fake categories, labels we should abandon. How could the profession survive the loss of face and public confidence that would surely result were it to embrace such notions?

Notes

1. INTRODUCTION

1. Isaiah Berlin, *The Hedgehog and the Fox: An Essay on Tolstoy's View of History*, 2nd ed. (Princeton, NJ: Princeton University Press, 2013).

2. Andrew Scull, *Decarceration: Community Treatment and the Deviant; A Radical View* (Englewood Cliffs, NJ: Prentice-Hall, 1977).

3. Erving Goffman, *Asylums: Essays on the Social Situation of Mental Patients and Other Inmates* (Garden City, NY: Doubleday, 1961).

4. Andrew Scull, *Museums of Madness: The Social Organization of Insanity in Nineteenth-Century England* (London: Allen Lane, 1979); Scull, ed., *Madhouses, Mad-Doctors and Madmen* (Philadelphia: University of Pennsylvania Press, 1981); Scull, *Social Order/Mental Disorder* (Berkeley: University of California Press, 1989).

5. Andrew Scull, *The Most Solitary of Afflictions: Madness and Society in Britain, 1700–1900* (London: Yale University Press, 1993); Scull, Nicholas Hervey, and Charlotte MacKenzie, *Masters of Bedlam: The Transformation of the Mad-Doctoring Trade* (Princeton: Princeton University Press 1996).

6. Jonathan Andrews and Andrew Scull, *Undertaker of the Mind: John Monro and Mad-Doctoring in Eighteenth-Century England* (Berkeley: University of California Press, 2001); Andrews and Scull, *Customers and Patrons of the Mad-Trade: The Management of Lunacy in Eighteenth Century London* (Berkeley: University of California Press, 2003).

7. Andrew Scull, "Desperate Remedies: A Gothic Tale of Madness and Modern Medicine," *Psychological Medicine* 17 (1987): 561–77; Scull, "Somatic Treatments and the Historiography of Psychiatry," *History of Psychiatry* 5 (1994): 1–12.

8. Andrew Scull, *Madhouse: A Tragic Tale of Megalomania and Modern Medicine* (London: Yale University Press, 2005).

9. Andrew Scull, *Hysteria: The Disturbing History* (Oxford: Oxford University Press, 2011).

10. Andrew Scull, *Madness in Civilization: A Cultural History of Insanity, from the Bible to Freud, and from the Madhouse to Modern Medicine* (London: Thames and Hudson; Princeton, NJ: Princeton University Press, 2015).

11. Karl Marx, *The Eighteenth Brumaire of Louis Bonaparte* (London: International Publishers, 1994), 1.

12. Charles Rosenberg, "The Crisis in Psychiatric Legitimacy," in G. Kriegman, R. D. Gardner, and D. W. Abse, eds., *American Psychiatry: Past, Present, and Future* (Charlottesville, VA: University of Virginia Press, 1975), 135–48.

13. Eric Caplan, *Mind Games: American Culture and the Birth of Psychotherapy* (Berkeley: University of California Press, 1998).

14. Paul Dubois, *The Psychic Treatment of Nervous Disorders* (New York: Funk and Wagnalls, 1904).

15. Jay Schulkin, *Curt Richter: A Life in the Laboratory* (Baltimore: Johns Hopkins University Press, 2005). Schulkin cowrote the article published in this volume as chapter 7 and has kindly allowed me to reprint it here.

16. William Laurence, "Surgery Used on the Soul-Sick," *New York Times*, June 6, 1937.

17. Andrew Abbott, *The System of Professions: An Essay on the Division of Expert Labor* (Chicago: University of Chicago Press, 1988).

18. Simon Baron-Cohen, *Mindblindness: An Essay on Autism and Theory of Mind* (Cambridge, MA: MIT Press, 1995); Baron-Cohen, *Autism and Asperger Syndrome: Facts* (Oxford: Oxford University Press, 2008); Baron-Cohen, *Zero Degrees of Empathy: A New Theory of Human Cruelty* (London: Allen Lane, 2011).

19. Simon Baron-Cohen, *The Essential Difference: Men, Women and the Extreme Male Brain* (London: Penguin, 2008).

20. Roger Smith, *Trial by Medicine: Insanity and Responsibility in Victorian Trials* (Edinburgh: Edinburgh University Press, 1981); Joel Eigen, *Mad-Doctors in the Dock: Defending the Diagnosis, 1760–1913* (Baltimore: Johns Hopkins University Press, 2016).

21. Karl Menninger, *The Crime of Punishment* (New York: Viking, 1968).

2. THE FICTIONS OF FOUCAULT'S SCHOLARSHIP

This chapter is a modified version of my review of *History of Madness*, by Michel Foucault, trans. Jonathan Murphy and Jean Khalfa, ed. Jean Khalfa (London: Routledge, 2006), which originally appeared in the *Times Literary Supplement* on May 21, 2007.

3. THE ASYLUM, THE HOSPITAL, AND THE CLINIC

This chapter is a revised version of a paper that originally appeared in Greg Eghigian, ed., *The Routledge History of Madness and Mental Health* (New York: Routledge, 2017), 101-14.

1. See Lawrence Conrad, "Arab-Islamic Medicine," in *Companion Encyclopedia of the History of Medicine*, vol. 1, ed. W. F. Bynum and R. S. Porter (London: Routledge, 1993), 676-727; Michael W. Dols, "Insanity and Its Treatment in Islamic Society," *Medical History* 31 (1987): 1-14; Dols, "The Origins of the Islamic Hospital: Myth and Reality," *Bulletin of the History of Medicine* 61 (1987): 367-90; Timothy S. Miller, *The Birth of the Hospital in the Byzantine Empire* (Baltimore: Johns Hopkins University Press, 1985); and Manfred Ullman, *Islamic Medicine* (Edinburgh: Edinburgh University Press, 1978).

2. Michael W. Dols, *Majnun: The Madman in Medieval Islamic Society* (Oxford: Clarendon Press, 1992).

3. W. Montgomery Watt, *The Influence of Islam on Medieval Europe* (Edinburgh: Edinburgh University Press, 1972).

4. For an excellent history of the asylum, which survives in the twenty-first century, see Jonathan Andrews, Asa Briggs, Roy Porter, Penny Tucker, and Keir Waddington, *The History of Bethlem* (London: Routledge, 1997).

5. The best general perspective on the trade in lunacy remains William Parry-Jones, *The Trade in Lunacy: A Study of Private Madhouses in England in the Eighteenth and Nineteenth Centuries* (London: Routledge, 1972). See also Roy Porter, *Mind Forg'd Manacles* (London: Athlone, 1987); and Leonard Smith, *Lunatic Hospitals in Georgian England* (London: Routledge 2014).

6. See Michel Foucault, *Madness and Civilization*, trans. Richard Howard (New York: Pantheon, 1965), chap. 2; and Foucault, *The History of Madness*, trans. Jean Khalfa and Jonathan Murphy (London: Routledge, 2006), chap. 2.

7. Jacques Tenon, *Memoires sur les hôpitaux de Paris* (Paris: Pierres, 1778), 85.

8. Colin Jones, "The Treatment of the Insane in Eighteenth and Early Nineteenth Century Montpellier," *Medical History*, 24 (1980): 371-90. To be sure, Tenon lists a handful of private madhouses in Paris on the Faubourg Saint-

Antoine and in Montmartre, but taken together these housed barely three hundred lunatics.

9. Sir G. E. Paget, *The Harveian Oration* (Cambridge: Deighton and Bell, 1866), 34–5.

10. David Rothman, *The Discovery of the Asylum: Social Order and Disorder in the New Republic* (Boston: Little, Brown, 1971).

11. The quotes are from the Scottish alienist William Alexander Francis Browne's book *What Asylums Were, Are, and Ought to Be* (Edinburgh: Black, 1837), 203, 213, but similar sentiments were voiced elsewhere. In the United States in the 1830s and 1840s, there emerged what historians have dubbed "the cult of curability," where estimates of the feasibility of cure were steadily bid up (and allegedly supported by asylum statistics) until the day when Dr. William Awl of Virginia announced he had cured 100 percent of those he had treated. (He was promptly renamed "Dr. Cure-Awl.")

12. George Mora, "Vincenzo Chiarugi (1759–1820) and His Psychiatric Reform in Florence in the Eighteenth Century," *Journal of the History of Medicine and the Allied Sciences* 14 (1959): 424–33.

13. See Anne Digby, *Madness, Morality and Medicine: A Study of the York Retreat, 1790–1914* (Cambridge: Cambridge University Press, 1985).

14. Dora Weiner, *Comprendre et soigner. Philippe Pinel et la medicine de l'esprit* (Paris: Fayard, 1999); Jan Goldstein, *Console and Classify: The French Psychiatric Profession in the Nineteenth Century* (Chicago: University of Chicago Press, 2001).

15. For analyses of these processes in France, see Goldstein, *Console and Classify;* and Ian Dowbiggin, *Inheriting Madness: Professionalization and Psychiatric Knowledge in Nineteenth Century France* (Berkeley: University of California Press, 1991). For Britain, see Andrew Scull, *The Most Solitary of Afflictions: Madness and Society in Britain, 1700–1900* (London: Yale University Press, 1993); and Scull, Charlotte MacKenzie, and Nicholas Hervey, *Masters of Bedlam: The Transformation of the Mad-Doctoring Trade* (Princeton: Princeton University Press, 1996). For Germany, Eric J. Engstrom's *Clinical Psychiatry in Imperial Germany* (Ithaca: Cornell University Press, 2003) is illuminating.

16. See Goldstein, *Console and Classify;* Dowbiggin, *Inheriting Madness;* Scull, *The Most Solitary of Afflictions;* Rothman, *The Discovery of the Asylum;* and Gerald Grob, *Mental Institutions in America: Social Policy to 1873* (New York: Free Press, 1973).

17. See David Gollaher, *Voice for the Mad: A Life of Dorothea Dix* (New York: Free Press, 1995).

18. Andrew Scull, "The Discovery of the Asylum Revisited: Lunacy Reform in the New American Republic," in *Madhouses, Mad-Doctors and Madmen: The Social History of Psychiatry in the Victorian Era*, ed. Andrew Scull (Philadelphia: University of Pennsylvania Press, 1981), 144–65.

19. "Lunatic Asylums," *Quarterly Review* 101 (1857): 353.

20. See, for example, David Wright and Peter Bartlett, eds., *Outside the Walls of the Asylum: The History of Care in the Community* (London: Bloomsbury, 2001); and Akihito Suzuki, *Madness at Home: The Psychiatrist, the Patient, and the Family in England, 1820-1860* (Berkeley: University of California Press, 2006).

21. See, for example, Joseph Melling and Bill Forsythe, eds., *Insanity, Institutions and Society: A Social History of Madness in Comparative Perspective* (London: Routledge, 1999); and David Wright, "Getting Out of the Asylum: Understanding the Confinement of the Insane in the Nineteenth Century," *Social History of Medicine* 10 (1997): 137-55.

22. Edward C. Spitzka, "Reform in the Scientific Study of Psychiatry," *Journal of Nervous and Mental Disease* 5 (1878): 201-29. For a useful discussion of these developments, see Bonnie Blustein, "'A Hollow Square of Psychological Science: American Neurologists and Psychiatrists in Conflict," in *Madhouses, Mad-Doctors and Madmen: The Social History of Psychiatry in the Victorian Age*, ed. Andrew Scull (Philadelphia: University of Pennsylvania Press, 1981), 241-70.

23. Silas Weir Mitchell, "Address before the Fiftieth Annual Meeting of the American Medico-Psychological Association," *Journal of Nervous and Mental Disease* 21 (1894): 413-37.

24. Henry Maudsley, *The Physiology and Pathology of Mind* (New York: Appleton, 1871), 432.

25. Gerald Grob, *Mental Institutions in America*, 238, 306-8, 258.

26. Andrew Scull, *Hysteria: The Disturbing History* (Oxford: Oxford University Press, 2011).

27. Jules Falret quoted in Ian Dowbiggin, "French Psychiatry, Hereditarianism, and Professional Legitimacy, 1840-1900," *Research in Law, Deviance, and Social Control* 7 (1985): 135-65.

28. York Retreat, *Annual Report*, 1904, Borthwick Institute Archives, York University, UK.

29. Charles G. Hill, "Presidential Address: How Can We Best Advance the Study of Psychiatry," *American Journal of Insanity* 64 (1907): 1-8.

30. Margo Horn, *Before It's Too Late: The Child Guidance Movement in the United States, 1922-1945* (Philadelphia: Temple University Press, 1989).

31. There were, in addition, private clinics to which the well-to-do flocked, attempting, like their counterparts in other countries, to avoid the stigma of being confined in an asylum. For a study of these enterprises and the tendency of their patients to seek physical diagnoses for what were often psychosomatic problems, see Edward Shorter, "Private Clinics in Central Europe, 1850-1933," *Social History of Medicine* 3 (1990): 159-95.

32. Susan Lamb, *Pathologist of the Mind* (Baltimore: Johns Hopkins University Press, 2015).

33. See chapter 7.

34. Representative examples include Joel Braslow, *Mental Ills, Bodily Cures* (Berkeley: University of California Press, 1997); Jack Pressman, *Last Resort: Psychosurgery and the Limits of Medicine* (Cambridge: Cambridge University Press, 1998); Andrew Scull, *Madhouse: A Tragic Tale of Megalomania and Modern Medicine* (New Haven, CT: Yale University Press, 2006); and Mical Raz, *The Lobotomy Letters: The Making of American Psychosurgery* (Rochester: University of Rochester Press, 2013).

35. See, for example, Waltraud Ernst, *Mad Tales from the Raj: Colonial Psychiatry in South Asia, 1800–58* (London: Anthem Press, 2010); Dolly McKinnon and Catherine Colebourne, *"Madness" in Australia: Histories, Heritage, and the Asylum* (St. Lucia, Queensland: University of Queensland Press, 2003); and Sloane Malone and Megan Vaughan, eds., *Psychiatry and Empire* (London: Palgrave, 2007).

36. See, for example, Jonathan Sadowsky, *Imperial Bedlam: Institutions of Madness in Colonial Southwest Nigeria* (Berkeley: University of California Press, 1999); Waltraud Ernst, *Colonialism and Transnational Psychiatry: The Development of an Indian Mental Hospital in British India, c. 1925–1940* (London: Anthem, 2013); Emily Baum, "'Spit, Chains and Hospital Beds': A History of Madness in Republican Bejing, 1912–1938" (PhD diss., University of California, San Diego, 2013); Claire Edington, "Getting Into and Getting Out of the Colonial Asylum: Families and Psychiatric Care in French Indochina," *Comparative Studies in Society and History* 25 (2013): 725–55; and Richard Keller, *Colonial Madness: Psychiatry in French North Africa* (Chicago: University of Chicago Press, 2007).

37. Akihito Suzuki, "The State, Family and the Insane in Japan, 1900–1945," in *The Confinement of the Insane: International Perspectives, 1800–1965*, ed. R. Porter and D. Wright (Cambridge: Cambridge University Press, 2003), 193–225.

38. F. Chapirreau, "La mortalité des maladies mentaux hospitalisés en France pendant la deuxième guerre mondiale," *L'Encéphale* 35 (2009): 121–28; Marc Masson and Jean-Michel Azorin, "La surmortalité des maladies mentaux à la lumière de l'Histoire," *L'Evolution psychiatrique* 67 (2002): 465–79.

39. Frank Wright, ed., *Out of Sight, Out of Mind* (Philadelphia: National Mental Health Foundation, 1947); Alfred Maisel, "Bedlam 1946," *Life* 20 (May 6, 1946): 102–16; Albert Deutsch, *The Shame of the States* (New York: Harcourt, Brace, 1948); Harold Orlans, "An American Death Camp," *Politics* 5 (1948): 162–68.

40. Alfred Stanton and Morris Schwartz, *The Mental Hospital* (New York: Basic Books, 1954); H. Warren Dunham and S. Kirson Weinberg, *The Culture of a State Mental Hospital* (Detroit: Wayne State University Press, 1960); Erving Goffman, *Asylums* (New York: Doubleday, 1961); Robert Perrucci, *Circle of Madness: On Being Insane and Institutionalized in America* (Englewood Cliffs, NJ: Prentice-Hall, 1974); Russell Barton, *Institutional Neurosis* (Bristol: Wright,

1965); John K. Wing and George W. Brown, *Institutionalism and Schizophrenia* (Cambridge: Cambridge University Press, 1970).

41. Ivan Belknap, *Human Problems of a State Mental Hospital* (New York: McGraw-Hill, 1956), xi, 212.

42. Thomas S. Szasz, *The Myth of Mental Illness* (New York: Harper and Row, 1961).

43. Enoch Powell, "Speech to the Annual Conference of the National Association for Mental Health," in *Report of the Annual Conference* (London: Mind, 1961).

44. Andrew Scull, *Decarceration: Community Treatment and the Deviant* (Englewood Cliffs, NJ: Prentice-Hall, 1977); Paul Lerman, *Deinstitutionalization and the Welfare State* (New Brunswick: Rutgers University Press, 1982); Stephen Rose, "Deciphering Deinstitutionalization: Complexities in Policy and Program Analysis," *Milbank Memorial Fund Quarterly* 57 (1979): 429–60; William Gronfein, "Psychotropic Drugs and the Origins of Deinstitutionalization," *Social Problems* 32 (1985): 437–54; Gerald Grob, *From Asylum to Community: Mental Health Care in Modern America* (Princeton, NJ: Princeton University Press, 1992).

45. Christopher Payne, *Asylum: Inside the Closed World of State Mental Hospitals* (Cambridge, MA: MIT Press, 2009).

4. A CULTURE OF COMPLAINT

A version of this chapter appeared in Jonathan Reinarz and Rebecca Wynter, eds., *Complaints, Controversies and Grievances in Medicine* (London: Routledge, 2014). I have revised and extended it for publication here.

1. See, for example, David Healy, *Mania* (Baltimore: Johns Hopkins University Press, 2008); Healy, *Pharmageddon* (Berkeley: University of California Press, 2012); Edward Shorter, *Before Prozac: The Troubled History of Mood Disorders in Psychiatry* (Oxford: Oxford University Press, 2008).

2. Roy Porter, *Mind Forg'd Manacles: A History of Madness in England from the Restoration to the Regency* (Harmondsworth: Penguin, 1990), 164–65.

3. See Andrew Scull, *The Most Solitary of Afflictions: Madness and Society in Britain, 1700–1900* (London: Yale University Press, 1993).

4. [Eliza Haywood], *The Distress'd Orphan; or, Love in a Mad-House*, 2nd ed. (London: printed for J. Roberts, 1726), 35. The book was published anonymously, but it was advertised as being written by, and clearly was written by, the prolific Eliza Haywood, novelist, actress, and editor of four-volume *The Female Spectator* (London: T. Gardner, 1744–46). One of her later novels has the wonderful title *The History of Miss Betsy Thoughtless* (Dublin: printed for Oliver Nelson, 1751) and is a reworking of the story of Betty Careless, a dissolute brothel keeper,

whose name the artist William Hogarth had depicted scratched on the banister rails of his Bedlam scene in *The Rake's Progress*. For a recent biography, see Kathryn King, *A Political Biography of Eliza Haywood* (London: Pickering and Chatto, 2012). Other late eighteenth-century novels with madhouse themes written by women include Mary Wollstonecraft's *Maria: or, The Wrongs of Women* (1798) and Charlotte Smith's *The Young Philosopher* (1798). My account in this chapter of the scandals and complaints that swirled around the trade in lunacy in the eighteenth century draws heavily on my earlier researches published in *The Most Solitary of Afflictions: Madness and Society in Britain, 1700–1900* (London: Yale University Press, 1993) and, more particularly, my book written with Jonathan Andrews, *Undertaker of the Mind: John Monro and Mad-Doctoring in Eighteenth-Century England* (Berkeley: University of California Press, 2001).

5. [Haywood], *The Distress'd Orphan*, 39–40.

6. Ibid., 40–43.

7. See Jonathan Andrews, "'In her Vapours [or] Indeed in her Madness'? Mrs Clerke's Case: An Early Eighteenth-Century Psychiatric Controversy," *History of Psychiatry*, 1 (1990): 125–43.

8. See Elizabeth Foyster, "Wrongful Confinement in Eighteenth-Century England: A Question of Gender?" (paper presented at Social and Medical Representations of the Links between Insanity and Sexuality conference, University of Wales, Bangor, July 1999). I am greatly indebted to Dr. Foyster for permitting me to quote from this paper.

9. Alexander Cruden, *The London Citizen Exceedingly Injured; or, A British Inquisition Display'd* (London: Cooper and Dodd, 1739).

10. Alexander Cruden, *The Adventures of Alexander the Corrector, with an Account of His Being Unjustly Sent to Chelsea, with an Account of the Chelsea Academies; or, The Private Places for the Confinement of Such as Are Supposed to Be Deprived of the Exercise of Their Reason* (London: printed for the author, 1754).

11. Anonymous, *A Full and True Account of the Whole Tryal, Examination, and Conviction of Dr. James Newton, who Keeps the Mad House at Islinstton [sic], for Violently Keeping and Misusing of William Rogers [. . .] by his Wife's Orders [. . .]* (London: printed by J. Benson, 1715).

12. Tobias Smollett, *The Adventures of Launcelot Greaves* (London: Coote, 1762). Smollett borrowed heavily from John Monro's *Remarks on Dr. Battie's Treatise on Madness* (London: Clarke, 1758) in constructing his images of treatment in a madhouse.

13. Daniel Defoe, *Augusta Triumphans* (London: Roberts, 1728).

14. Robert Baker, *A Rehearsal of a New Ballad-opera Burlesqu'd, Call'd The Mad-house, After the Manner of Pasquin, As it is now Acting at the Theatre-Royal in Lincoln's-Inn-Fields, By a Gentleman of the Inner-Temple* (London: printed for T. Cooper, 1737).

15. Cf. Allan Ingram, ed., *Voices of Madness* (Stroud, Gloucestershire: Sutton, 1997); *Proposals for Redressing Some Grievances Which Greatly Affect the Whole Nation* (London: Johnson, 1740); and "A Case Humbly Offered to the Consideration of Parliament," *Gentleman's Magazine*, 33 (1763): 25–26.

16. *A Report from the Committee Appointed to Enquire into the State of the Private Madhouses in This Kingdom* (London: Whiston, 1763), 5.

17. Porter, *Mind Forg'd Manacles*, 151–52.

18. J. T. Perceval, *A Narrative of the Treatment Received by a Gentleman during a State of Mental Derangement*, 2 vols. (London: Effingham, Wilson, 1838–40).

19. Ibid.

20. Quoted in John Conolly, *A Remonstrance with the Lord Chief Baron Touching the Case of Nottidge versus Ripley* (London: Churchill, 1849).

21. See the discussions of this case (and the Ruck case, which follows) in Andrew Scull, *Social Order/Mental Disorder* (Berkeley: University of California Press, 1989), 201–4; and, with much more circumstantial detail, in Sarah Wise, *Inconvenient People: Lunacy, Liberty, and the Mad-Doctors in Victorian England* (London: Bodley Head, 2012), 94–129, 267–77. Also very useful for the Ruck case is Akihito Suzuki's splendid *Madness at Home: The Psychiatrist, the Patient, and the Family in England, 1820–1860* (Berkeley: University of California Press, 2006), 144–46.

22. See Virginia Blain, "Rosina Bulwer Lytton and the Rage of the Unheard," *Huntington Library Quarterly* 53 (1990): 210–36.

23. See Rosina Bulwer Lytton's *A Blighted Life: A True Story* (London: London Publishing Office, 1880) for her polemical account of her travails, and Sarah Wise, *Inconvenient People*, 208–51, for a more balanced assessment of the case.

24. For contemporary commentary from the psychiatric perspective, see "Report on the Ruck Case," *Journal of Mental Science*, 4 (1858): 131.

25. For a contemporary report on this inquisition in lunacy, as it was called, see "The Windham Case," *Times* (London), December 17, 1861.

26. In addition to Sarah Wise's work, see Roy Porter, Helen Nicholson, and Bridgett Bennett, eds., *Women, Madness and Spiritualism* (London: Routledge, 2003), for examples of Lowe's and Weldon's complaints.

27. On this phenomenon, see Alison Winter, *Mesmerized: Powers of Mind in Victorian Britain* (Chicago: University of Chicago Press, 1998); and Alex Owen, *The Darkened Room: Women, Power, and Spiritualism in Late Victorian England* (Chicago: University of Chicago Press, 2004).

28. The overlap between Georgina Weldon and Mrs. Jellyby of Dickens's *Bleak House* is extraordinary, whether one looks to the women's marital relations, their treatment of their children, their obsession with "philanthropy," or the squalor in which they lived. But there is a further historical connection which is distinctly odd: The leasehold of Tavistock House, Weldon's home during her campaigns,

had been purchased and extensively renovated by Charles Dickens in 1851, and he had planned to live there for the rest of his life before changing his mind and selling the place in 1860 in the aftermath of the breakup of his marriage. And the first novel Dickens wrote on moving in was *Bleak House*.

29. Janet Frame, *An Autobiography*, 3 vols. (Toronto: Women's Press, 1999).

30. For discussions of madness and the movies, see Andrew Scull, *Madness in Civilization: A Cultural History of Insanity, from the Bible to Freud, and from the Madhouse to Modern Medicine* (London: Thames and Hudson; Princeton, NJ: Princeton University Press, 2015), 351–57; and (through a psychoanalytic lens) Krin Gabbard and Glen Gabbard, *Psychiatry and the Cinema* (Chicago: University of Chicago Press, 1987).

31. Ivan Belknap, *Human Problems of a State Mental Hospital* (New York: McGraw Hill, 1956); H. W. Dunham and S. K. Weinberg, *The Culture of the State Mental Hospital* (Detroit: Wayne Sate University Press, 1960); Erving Goffman, *Asylums* (New York: Doubleday, 1961).

32. See, for example, Aaron, T. Beck, "The Reliability of Psychiatric Diagnoses: A Critique of Systematic Studies," *American Journal of Psychiatry*, 119 (1962): 210–16; and Aaron T. Beck, C. H. Ward, M. Mendelson, J. Mock, and J. K. Erbaugh, "Reliability of Psychiatric Diagnoses: A Study of Consistency of Clinical Judgments and Ratings," *American Journal of Psychiatry*, 119 (1962): 351–57.

33. John E. Cooper, R. E. Kendell, and B. J. Gurland, *Psychiatric Diagnosis in New York and London: A Comparative Study of Mental Hospital Admissions* (London: Oxford University Press, 1972).

34. Scornfully, lawyers dismissed psychiatric claims to expertise, pointing out that their diagnostic competence was essentially nonexistent. See Bruce Ennis and Thomas Litwack, "Psychiatry and the Presumption of Expertise: Flipping Coins in the Courtroom," *California Law Review*, 62 (1974): 693–752.

35. David Rosenhan, "On Being Sane in Insane Places," *Science* 179 (January 19, 1974): 250–58. Thanks to the work of the New York journalist Susannah Cahalan, there are now serious reasons to doubt Rosenhan's work, which may have been largely faked.

36. Cf. Robert Spitzer and Joseph Fleiss, "A Re-Analysis of the Reliability of Psychiatric Diagnosis," *British Journal of Psychiatry* 125 (1974): 341–47.

37. Linda Mulcahy has, of course, argued that many medical complainants are similarly labeled as "sick," which challenges the validity of their complaints. See L. Mulcahy, *Disputing Doctors: The Socio-Legal Dynamics of Complaints about Medical Care* (Maidenhead: Open University Press, 2003), 112.

38. H. Kutchins and S. A. Kirk, *Making Us Crazy: The Psychiatric Bible and the Creation of Mental Disorders* (New York: Free Press, 1997).

39. A. V. Horwitz and J. C. Wakefield, *All We Have to Fear: Psychiatry's Transformation of Natural Anxiety into Mental Disorder* (Oxford: Oxford University

Press, 2012); David Healy, *Mania: A Short History of Bipolar Disorder* (Baltimore: Johns Hopkins University Press, 2008).

40. A. Johnson, "Under Criticism, Drug Maker Lilly Discloses Funding," *Wall Street Journal*, May 1, 2007, www.wsj.com/articles/SB117798677706987755.

41. Benedict Carey, "New Definition of Autism Will Exclude Many, Study Suggests," *New York Times*, January 19, 2012, www.nytimes.com/2012/01/20 /health/research/new-autism-definition-would-exclude-many-study-suggests. html; Carey, "Psychiatry Manual Drafters Back Down on Diagnoses," *New York Times*, May 8, 2012, www.nytimes.com/2012/05/09/health/dsm-panel-backs-down-on-diagnoses.html.

42. Cf. Allen Frances, "*DSM-V* Badly Off-Track," *Psychiatric Times*, June 26, 2009; and Robert Spitzer, "APA and *DSM-V:* Empty Promises," *Psychiatric Times*, July 2, 2009.

43. Alan F. Schatzberg, James H. Scully, David J. Kupfer, and Darrel A. Regler "Setting the Record Straight: A Response to Frances [*sic*] Commentary on *DSM-V*," *Psychiatric Times*, July 1, 2009.

44. Both quoted in Pam Bellick and Benedict Carey, "Psychiatry's Guide Is Out of Touch with Science, Experts Say," *New York Times*, May 6, 2013, www .nytimes.com/2013/05/07/health/psychiatrys-new-guide-falls-short-experts-say .html.

45. Quoted in Gary Greenberg, *The Book of Woe: The* DSM *and the Unmaking of Psychiatry* (New York: Blue Rider Press, 2013).

5. PROMISES OF MIRACLES

This essay was originally published on September 1, 2017, as "God, Money, Health and Happiness" on the *Times Literary Supplement* online, www.the-tls .co.uk/articles/public/god-money-health-happiness-christian-science.

1. Mary Baker Eddy, *Science and Health with Key to the Scriptures* (Boston: Stewart, 1912), xi.

2. Mark Twain, *Christian Science* (New York: Harper and Brothers, 1907), 205.

3. Mark Twain, "Christian Science-II," *North American Review* 554 (January, 1903): 2.

4. See John Harvey Kellogg, *Autointoxication or Intestinal Toxemia* (Battle Creek, MI: Modern Medicine Publishing Company, 1918); Kellogg, *Colon Hygiene, Comprising New and Important Facts Concerning the Physiology of the Colon and Practical and Successful Methods of Combatting Intestinal Inactivity and Toxemia* (Battle Creek, MI: Good Health Publishing Company, 1915).

5. Barbara Sicherman, "The Quest for Mental Health in America, 1880–1917," (Ph.D. diss., Columbia University, 1967), 69–270.

6. Charles L. Dana's discussion of "Rest Treatment in Relation to Psychotherapy," by Silas Weir Mitchell, *Transactions of the American Neurological Association* 34 (1938): 217.

7. See the discussion in Eric Caplan, *Mind Games: American Culture and the Birth of Psychotherapy* (Berkeley: University of California Press, 1998), chap. 6.

8. Sigmund Freud, interview with Adelbert Albrecht, *Boston Evening Transcript*, September 11, 1909.

9. The best discussion of Scientology is Lawrence Wright, *Going Clear: Scientology, Hollywood, and the Prison of Belief* (New York: Knopf, 2013).

6. BURYING FREUD

This chapter is a modified version of my review of *Freud: The Making of an Illusion*, by Frederick Crews (London: Profile Books, 2017), which originally appeared in *Arete*, no. 54 (Winter 2017): 67–79.

1. Joseph Shaw Bolton, "The Myth of the Unconscious Mind," *Journal of Mental Science* 72 (1926): 30, 38; Charles Mercier, "Psychoanalysis," *British Medical Journal* ii (1916): 897.

2. William James to Theodore Flournoy, September 28, 1909; William James to Mary Calkins, September 29, 1909, both quoted in Nathan G. Hale Jr., *Freud and the Americans: The Beginning of Psychoanalysis in the United Sates, 1876–1917* (Oxford: Oxford University Press), 19.

3. Richard Wollheim, *Sigmund Freud* (Cambridge: Cambridge University Press 1981), 252.

4. Christopher Bollas, *The Freudian Moment*, 2nd ed. (London: Karnac, 2007), 2.

5. Adolf Grunbaum, *The Foundations of Psychoanalysis: A Philosophical Critique* (Berkeley: University of California Press, 1984).

6. Frank Cioffi, *Freud and the Question of Pseudoscience* (Chicago: Open Court, 1998), 17.

7. Jeffrey Masson, *The Assault on Truth: Freud's Suppression of the Seduction Theory* (New York: Farrar, Straus and Giroux, 1984).

8. Erik Erikson, quoted in Patrick Mahony, *Freud's Dora: A Psychoanalytic, Historical, and Textual Study* (New Haven: Yale University Press, 1996), 148–49. Erikson goes on to describe Ida Bauer's treatment at Freud's hands as "one of the great psychotherapeutic disasters; one of the most remarkable exhibitions of a clinician's published rejection of his patient; spectacular, though tragic, evidence of sexual abuse of a young girl and her own analyst's exoneration of that abuse; an eminent case of forced associations, forced remembering, and perhaps several forced dreams."

7. PSYCHOBIOLOGY, PSYCHIATRY, AND PSYCHOANALYSIS

This chapter first appeared as an article by the same name coauthored with Jay Schulkin, originally published in *Medical History* 53 (2009): 5–36. I am grateful to Jay for giving me permission to reprint our collaboration, in a slightly modified form, here.

1. T. Lidz, "Adolf Meyer and the Development of American Psychiatry," *American Journal of Psychiatry*, 123 (1966): 320–32.

2. Cf. Michael Gelder, "Adolf Meyer and His Influence on British Psychiatry," in *150 Years of British Psychiatry 1841–1991*, ed. G. E. Berrios and H. Freeman (London: Gaskell, 1991), 419–35.

3. Silas Weir Mitchell, "Address before the Fiftieth Annual Meeting of the American Medico-Psychological Association," *Journal of Nervous and Mental Disease* 21 (1894): 443–73.

4. Adolf Meyer to Alden Blumer, 23 October 1894, Meyer Papers, Series I/355, Alan Mason Chesney Medical Archives of The Johns Hopkins Medical Institutions, Baltimore, MD (hereafter cited as CAJH).

5. As Meyer himself recalled, "I found the medical staff . . . hopelessly sunk into routine and perfectly satisfied with it. . . . A bewildering multiplicity of cases stared me in the face. It would have been the easiest thing for me to settle into the traditions—I had to make autopsies at random on cases without any decent clinical observation, and examinations of urine and sputum of patients whom I did not know, and for physicians who merely filed the reports. . . . Whenever I tried to collect my results, I saw no safe clinical and general medical foundation to put my findings on." Adolf Meyer, "Aims and Plans of the Pathological Institute for the New York State Hospitals," in *The Collected Papers of Adolf Meyer*, 4 vols., ed. Eunice E Winters (Baltimore: Johns Hopkins University Press, 1950–52), 2:93.

6. Eunice E. Winters, "Adolf Meyer's Two and a Half Years at Kankakee," *Bulletin of the History of Medicine* 40 (1966): 441–58.

7. T. Lidz, "Adolf Meyer," 323; Ruth Leys, "Meyer, Watson, and the Dangers of Behaviorism," *Journal of the History of the Behavioral Sciences* 20 (1984): 128–49.

8. Winters, *Collected Papers of Adolf Meyer*, 2:28; see also Ruth Leys and Rand B Evans, eds., *Defining American Psychology: The Correspondence between Adolf Meyer and Edward Bradford Titchner* (Baltimore: Johns Hopkins University Press, 1990).

9. William James, *Pragmatism* (New York: Meridian, 1958; first published 1907).

10. Gerald Grob, *The State and the Mentally Ill: A History of the Worcester State Hospital in Massachusetts, 1830–1920* (Chapel Hill: University of North Carolina Press, 1966), 287, 297–98.

11. For Van Gieson's vision of the Pathological Institute's future, see his "Remarks on the Scope and Organization of the Pathological Institute of the New York State Hospitals," *State Hospitals Bulletin* 1 (1896): 255–74, 407–88.

12. Gerald Grob provides a valuable overview of Van Gieson's tenure and professional demise in his *Mental Illness and American Society 1875–1940* (Princeton, NJ: Princeton University Press, 1983), 127–9.

13. See the useful discussions in ibid., 128–31; and Ruth Leys, "Adolf Meyer: A Biographical Note," in Leys and Evans, *Defining American Psychology*, 43–6.

14. Frank G. Ebaugh, "Adolf Meyer's Contribution to Psychiatric Education," supplement, *Bulletin of the Johns Hopkins Hospital* 89 (1951): 64–72, 71.

15. For a discussion of Meyer's international influence, see Michael Gelder, "Adolf Meyer and his Influence on British Psychiatry," in Berrios and Freeman, *150 Years of British Psychiatry*, 419–35.

16. Smith Ely Jelliffe to Harry Stack Sullivan, 1 June 1937, Jelliffe Papers, Library of Congress, Washington, DC.

17. For discussions of Meyer's complicated relationship with Freud and psychoanalysis, see Ruth Leys, "Meyer's Dealings with Jones: A Chapter in the History of the American Response to Psychoanalysis," *Journal of the History of the Behavioral Sciences* 17 (1981): 445–65; and Nathan G. Hale Jr., *The Rise and Crisis of Psychoanalysis in the United States: Freud and the Americans, 1917–1985* (New York: Oxford University Press, 1995), 168–72.

18. Thomas Turner, for example, in a generally hagiographic account of the Hopkins faculty in these years, judges that "Meyer seems to have done very little research in the accepted sense after coming to Hopkins" and pronounces himself unable to discern "any direct contribution [Meyer made] to knowledge in the field"—a damning assessment of a Hopkins professor. See Thomas B. Turner, *Heritage of Excellence: The Johns Hopkins Medical Institutions, 1914–1947* (Baltimore: Johns Hopkins University Press, 1974), 441–44.

19. Decades later, Richter reported that Robert Yerkes (who had given him the only A grade he earned at Harvard) had urged him to read Watson's book *Animal Eduction*, an intellectual encounter that prompted him to move to Hopkins. See C. Richter, "It's a Long Way to Tipperary, the Land of My Genes," in *Leaders in the Study of Animal Behavior: Autobiographical Perspectives*, ed. Donald A Dewsbury (Lewisburg, PA: Bucknell University Press, 1985), 369.

20. C. A. Logan, "The Altered Rationale for the Choice of a Standard Animal in Experimental Psychology: Henry H. Donaldson, Adolf Meyer and the Albino Rat," *Hisory of Psychology* 2 (1999): 3–24.

21. On these differences, see Leys, "Meyer, Watson, and the Dangers of Behaviorism."

22. This was a feature of Meyer's character that Phyllis Greenacre attributed in part to his Zwinglian upbringing (Phyllis Greenacre, interview by Andrew Scull, New York City, 22 December 1983). It is also discussed in passing in Leys,

"Meyer's Dealings with Jones," which includes a claim that "sexuality was an area of personal tension for Meyer during these years" (456).

23. John Watson to A. Meyer, 13 August 1920; A. Meyer to J. Watson, 17 August 1920; J. Watson to A. Meyer, 18 August 1920; assorted notes, Meyer Papers, Series I/3974/20, CAJH.

24. A. Meyer to Frank Goodnow, September 29, 1920, Series III/11, Johns Hopkins University Archives, Sheridan Libraries, Baltimore, MD.

25. A. Meyer to Robert Levy, 6 March 1922, Meyer Papers, Series I/2341/1, CAJH.

26. A more benign interpretation of Meyer's actions in the case is offered in Leys, "Meyer's Dealings with Jones," 455–56, where Meyer is described as having "sympathized" with Watson (though deploring his sexual misbehavior), and it is claimed that Meyer "hated to lose [Watson]." The misrepresentations to Levy are explained away as an indication of Meyer's "ambivalence." This interpretation strikes me as strained, given Meyer's proactive role in securing Watson's dismissal and the long-standing intellectual disagreements between the two men. I note, too, that Leys's discussion of Meyer censoring a paper by Jones on Freud's psychology and blocking a possible appointment for Jones at Hopkins reveals a similar pattern of double-dealing and deceit.

27. In appointing Richter, Meyer passed over an application from the far more senior and prominent Robert Yerkes, who had taught Richter at Harvard. See Kerry W. Buckley, *Mechanical Man: John Broadus Watson and the Beginnings of Behaviorism* (New York: Guilford Press, 1989); and A. Meyer to J. Watson, 12 April 1921, Meyer Papers, Series I/3974/21, CAJH. Perhaps Meyer thought he could more readily dominate the younger man. Significantly, Richter's appointment led to the Psychological Laboratory being renamed the Psychobiological Laboratory. For further elaboration of this point, see Jay Schulkin, *Curt Richter: A Life in the Laboratory* (Baltimore: Johns Hopkins University Press, 2005), 16–19.

28. A. Meyer to Phyllis Greenacre, undated (probably late summer 1919), Meyer Papers, Series XV, CAJH.

29. On the Hopkins policy prohibiting marriages between junior members of staff, on pain of forced resignation, see T. Turner, *Heritage of Excellence*, 237–38. Officially, the policy was still in place at the outbreak of World War II.

30. P. Greenacre to A. Meyer, 14 August 1919, Meyer Papers, Series XV, CAJH.

31. A. Meyer to P. Greenacre, 1 and 24 July 1919, CAJH Series XV,

32. A. Meyer to P. Greenacre, undated [1919]. Meyer Papers, Series XV, CAJH.

33. P. Greenacre to A. Meyer, 14 August 1919, Meyer Papers, Series XV, CAJH.

34. Meyer to Greenacre, undated, Meyer Papers, Series XV, CAJH.

35. P. Greenacre to A. Meyer, 8 September 1919, Meyer Papers, Series XV, CAJH.

36. A. Meyer to P. Greenacre, undated, Meyer Papers, Series XV, CAJH.

37. Quoted in Regina Morantz-Sanchez, "Dorothy Reed Mendenhall," in *American National Biography,* online edition, ed. John A. Garraty and Mark C. Carnes (New York: Oxford University Press, 2000), www.anb.org/abstract/10.1093/anb/9780198606697.001.0001/anb-9780198606697-e-1200609.

38. P. Greenacre to A. Meyer, 5 January 1922, Meyer Papers, Series XV, CAJH.

39. Phyllis Greenacre, interview by Andrew Scull, New York City, 22 December 1983. Sixty years and more after these events, Meyer's obstructionism still produced a visible emotional reaction in Greenacre. She had earlier given to Ruth Leys a fuller account of Meyer's repeated interventions to block the paper's publication. These actions continued into the late 1930s, despite his description of it in a meeting of his staff "as the best piece of work to come out of the clinic". Further fueling Greenacre's sense of grievance, having said that, Meyer promptly attributed the paper to Ruth Fairbank. Phyllis Greenacre, interview by Ruth Leys, New York City, 16 June 1982. I am grateful to Dr. Leys for permission to quote from her notes on this interview.

40. A. Meyer to P. Greenacre, undated [July 1919], Meyer Papers, CAJH Series XV.

41. Quotations are from Phyllis Greenacre, interview by Ruth Leys, New York City, 16 June 1982. Greenacre's memories were equally bitter when she spoke of these matters in an interview with Andrew Scull in December 1983.

42. P. Greenacre to A. Meyer, 5 January 1922, Meyer Papers, Series XV, CAJH.

43. Richter's personal closeness to Meyer is evident in an autobiographical talk about his years at Hopkins that he gave to medical residents during the 1973-74 academic year. See "Reminiscences," unpublished paper, Richter Papers, CAJH, Adolf Meyer. The couple's frequent weekend trips to dine with the Meyers were confirmed by Richter's son, Peter Richter, in an interview with Andrew Scull in Garrison, New York, on 15 August 1996.

44. See, for example, the discussion in A. McGehee Harvey, *Adventures in Medical Research: A Century of Discovery at Johns Hopkins* (Baltimore: Johns Hopkins University Press, 1976).

45. See Paul Rozin, "The Compleat Psychobiologist," in *The Psychobiology of Curt Richter,* ed. Elliott M. Blass (Baltimore: York Press, 1976), xv–xxviii. Relevant work by Richter includes Richter, "A Behavioristic Study of the Activity of the Rat," *Comparative Psychology Mongraphs* 1 (1922): 1–55; Richter, "Some Observations on the Self-Stimulation Habits of Young Wild Animals," *Archives of Neurology and Psychiatry* 13 (1925): 724–28; Richter, "Animal Behavior and Internal Drives," *Quarterly Review of Biology* 2 (1927): 307–43; Richter, "The Electrical Skin Resistance," *Archives of Neurology and Psychiatry* 19 (1928): 488–508; Richter, "The Grasping Reflex in the New-Born Monkey," *Archives of Neurology and Psychiatry* 26 (1931): 784–90; Richter, "The Grasp Reflex of the New-Born Infant," *American Journal of the Diseases of Childhood* 48 (1934):

327–32; Richter, "Cyclic Manifestations in the Sleep Curves of Psychotic Patients," *Archives of Neurology and Psychiatry* 31 (1934): 149–51; Richter, "Increased Salt Appetite in Adrenalectomized Rats," *American Journal of Physiology* 115 (1936): 155–61; Richter, "Total Self Regulatory Functions in Animals and Human Beings," *Harvey Lectures,* 1942–43, series 38, pp. 63–103; Richter, "The Use of the Wild Norway Rat for Psychiatric Research," *Journal of Nervous and Mental Diseases* 110 (1949): 379–86; Richter, "Diurnal Cycles of Man and Animals," *Science* 128 (1958): 1147–48; Richter, "The Phenomenon of Unexplained Sudden Death in Animals and Man," in *Physiological Bases of Psychiatry,* compiled and edited by W. Horsley Gantt (Springfield, IL: Thomas, 1958), 302–13 (paper read at the twenty-fifth anniversary celebration of the Pavlovian Laboratory, Phipps Psychiatric Clinic, Johns Hopkins Hospital); Richter, "Biological Clocks in Medicine and Psychiatry: Shock-Phase Hypothesis," *Proceedings of the National Academy of Science* 46 (1960): 1506–30; Richter, *Biological Clocks in Medicine and Psychiatry* (Springfield, IL: Thomas, 1965).

46. P. Greenacre to A. Meyer, 5 January 1922, Meyer Papers, Series XV, CAJH.

47. Ibid.

48. P. Greenacre to A. Meyer, 22 August 1922, Meyer Papers, Series XV, CAJH.

49. Stanley McCormick had had a psychotic breakdown some months after his marriage. Diagnosed as a paranoid schizophrenic, he was to remain confined for the rest of his life, much of the time in a family mansion in California. Meyer had first been consulted on the case in 1906. For him, and for several other psychiatrists, McCormick provided the opportunity for an almost endless stream of lucrative consultations stretching over four decades.

50. A. Meyer to P. Greenacre, 24 July 1924, Meyer Papers, Series XV, CAJH.

51. P. Greenacre to A. Meyer, 18 July 1924, Meyer Papers, Series XV, CAJH; italics in the original.

52. A. Meyer to P. Greenacre, 29 July 1924, Meyer Papers, Series XV, CAJH. A notation on this document indicates that it was "not sent." It does serve as an indicator, however, of Meyer's worries in the face of Greenacre's mounting unhappiness about her stalled career, and it seems likely that an alternate version of this document was dispatched to Greenacre, for a key proposal made later in this draft was implemented a few weeks later.

53. Ibid. For a detailed examination of the entire focal sepsis episode, see Andrew Scull, *Madhouse: A Tragic Tale of Megalomania and Modern Medicine* (New Haven, CT: Yale University Press, 2005).

54. Henry A. Cotton, *The Defective, Delinquent, and Insane* (Princeton, NJ: Princeton University Press, 1921).

55. A. Meyer to P. Greenacre, 22 July 1924, Meyer Papers, Series XV, CAJH; A. Meyer to Henry Cotton, 11 Septempter 1924, Meyer Papers, Series I/767/24,

CAJH; Phyllis Greenacre, interview by Andrew Scull, New York City, 22 December 1983.

56. Phyllis Greenacrce, "Trenton State Hospital Survey, 1924–1926" (unpublished typescript), 16, 20–4; italics in the original.

57. See J. Schulkin, *Curt Richter*, 101–8.

58. P. Greenacre to A. Meyer, 10 September 1928, Meyer Papers, Series XV, CAJH.

59. A. Meyer to Hermann Meyer, 27 October 1927, Meyer Papers, Series IV/3/237, CAJH.

60. Curt Richter to his mother, Marta Richter, 3 February 1930, Richter Papers, Correspondence (Family), CAJH. See also C. Richter to M. Richter, 14 June 1930, Richter Papers, Correspondence (Family), CAJH.

61. Adolf Meyer, manuscript notes on Curt Richter, dated May 1928, Meyer Papers, Series XV, CAJH.

62. A. Meyer to H. Meyer, 27 October 1927, Meyer Papers, Series IV/3/239, CAJH.

63. A. Meyer to H. Meyer, 17 November 1927, Meyer Papers, Series IV/3/240, CAJH.

64. A. Meyer to H. Meyer, 12 December 1927, Meyer Papers, Series IV/3/240, CAJH.

65. P. Greenacre to Mrs. Meyer, 3 January 1928; P. Greenacre to A. Meyer, 17 January 1928, Meyer Papers, Series XV, CAJH.

66. P. Greenacre to A. Meyer, 29 February 1928, Meyer Papers, Series XV, CAJH.

67. A. Meyer to P. Greenacre, 20 February 1928, Meyer Papers, Series XV, CAJH.

68. A. Meyer to P. Greenacre, 15 June 1928, Meyer Papers, Series XV, CAJH.

69. Greenacre's letters to Meyer included copies of some of Richter's letters to her, as she provided him with a blow-by-blow account of their disputes. See P. Greenacre to A. Meyer, 17 January 1928, 29 February 1928, 6 March 1928, 17 April 1928, 15 May 1928, 10 and 19 September 1928, 2 and 25 October 1928, 3 (telegram) and 20 June 1929, 18 and 21 June 1920; C. Richter to P. Greenacre, 23 August 1928; and P. Greenacre to C. Richter, 13 September 1928, all in the Meyer Papers, Series XV, CAJH. There were a number of meetings between Greenacre and Meyer about these matters, and at least one three-way meeting with Richter at which Meyer sought, unsuccessfully, to bring matters to a conclusion.

70. C. Richter to A. Meyer, 26 August 1929, Meyer Papers, Series XV, CAJH.

71. T. Turner, *Heritage of Excellence*, 268 (where he attributes the Chinese lecture story to Richter), 441–44; Bertram N. Bernheim, *Story of the Johns Hopkins* (New York: McGraw-Hill, 1948), chap. 13. Then there is the deafening silence about Meyer in A. McGehee Harvey's *Adventures in Medical Research* (Balti-

more: Johns Hopkins University Press, 1976), a lengthy hymn of praise to all the medical breakthroughs pioneered at the university.

72. Greenacre articulated this sentiment in interviews with both Andrew Scull (New York City, 22 December 1983) and Ruth Leys ("Impressions of My Evening with Phyllis Greenacre," unpublished manuscript, 16 June 1982), and without being aware of his mother's comments, Peter Richter made the same point in an interview with Andrew Scull (15 August 1996).

73. Adolf Meyer, manuscript note about Phyllis Greenacre, undated [1928], Meyer Papers, Series XV, CAJH.

74. A. Meyer to P. Greenacre, 20 February 1928, Meyer Papers, Series XV, CAJH.

75. P. Greenacre to A. Meyer, 29 February 1928, Meyer Papers, Series XV, CAJH.

76. P. Greenacre to A. Meyer, 17 April 1928, Meyer Papers, Series XV, CAJH.

77. A. Meyer to P. Greenacre, 15 June 1928, Meyer Papers, Series XV, CAJH.

78. Ibid.

79. P. Greenacre to A. Meyer, 10 September 1928, Meyer Papers, Series XV, CAJH.

80. See Fritz Wittels, *Freud and His Time* (New York: Liveright, 1931).

81. The sessions with Jacobson went very badly, and Greenacre finally terminated the analysis. Peter Richter, interview by Andrew Scull, 4 February 1996.

82. P. Greenacre to A. Meyer, 13 December 1930, Meyer Papers, Series XV, CAJH.

83. Ibid.

84. P. Greenacre to A. Meyer, 18 September 1931, Meyer Papers, Series XV, CAJH. Greenacre asserted many years later that when she had left Baltimore, Meyer "told her at that time that he had not treated her correctly. She felt that this was true, and that he would therefore do anything for her" (Ruth Leys, "Impressions of My Evening with Phyllis Greenacre," 16 June 1982).

85. Greenacre commented at length about Meyer's dismay at her embrace of Freud, of whom he became increasingly critical (and jealous) in the later stages of his own career, in her interview with Ruth Leys (New York City, 16 June 1982) and Andrew Scull (New York City, 22 December 1983), and noted that a number of Meyer's most talented students had emulated her. For discussions of Meyer's complicated relationship with Freud and psychoanalysis, see Leys, "Meyer's Dealings with Jones"; and Hale, *Rise and Crisis of Psychoanalysis*, esp. 168-72.

86. See, for example, John Frosch, "The New York Psychoanalytical Civil War," *Journal of the American Psychoanalytical Association* 39 (1991): 1037-64.

87. David James Fisher, review of *Unfree Associations: Inside Psychoanalytic Institutes,* by Douglas Kirsner, *American Imago* 59 (2002): 213.

88. Manuel Furer, quoted in Douglas Kirsner, *Unfree Associations: Inside Psychoanalytic Institutes* (London: Process Press, 2000), 27.

89. See, for example, Phyllis Greenacre, *Trauma, Growth, and Personality* (New York: Norton, 1952).

90. Phyllis Greenacre, *Swift and Carroll* (New York: International Universities Press, 1955); Greenacre. *The Quest for the Father: A Study of the Darwin–Butler Controversy as a Contribution to the Understanding of the Creative Individual* (New York: International Universities Press, 1963).

91. Fisher, review of *Unfree Associations*, 212.

92. Arnold A Rogow, *The Psychiatrists* (New York: Putnam, 1970), 109. Greenacre was the highest-ranking analyst in the world who was not either a European or a European refugee.

93. This is not idle speculation. In 2017, the Nobel Prize in Physiology or Medicine was awarded to three Americans, Jeffrey Hall, Michael Robash, and Michael Young, for their discoveries of molecular mechanisms controlling the circadian rhythm, a belated recognition of the importance of Richter's discoveries.

94. In other contexts, Nathan Hale. Jr. has spoken of Meyer's "personal failings, . . . notably his ambivalence and paralyzing caution" (*Rise and Crisis of Psychoanalysis*, 168); and Ruth Leys has discussed his dislike of "conflict and contention of any kind" and his "intellectual timidity that all too often . . . made him incapable of acting decisively when controversial matters were at stake." ("Meyer's Dealings with Jones," 451). For her part, Phyllis Greenacre adduced his horror of airing dirty professional laundry in public and his loyalty to the weakest of his disciples as possible spurs to silence (Greenacre, interview by Andrew Scull, New York City, 22 December 1983). All these factors may help us understand Meyer's behavior. None of them, it goes without saying, excuses it.

95. Phyllis Greenacre, *Emotional Growth* (New York: International University Press, 1971), xxii.

96. For a discussion of Meyer's invention of the "life chart" and its relationship to his psychiatry, see Ruth Leys, "Types of One: Adolf Meyer's Life Chart and the Representation of Individuality," *Representations* 34 (Spring 1991): 1–28.

97. Adolf Meyer, "The Scope and Teaching of Psychobiology," in *The Commonsense Psychiatry of Dr. Adolf Meyer*, ed. Alfred Lief (New York: McGraw–Hill, 1948), 436.

98. On the Rockefeller initiative, see Donald Fleming, "The Full Time Controversy," *Journal of Medical Education* 30 (1955): 398–406. Harvey Cushing, the pioneering neurosurgeon, was another prominent medical academic who objected fiercely to the Rockefeller proposals.

99. Adolf Meyer, 20 November 1947, quoted in Hale, *Rise and Crisis of Psychoanalysis*, 167–68.

100. See Philip Pauly, "Psychology at Hopkins: Its Rise and Fall," *Johns Hopkins Magazine* 30 (December 1979): 36–41.

101. See Leys, "Meyer's Dealings with Jones," 448–50, 454–56.

102. Schulkin, *Curt Richter*, 136–37.

103. C. Fred Alford, *Whistleblowers: Broken Lives and Organizational Power* (Ithaca, NY: Cornell University Press, 2001); David Rothman, *Strangers at the Bedside* (New York, Basic Books, 1991), 70–84; Robert Bell, *Impure Science: Fraud, Compromise, and Political Influence in Scientific Research* (New York: Wiley, 1992).

8. MANGLING MEMORIES

This chapter is a modified version of "Losing Their Minds," my review of *Patient H.M.: A Story of Memory, Madness and Family Secrets,* by Luke Dittrich (London: Chatto and Windus, 2016), which originally appeared in the *Times Literary Supplement* on January 4, 2017.

1. Dittrich, *Patient H.M.*, 214.

2. Ibid., 215, 216; italics in the original.

3. Ibid., 68.

9. CREATING A NEW PSYCHIATRY

I would like to acknowledge a grant-in-aid from the Rockefeller Foundation to support my work in the Rockefeller Foundation Archives, and to thank Tom Rosenbaum in particular for his wonderful assistance in locating relevant materials. The archives have kindly granted permission to quote from their records. An earlier version of this chapter was published as "Creating a New Psychiatry: On the Origins of Non-Institutional Psychiatry in the USA, 1900–50," in *History of Psychiatry* 29 (2018): 389–408.

1. Gerald Grob, *Mental Institutions in America: Social Policy to 1875* (New York: Free Press, 1973); David Rothman, *The Discovery of the Asylum* (Boston: Little, Brown, 1971).

2. Andrew Scull, "The Mental Health Sector and the Social Sciences in Post-World War II USA, Part I: Total War and Its Aftermath," *History of Psychiatry* 22 (2011): 3–19; and Scull, "The Mental Health Sector and the Social Sciences, Part II: The Impact of Federal Funding and the Drugs Revolution," *History of Psychiatry* 22 (2011): 268–84.

3. See Andrew Scull, *Hysteria: The Biography* (Oxford: Oxford University Press, 2009), chap. 5.

4. Eric Caplan, *Mind Games: American Culture and the Birth of Psychotherapy* (Berkeley: University of California Press, 2001).

5. Franklin Ebaugh, "The Crisis in Psychiatric Education," (chairman's address read before the Section on Nervous and Mental Diseases, American

Medical Association, New Orleans, May 12, 1932), transcript in the Commonwealth Fund Mental Hygiene Program Files, box 17, folder MH 271, Rockefeller Foundation Archives, Tarrytown, New York.

6. For sympathetic discussions of the life chart (more sympathetic than I can muster), see Ruth Leys, "Types of One: Adolf Meyer's Life Chart and the Representation of individuality," *Representations* 34 (Spring 1991): 1-28; Susan Lamb, *Pathologist of the Mind: Adolf Meyer and the Origins of American Psychiatry* (Baltimore: Johns Hopkins University Press, 2014), 23, 151; and Lamb, "Social Skills: Adolf Meyer's Revision of Clinical Skill for the New Psychiatry of the Twentieth Century," *Medical History* 59 (2015): 443-64.

7. Adolf Meyer, "The Scope and Teaching of Psychobiology," in *The Commonsense Psychiatry of Dr. Adolf Meyer*, ed. Alfred Lief (New York: McGraw-Hill, 1948), 436.

8. Phyllis Greenacre, *Emotional Growth* (New York: International University Press, 1971), xxii.

9. Adolf Meyer, "The Role of Mental Factors in Psychiatry" (1908), reprinted in *The Collected Papers of Adolf Meyer*, vol. 2, ed. Eunice E. Winters (Baltimore: Johns Hopkins University Press), 586.

10. William James, *Talks to Teachers on Psychology*, quoted in Eric Caplan, *Mind Games: American Culture and the Birth of Psychotherapy* (Berkeley: University of California Press, 1998), 99. *Talks to Teachers on Psychology* was a course of lectures first delivered in the early 1890s.

11. William B. Carpenter, *Principles of Mental Physiology* (New York: Appleton, 1875), quoted in William James, "Habit," *Popular Science Monthly* 30 (1886-87): 437.

12. Clifford Beers, *A Mind That Found Itself* (New York: Longmans, Green, 1908).

13. The Commonwealth Fund was set up by Mary Harkness, the widow of Stephen Harkness, John D. Rockefeller's silent partner in Standard Oil. It was the first major foundation established by a woman.

14. See Margot Horn, *Before It's Too Late: The Child Guidance Movement in the United States, 1922-1945* (Philadelphia: Temple University Press, 1989).

15. On these developments, see Gerald Grob, *Mental Illness and American Society 1875-1940* (Princeton: Princeton University Press, 1983), 234-65. Privately, some leading psychiatrists were scornful about the very notion of mental hygiene. Maxwell Gitelson, an early convert to psychoanalysis, commented that mental hygiene's "capacity for creating a need has developed far in advance of its capacity for meeting the developed need." Gitelson to Earle Saxe, 19 December 1939, Gitelson Papers, Library of Congress, Washington, DC. Even Adolf Meyer, whose ideas underpinned the movement, grew skeptical (at least in private), complaining of "the unfortunate noise and propaganda that has become necessary to maintain the salaries and professionalism of so many half-doctors and new 'pro-

fessions' under the name of mental hygiene, and under the praise of unattainable panaceas." Meyer to W. G. Morgan, 2 July 1930, quoted in Grob, *Mental Illness and American Society,* 165. Meyer had expressed similar doubts three years earlier. See Meyer to Abraham Flexner, 20 April 1927, Meyer Papers, Series I, CAJH.

16. Frederick Brown, "General Hospital Facilities for Mental Patients," *Mental Hygiene* 15 (1931), 378–84.

17. Alan Gregg, diary, 6 and 8 May 1931, 21 October 1931, 20 June 1935, 3 July 1935, 15 October 1935, Rockefeller Foundation Archives. Under Gregg, NCMH's pleas for funding generally fell on deaf ears.

18. Howard S. Berliner, *A System of Scientific Medicine: Philanthropic Foundations in the Flexner Era* (New York: Tavistock, 1985); Richard Brown, *Rockefeller Medicine Men: Medicine and Capitalism in America* (Berkeley: University of California Press, 1979); Kenneth Ludmerer, *Learning to Heal: The Development of American Medical Education* (New York: Basic Books, 1985), chap. 10. The minutes of a staff conference held in 1930 reveal that the General Education Board had spent $77 million over the course of seventeen years on revamping medical education in the United States. See minutes of General Education Board staff conference, 13 January 1930, RG 3, Series 906, box 1, folder 4, Rockefeller Foundation Archives.

19. Thomas Duffy, "The Flexner Report—100 Years Later," *Yale Journal of Biology and Medicine* 84 (2011): 269–76.

20. I borrow this metaphor from the eminent US science journalist and agent provocateur Daniel S. Greenberg, who spoke of the period before World War II as one where "science was an orphan, . . . [and] there was a mutual aloofness between the federal government and the most influential and creative segments of the scientific community." *The Politics of Pure Science,* 2nd ed. (Chicago: University of Chicago Press, 1999), 51.

21. David Edsall, "Memorandum Regarding Possible Psychiatric Developments," 3 October 1930, RG 3, Series 906, box 2, folder 19, Rockefeller Foundation Archives.

22. See Gregg, diary, 22 January 1931, 24 February 1931, 30 March 1931, 4, 5, 6, and 8 May 1931, 21 October 1931, 28 October 1931, 4 November 1931, 18 December 1931.

23. Warren Weaver's biographical memoir of his colleague suggests that Mason's interest in psychiatry played some role in the Rockefeller Foundation's decision to focus on this specialty. See *Max Mason 1877–1961, A Biographical Memoir* (Washington, DC: National Academy of Sciences, 1964). See also Wilder Penfield, *The Difficult Art of Giving: The Epic of Alan Gregg* (Boston: Little, Brown, 1967), 224; and William H. Schneider, "The Model Foundation Officer: Alan Gregg and the Rockefeller Foundation Medical Division," *Minerva* 41 (2003); 155–66. Schneider suggests that other foundation officers lent their support because of mental illness in their families.

24. The double murder and suicide was front-page news in the *New York Times* the following day. Fosdick traveled a great deal in the course of his work, and the paper reported that he generally stayed in a New York hotel when in town. The family had been gathered together for the Easter holidays. Fosdick slept through the shootings, only to discover the bodies on the morning of April 4. Diagnosed as manic depressive, Winifred Fosdick reportedly "had been deranged for ten years" (the age of her young son) but lived next door to her parents and was being treated on an outpatient basis by a local Montclair doctor, Victor Seidler ("Mrs. Fosdick Kills Two Children and Self," *New York Times*, April 5, 1932). Fosdick's autobiography is largely bereft of references to his private life. The exception is a brief aside in which he acknowledges losing his wife and two children "in a moment of manic violence. The letters which my wife left behind her showed a mind completely out of touch with reality; she was far more ill than we realized even in the anxious years that preceded her death. . . . It takes time to recover from such a blow—if indeed one ever recovers." *Chronicle of a Generation: An Autobiography* (New York: Harper and Brothers, 1958).

25. That not all the trustees were convinced that this decision was a good one is hinted at in the 1934 report of the appraisal committee, which bluntly stated: "In this field, as in all other in which the Foundation is engaged, the Trustees would expect officers to give them definite warning when, in their opinion, the threshold of diminishing returns is reached in relation to a particular approach. Definite sailing directions can always be changed if the course proves to be unwise." "Medical Sciences—Program and Policy—Psychiatry," RG 3, Series 906, box 2, folder 19, Rockefeller Foundation Archives. Such doubts would resurface in more pointed form after World War II and toward the end of Gregg's tenure as director.

26. See Alan Gregg, "The New Program for Intensive Development Is in the Field of Psychiatry and Neurology," memorandum, RG 3, Series 906, box 1, folder 4, Rockefeller Foundation Archives.

27. Alan Gregg, "The Emphasis on Psychiatry," Trustees Confidential Memorandum, October 1943, RG 3, Series 906, box 2, folder 18, Rockefeller Foundation Archives.

28. Staff conference minutes, 7 October 1930, RG 3, Series 906, box 1, folder 4, Rockefeller Foundation Archives.

29. Susan Lamb and the late Jack Pressman have been particularly prominent exponents of the view that Adolf Meyer was the major influence here. See Jack Pressman, *Last Resort: Psychosurgery and the Limits of Medicine* (Cambridge: Cambridge University Press, 1998), 18–46; Pressman, "Psychiatry and Its Origins," *Bulletin of the History of Medicine* 71 (1997): 129–39; Pressman, "Psychosomatic Medicine and the Mission of the Rockefeller Foundation," in *Greater Than the Parts: Holism in Biomedicine, 1920–1950,* ed. Christopher Lawrence and George Weisz (New York : Oxford University Press, 1998), 189–208; Susan Lamb, *Pathologist of the Mind;* and Lamb, "Social Skills."

30. Johns Hopkins University Psychiatry, Grant in Aid, 5 December 1933, RG 1.1, Series 200, box 95, folder 1144, Rockefeller Foundation Archives.

31. That the foundation did not think much of what Meyer had accomplished is confirmed in an internal memorandum written in the late 1940s, which commented that "the prestige of psychiatry, which had never been very high, declined almost to a disappearing point during the Twenties and Thirties." Robert S. Morison, memorandum to President Chester Barnard, 30 September 1948, RG 3, Series 906, box 2, folder 18, Rockefeller Foundation Archives.

32. On Richter, see Jay Schulkin, *Curt Richter: A Life in the Laboratory* (Baltimore: Johns Hopkins University Press, 2005). On his relations with Adolf Meyer, see chapter 7. Richter was nominated for a Nobel Prize and arguably should have won. The Nobel committee eventually recognized the importance of the circadian rhythm by awarding the 2017 Prize in Physiology or Medicine to Jeffrey Hall, Michael Rosbash, and Michael Young for uncovering the molecular mechanisms that control it.

33. Gregg, diary, 30 June 1932. The files on Johns Hopkins Psychiatry record that from 1933 to 1939, Hopkins psychiatry received a total of $194,800, almost all of it allocated to Gantt, Richter, and Kanner, summarized in a memorandum dated, 1 July 1939, RG 1.1, Series 200A, Series 200, box 95, folder 1144, Rockefeller Foundation Archives. Gantt's attempts to "cure" his neurotic dogs were, sad to say, useless.

34. Alan Gregg to Francis Blake, dean of Yale Medical School, 3 December 1942, RG 1.1, Series 200, box 120, folder 1484, Rockefeller Foundation Archives. Beginning in 1938, the foundation offered a further endowment of $1,500,000 to Yale on condition that it funded a fifty-bed psychopathic hospital for use as a teaching hospital. Yale temporized for years, and the foundation eventually lost patience and withdrew the offer.

35. Gregg to Meyer, 2 June 1941, RG 1.1, Series 200, box 95, folder 1145, Rockefeller Foundation Archives.

36. Jerome D. Frank, "Impressions of Half a Century at Hopkins," *Maryland Psychiatrist* 22 (1995): 1.

37. R.A. Lambert, diary, 1948, RG 1.1, Series 200, box 120, folder 1487, Rockefeller Foundation Archives.

38. Alan Gregg, "The Emphasis on Psychiatry," confidential memorandum to the Trustees, October 1943, RG 3, Series 906, box 2, folder 18, Rockefeller Foundation Archives.

39. Robert Morison, "The Alan Gregg Lecture 1964: Some Illness of Mental Health," *Journal of Medical Education* 39 (1964): 985–86.

40. The recipients included the laboratory of Otmar von Verschuer, one of whose employees was Josef Mengele; and Ernst Rüdin, one of the architects of Hitler's plans for mass sterilization and later extermination of the mentally ill, whose activities were largely funded by the Rockefeller Foundation all the way

up to 1939. Rüdin somehow escaped being tried at Nuremberg (lesser figures who had participated in psychogenocide were tried and convicted). He was allowed to continue his career as a prominent psychiatrist and was treated as an honorable contributor to psychiatric genetics. The term "psychogenocide," incidentally, an apt label, was coined by the Belgian psychiatrist Erik Thys. See his *Psychogenocide: Psychiatrie, kunst en massamoord onder de Nazi's* (Antwerp: EPO, 2015).

41. Gregg, diary, 28 May 1935.

42. Staff Conference, Ocotber 7, 1930, RG 3, Series 906, box 1, folder 4, Rockefeller Foundation Archives.

43. Alexander himself termed the visit a "fiasco." See Franz Alexander, "Psychoanalytic Training in the Past, the Present, and the Future," address to the Association of Candidates of the Chicago Institute for Psychoanalysis, transcript, Chicago Institute for Psychoanalysis Archives, McLean Library, p. 4. On the "hostility of men in the Medical Faculty in Chicago" and the sense of relief when Alexander's year at the university came to an end, see Gregg, diary, 8 May 1931. Theodore Brown writes that Alexander "soon discovered that the social climate during the extended stay was to be shockingly different from the cordial welcome he had initially received. The medical faculty proved particularly hostile." "Alan Gregg and the Rockefeller Foundation's Support of Franz Alexander's Psychosomatic Research," *Bulletin of the History of Medicine* 61 (1987): 169. Funding for Alexander's year in Boston at the Judge Baker Foundation was underwritten by the Rosenwald Fund, which was headed by his patient Alfred Stern, Julius Rosenwald's son-in-law.

44. Douglas Kirsner, "On the Make: The Chicago Psychoanalytic Institute," in *Unfree Associations: Inside Psychoanalytic Institutes* (London: Process Press, 2000), 108–38.

45. Gregg, diary, 4 April 1932, RG 12, FA392, Rockefeller Foundation Archives. Max Mason, the president of the foundation, attended the meeting with Stern and Alexander. Gregg had made the same point about the need for a university affiliation for the institute three months earlier (see Gregg, diary, 14 February 1933). At that meeting, Gregg had also indicated that it was far from clear to him whether psychoanalysts "know enough to have something definitely to contribute to the study of somatic diseases."

46. Gregg's draft authorization when he submitted his recommendation to fund the institute makes this abundantly clear, emphasizing the institute's promised focus on "the correlation of medical and physiological problems with the findings of psychoanalysis." "Authorizing Resolution," RG 1.1, Series 216, box 3, folder 28, Rockefeller Foundation Archives, p. 4. For a detailed account of this episode, see Brown, "Alan Gregg and the Rockefeller Foundation's Support of Franz Alexander's Psychosomatic Research," 155–182. I have supplemented this with my own research in the Rockefeller Foundation Archives. Gregg's diary

entries for January 2 and February 4, 1934, document the meetings that led ultimately to his recommendation to the trustees that they provide support.

47. Theodore Brown notes "Alexander's not always subtle reorientation during
his courtship of Gregg" as documented in a series of letters to him. "Alan Gregg
and the Rockefeller Foundation's Support of Franz Alexander's Psychosomatic
Research," 172–73. The opportunism was characteristic of the man.

48. Stern helped to reassure Gregg on this front, writing that the institute
proposed to focus its research efforts on gastrointestinal disorders and on "psychological factors involved in ailments of the respiratory tract, hypertension,
endocrine gland disturbances, and skin disorders." Stern to Gregg, 26 June 1934,
RG 1.1. Series 216, box 3, folder 27, Rockefeller Foundation Archives.

49. Gregg, diary, 2 January 1934. On Alexander's efforts to legitimize the
institute and make possible "a more liberal and friendly interchange between
internal medicine and [the] Psychoanalytic Institute," see Gregg, diary, 15 October 1935. When Alexander threatened to move away from the emphasis on psychosomatic medicine, Gregg was quick to warn Stern that he was unhappy with
this prospect. See Stern to Gregg, 15 August 1936, RG 1.1, Series 216, box 3, folder
31, Rockefeller Foundation Archives. When Alexander once again sought to
engage with the political and sociological dimensions of psychoanalysis in 1938,
Stern did not wait to hear from Gregg, immediately sending Alexander a letter of
reproof and copying Gregg on the correspondence. Gregg was quick to voice his
gratitude and concurrence. Stern to Alexander (Gregg copied), 7 November
1938; Gregg to Stern 9 November 1938, RG 1.1, Series 216, box 3, folder 35, Rockefeller Foundation Archives.

50. Gregg, diary, 2 November 1937. He had earlier communicated his disquiet
directly to Alexander. See Gregg to Alexander, 24 March 1937, RG 1.1, Series 216,
box 3, folder 32, Rockefeller Foundation Archives.

51. R. A. Lambert to D. P. O'Brien, 22 August 1939; D. P. O'Brien to R. A. Lambert, 30 August 1939, RG 1.1, Series 216, box 3, folder 37, Rockefeller Foundation
Archives.

52. Stern had subsequently married Dodd and moved to New York, loosening
his ties to Alexander. His new wife had had a remarkable time in Berlin, sleeping
with, among others, the first head of the Gestapo, the French ambassador, and
the chief Russian spy in Berlin, with whom she had been besotted. In the months
leading up to her marriage to Stern, she had carried on an affair with the Hollywood director Sidney Kauffman, and her exotic love life did not diminish after
she was married. In Berlin, she had become a Soviet spy, and she subsequently
recruited the hapless Stern to the cause. Both of them were forced to flee the
United States in the McCarthy years, first to Mexico and then, on passports
bought from Paraguay, to Prague, where they both died in exile decades later.

53. Gregg, diary, 31 October 1941. Gregg had earlier voiced his unhappiness
with Alexander's lifestyle and salary. In a conversation with Stern, he expressed

his dismay with unnamed psychoanalysts who ought to be "prepared to further what they regard as the cause by a larger measure of personal sacrifice in point particularly of salaries." The foundation would not provide "permanent maintenance" for such people. Stern was no longer closely associated with the institute by that point, but he indicated that he concurred with Gregg's assessment. Gregg, diary, 8 December 1938.

54. Gregg, diary, 15 February 1934, 4 March 1934.

55. On Weaver, see Robert Kohler, "The Management of Science: The Experience of Warren Weaver and the Rockefeller Foundation Programme in Molecular Biology," *Minerva* 14 (1976), 279–306; and Pnina Abir-Am, "The Rockefeller Foundation and the Rise of Molecular Biology," *Nature Reviews Molecular Cell Biology* 3 (2002), 65–70. Weaver was Mason's protégé, and Abir-Am notes their close ties allowed Weaver to intrude on territory Gregg thought was rightfully his and to adopt the policy of granting many small and short-term grants—something Gregg dismissed as distributing "chicken feed." It was chicken feed that had massive and lasting effects on the shape of the biological sciences.

56. Mina Rees, *Warren Weaver, July 17, 1894–November 24, 1978: A Biographical Memoir* (Washington, DC: National Academy of Sciences, 1987), 504.

57. Jack Pressman, "Psychosomatic Medicine and the Mission of the Rockefeller Foundation," in *Greater Than the Parts: Holism in Scientific Medicine, 1920–1950,* ed. Christopher Lawrence and George Weisz (New York: Oxford University Press, 1998), 202.

58. Robert S. Morison, interoffice memorandum, 3 February 1947, RG 3, Series 906, box 1, folder 5, Rockefeller Foundation Archives. See also his interoffice memorandum for January 24, 1947, which lamented the fact that the problem of nervous and mental disease was so large and intractable, and noted that it was not clear what the foundation should support in order to make progress. Morison suggested that the Rockefeller Foundation should, rather than throw in the towel, seek out the "best men" in different areas and fund their research, a belated recognition, perhaps, of the success of Warren Weaver's approach in the Division of Natural Sciences.

59. Chester Barnard to Alan Gregg and Robert S. Morison, 5 August 1948, RG 3, Series 906, box 2, folder 18, Rockefeller Foundation Archives.

60. Chester Barnard to Alan Gregg and Robert S. Morison, 9 August 1948, RG 3, Series 906, box 2, folder 18, Rockefeller Foundation Archives.

61. Robert S. Morison, memorandum to Chester Barnard (also read by Alan Gregg), 30 September 1948, RG 3, Series 906, box 2, folder 18, Rockefeller Foundation Archives.

62. Ibid.

63. Ronald Bayer, *Homosexuality and American Psychiatry: The Politics of Diagnosis* (Princeton: Princeton University Press, 1981).

64. Robert S. Morison, memorandum, 26 August 1948, RG 1.1, Series 200, box 117, folder 1442, Rockefeller Foundation Archives.

65. Robert S. Morison, interview with S. Bernard Wortis, 8 October 1948, Morison diary, RG 12, box 334, Rockefeller Foundation Archives. See also Morison's report of his interview with Jurgen Ruesch, Langley Porter Clinic, San Francisco: "Like so many of his generation of psychiatrists (about my age) he is intellectually brilliant, discouragingly smug, and fails utterly to understand the scientific method. I had a lot of fun talking to him though I am tired of hearing that it is impossible to validate psychotherapy." Morison, diary, 17 November 1948.

66. Robert S. Morison, internal memorandum, 11 April 1951, RG 3, Series 906, box 1, folder 5, Rockefeller Foundation Archives.

67. Gerald Grob, *Mental Illness and American Society, 1875–1940* (Princeton: Princeton University Press, 1983), xi.

10. SHRINKS

The chapter is based on "Shrink-Wrapped," my review of *Shrinks: The Untold Story of Psychiatry*, by Jeffrey A. Lieberman with Ogi Ogas (London: Weidenfeld and Nicolson, 2015), originally published in the *Times Literary Supplement* on June 8, 2016.

1. See, for example, Joel Braslow, *Mental Ills and Bodily Cures: Psychiatric Treatment in the First Half of the Twentieth Century* (Berkeley: University of California Press 1997); German Berrios, *The History of Mental Symptoms: Descriptive Psychopathology since the Nineteenth Century* (Cambridge: Cambridge University Press, 1996); David Healy, *The Antidepressant Era* (Cambridge, MA: Harvard University Press, 1999); and George Makari, *Revolution in Mind: The Creation of Psychoanalysis* (New York: Harper, 2008).

2. Lieberman with Ogas, *Shrinks*, 12.

3. Ibid., 39.

4. Ibid., 73.

5. Ibid., 77.

6. Ibid., 96.

7. Ibid., 292.

8. See my discussion of this deeply flawed study in chapter 17.

9. Both men are quoted in Pam Bellick and Benedict Carey, "Psychiatry's Guide Is Out of Touch with Science, Experts Say," *New York Times,* May 6, 2013. For further discussion of these intraprofessional squabbles, see my detailed discussion of the *DSM* revolution in chapter 17.

10. "Lieberman, Insel Issue Joint Statement about DSM-5 and RDoC," Alert (blog), *Psychiatric News,* May 14, 2013, http://alert.psychnews.org/2013/05/lieberman-insel-issue-joint-statement.html.

11. Lieberman, *Shrinks,* 310.

12. See G. Reynolds, "Metabolic and Cardiovascular Risks Associated with Antipsychotics: Review of the Evidence," *Therapeutic Advances in Psychopharmacology* 7 (2017): 6–8.

13. Glen Spielmans and Peter Parry prefer to call it "marketing-based medicine." See their paper, "From Evidence-Based Medicine to Marketing-Based Medicine: Evidence from Internal Industry Documents," *Bioethical Inquiry* 7 (2010): 13–29.

14. In a footnote to the 2005 article reporting the results of the CATIE study, Lieberman reports receiving research funding from AstraZeneca Pharmaceuticals, Bristol-Myers Squibb, GlaxoSmithKline, Janssen Pharmaceutica, and Pfizer, and "consulting and educational fees" from AstraZeneca Pharmaceuticals, Bristol-Myers Squibb, Eli Lilly, Forest Pharmaceuticals, GlaxoSmithKline, Jannsen Pharmaceutica, Novartis, Pfizer, and Solvay. On such foundations are academic careers in psychiatry now built. J. Lieberman, T. S. Stroup, J. McEvoy, M. Swarz, R. Rosenheck, D. Perkins, R. Keefe, S. Davis, C. Davis, B. Lebowitz, S. Severe, and J. K. Hsaio, "Effectiveness of Antipsychotic Drugs in Chronic Schizophrenia," *New England Journal of Medicine* 353 (2005): 1209–23.

15. In their discussion, the study's authors conclude that "the proportion of patients with extrapyramidal symptoms did not differ significantly among those who received first-generation and second-generation drugs in our study." Lieberman et al., "Effectiveness of Antipsychotic Drugs," 1218.

16. The rate at which patients discontinued treatment should not have come as a surprise since, as the authors note, "the rates are generally consistent with those previously observed" (Lieberman et al., "Effectiveness of Antipsychotic Drugs," 1215, 1218). See K. Wahlbeck, A. Tuunainen, A. Ahokas, and S. Leucht, "Dropout Rates in Randomized Antipsychotic Drug Trials," *Psychopharmacology* 155 (2001): 230–33.

17. Lieberman et al., "Effectiveness of Antipsychotic Drugs," 1210.

18. Ibid., 1215, 1218.

19. Peter Tyrer and Tim Kendall, "The Spurious Advance of Antipsychotic Drug Therapy," *Lancet* 373 (2009): 4–5. For the study, see S. Leucht, C. Corves, D. Arbter, R. Engel, C. Li, and J. Davis, "Second-Generation Versus First-Generation Antipsychotic Drugs for Schizophrenia: A Meta-Analysis," *Lancet* 373 (2009): 31–41.

20. Steven Hyman, "Cognition in Neuropsychiatric Disorders: An Interview with Steven E. Hyman," *Trends in Cognitive Sciences* 16 (2012): 4. Compare with the official statement issued by David Kupfer, the chair of the *DSM* Task Force, to accompany the release of *DSM 5:* "In the future, we hope to identify disorders using biological and genetic markers that provide precise diagnoses that can be delivered with complete reliability and validity. Yet this promise, which we have anticipated since the 1970s, remains disappointingly distant. We have been tell-

ing patients for several decades that we are waiting for biomarkers. We're still waiting." "Statement by David Kupfer, MD," news release, American Psychiatric Association, May 3, 2013, www.madinamerica.com/wp-content/uploads/2013 /05/Statement-from-dsm-chair-david-kupfer-md.pdf.

21. J. F. Hayes, L. Matson, K. Waters, M. King, and D. Osborn, "Mortality Gap for People with Bipolar Disorder and Schizophrenia: UK-Based Cohort Study 2000–2014," *British Journal of Psychiatry* 211 (2017): 175–81. Hayes and his colleagues report that the gap between the seriously mentally ill and the general population has worsened over time. See also T. M. Laursen, "Life Expectancy among Persons with Schizophrenia or Bipolar Affective Disorder," *Schizophrenia Research* 131 (2011): 101–4; S. Saha, D. Dent, and J. McGrath, "A Systematic Review of Mortality in Schizophrenia: Is the Mortality Gap Worsening over Time?" *Archives of General Psychiatry* 64 (2007): 1123–31; and S. Brown, "Excess Mortality of Schizophrenia: A Meta-Analysis," *British Journal of Psychiatry* 171 (1997): 502–8.

11. THE HUNTING OF THE SNARK

This chapter is a modified version of my review of *The Intentional Brain: Motion, Emotion, and the Development of Modern Neuropsychiatry*, by Michael R. Trimble (Baltimore: Johns Hopkins University Press, 2016), originally published in *Brain* 140 (2017): 1166–69.

1. In the words of Frankwood E. Williams, director of the National Committee for Mental Hygiene, which had established the Committee for Organizing Psychiatric Units for Base Hospitals in World War I, "The name grew not out of a medical need but a political one. The term had only political significance to those of us who used it first in the war work or in connection with war work. I do not think that any of us felt that it represented anything that existed at the time in medicine or had any idea that its use would continue beyond the war or that men would come to call themselves 'Neuropsychiatrists' and I think that some of us were somewhat chagrined when after the war some comparatively few men did continue the use of the term in reference to their practice, for it did not seem to us then and does not seem to me now that there is any justification for the term medically." Williams to Frank Norbury, 14 November 1935, American Foundation for Mental Hygiene Papers, quoted in Gerald Grob, *Mental Illness and American Society, 1875–1940* (Princeton: Princeton University Press, 1983), 279–80. The political problem Williams refers to was the reluctance or refusal of neurologists to associate with things labeled "psychiatry."

2. Trimble, *Intentional Brain*, 41.

3. Ibid., 88.

4. Ibid., 208–9.

5. Ibid., xiii.
6. Ibid.
7. Ibid.
8. Ibid., 252.
9. Ibid., 283.
10. Ibid.
11. Ibid.
12. Ibid.
13. Ibid.

12. CONTENDING PROFESSIONS

The chapter is a revised version of my article "Contending Professions: Sciences of the Brain and Mind in the United States, 1850–2013," originally published in *Science in Context* 28 (2015): 131–61.

1. David Rothman, *The Discovery of the Asylum: Social Order and Disorder in the New Republic* (Boston: Little, Brown, 1971); Gerald Grob, *Mental Institutions in America: Social Policy to 1875* (New York: Free Press, 1973); Grob, *Mental Illness and American Society, 1875–1940* (Princeton: Princeton University Press, 1983).

2. Andrew Scull, "The Discovery of the Asylum Revisited: Lunacy Reform in the New American Republic," in *Madhouses: Mad-Doctors, and Madmen: The Social History of Psychiatry in the Victorian Era,* ed. Andrew Scull (Philadelphia: University of Pennsylvania Press, 1981), 144–65.

3. Gerald Grob, *The State and the Mentally Ill: A History of Worcester State Hospital in Massachusetts* (Chapel Hill, NC: University of North Carolina Press, 1966).

4. David Gollaher, *Voice for the Mad: The Life of Dorothea Dix* (New York: Free Press, 1995).

5. Andrew Scull, *The Asylum as Utopia: W.A.F. Browne and the Mid-Nineteenth Century Consolidation of Psychiatry* (London: Routledge, 1991).

6. David Rothman, *Conscience and Convenience: The Asylum and Its Alternatives in Progressive America* (Boston: Little, Brown, 1980); Grob, *Mental Illness and American Society;* Ellen Dwyer, *Homes for the Mad: Life inside Two Nineteenth-Century Asylums* (New Brunswick, NJ: Rutgers University Press, 1987).

7. Ian Dowbiggin, *Keeping America Sane: Psychiatry and Eugenics in the United States and Canada 1880–1940* (Ithaca, NY: Cornell University Press, 1997).

8. Silas Weir Mitchell, "Address before the Fiftieth Annual Meeting of the American Medico-Psychological Association, Held in Philadelphia, May 16, 1894," *Journal of Nervous and Mental Disease* 21 (1894): 431.

9. Grob, *Mental Illness and American Society*, 201–33.

10. Dowbiggin, *Keeping America Sane*, 34–58.

11. Edward Spitka, "Reform in the Scientific Study of Psychiatry," *Journal of Nervous and Mental Disease* 5 (1878): 200, 229.

12. William Alexander Hammond, "The Non-Asylum Treatment of the Insane," *Transactions of the Medical Society of New York* (1879): 280, 297.

13. Mitchell, "Address," 413–37.

14. Andrew Scull, *The Insanity of Place/The Place of Insanity: Essays on the History of Psychiatry* (London: Routledge, 2006), 129–49.

15. Harry Brunius, *Better for All the World: The Secret History of Forced Sterilization and America's Quest for Racial Purity* (New York: Knopf, 2006).

16. Joel Braslow, *Mental Ills and Bodily Cures: Psychiatric Treatment in the First Half of the Twentieth Century* (Berkeley: University of California Press, 1997), 54–70.

17. Eric Engstrom, *Clinical Psychiatry in Imperial Germany: A History of Psychiatric Practice* (Ithaca, NY: Cornell University Press, 2003), 140–46.

18. Richard Noll, *American Madness: The Rise and Fall of Dementia Praecox* (Cambridge MA: Harvard University Press 2011), 49–73.

19. Dowbiggin, *Keeping America Sane*, 51–54; Grob, *Mental Illness and American Society*, 127–29.

20. Grob, *Mental Illness and American Society*, 188–89; Braslow, *Mental Ills and Bodily Cures*, 72–74.

21. Hideo Noguchi and J. W. Moore, "A Demonstration of Treponema Pallidum in the Brain in Cases of General Paralysis," *Journal of Experimental Medicine* 17 (1913): 232–38.

22. Andrew Scull, *Madhouse: A Tragic Tale of Megalomania and Modern Medicine* (London: Yale University Press, 2005).

23. Andrew Scull, "Focal Sepsis and Psychiatry: The Career of Thomas Chivers Graves, B.Sc., MD, FRCS, MRCVS (1883–1964)," in *150 Years of British Psychiatry*, vol. 2, *The Aftermath*, ed. H. Freeman and G. Berrios (London: Athlone, 1996), 517–36.

24. Magda Whitrow, *Julius Wagner-Jauregg (1857–1940)* (London: Smith-Gordon, 1993); Braslow, *Mental Ills and Bodily Cures*, 71–94.

25. Andrew Scull, "Somatic Treatments and the Historiography of Psychiatry," *History of Psychiatry* 5 (1994): 1–12.

26. Deborah Doroshaw, "Performing a Cure for Schizophrenia: Insulin Coma Therapy on the Wards," *Journal of the History of Medicine and Allied Sciences* 62 (2007): 213–43.

27. Ladislas Meduna, "The Use of Metrazol in the Treatment of Patients with Mental Diseases," *Convulsive Therapy* 6 (1990): 287–98.

28. Eliot Valenstein, *Great and Desperate Cures: The Rise and Decline of Psychosurgery and Other Radical Treatments for Mental Illness* (New York: Basic

Books, 1986); Jack Pressman, *Last Resort: Psychosurgery and the Limits of Medicine* (Cambridge: Cambridge University Press, 1998); Jack El Hai, *The Lobotomist* (New York: Wiley, 2005).

29. Edward Shorter and David Healy, *Shock Therapy: A History of Electroconvulsive Treatment in Mental Illness* (New Brunswick, NJ: Rutgers University Press, 2007).

30. See Andrew Scull, "The Mental Health Sector and the Social Sciences in Post-World War II USA, Part I: Total War and Its Aftermath," *History of Psychiatry* 22 (2011): 3-19; and Scull, "The Mental Health Sector and the Social Sciences, Part II: The Impact of Federal Funding and the Drugs Revolution," *History of Psychiatry* 22 (2011): 268-84.

31. Margo Horn, *Before It's Too Late: The Child Guidance Movement in the United States, 1922-1945* (Philadelphia: Temple University Press, 1989); L. Zenderland, *Measuring Minds: Henry Herbert Goddard and the Origins of American Intelligence Testing* (New York: Cambridge University Press, 1998).

32. C. Dana, "Psychiatry and Psychology," *Medical Record* 91 (1917): 265-67; C. A. Dickinson et al., "The Relation between Psychiatry and Psychology: A Symposium," *Psychological Exchange* 2 (1933): 149-61; Grob, *Mental Illness and American Society*, 243-65; Ingrid Farreras, "Before Boulder: Professionalizing Clinical Psychology, 1896-1949" (PhD diss., University of New Hampshire, 2001), chaps. 1, 2.

33. Sonu Shamdasani, "Psychotherapy 1909: Notes on a Vintage," in *After Freud Left: A Century of Psychoanalysis in America*, ed. J. C. Burnham (Chicago: University of Chicago Press, 2012), 31-47; R. Skues, "Clark Revisited: Reappraising Freud in America," in Burnham, *After Freud Left*, 49-84.

34. George Makari, *Revolution in Mind: The Creation of Psychoanalysis* (London: Duckworth, 2008), 468-83.

35. For general commentary on the forced emigration of Jewish medics and scientists, including psychoanalysts, from Nazi Germany, see Mitchell G. Ash and Alfons Söllner, *Forced Migration and Scientific Change: Emigré German-Speaking Scientists and Scholars after 1933* (Cambridge: Cambridge University Press, 1996). Also useful, although less focused on forced migration, with the exception of Paul Weindling's chapter, is V. Roelcke, P. Weindling, and L. Westwood, eds., *International Relations in Psychiatry: Britain, Germany, and the United States to World War II* (Rochester, NY: University of Rochester Press, 2010).

36. J. Capshew, "Psychology on the March: American Psychologists and World War II" (PhD diss., University of Pennsylvania, 1986).

37. R. M. Yerkes, "Psychology and Defense," *Proceedings of the American Philosophical Society* 84 (1941): 527-42; K. M. Dallenbach, "The Emergency Committee in Psychology, National Research Council," *American Journal of Psychology* 59 (1946): 496-582.

38. Ben Shephard, *A War of Nerves: Soldiers and Psychiatrists in the Twentieth Century* (Cambridge, MA: Harvard University Press, 2001), 327.

39. Gerald Grob, "World War II and American Psychiatry," *Psychohistory Review* 19 (1990): 41–69; Shephard, *War of Nerves*.

40. F. D. Jones, *Military Psychiatry since World War II* (Washington, DC: American Psychiatric Press, 2000).

41. Gerald Grob, *The Mad among Us* (New York: Free Press, 1994), 193–94.

42. Grob, "World War II and American Psychiatry."

43. Ellen Herman, *The Romance of American Psychology* (Berkeley: University of California Press 1995), 84, 92.

44. Daniel S. Greenberg, *The Politics of Pure Science* (Chicago: University of Chicago Press, 1999); T. Appel, *Shaping Biology: The National Science Foundation and American Biological Research, 1945–1975* (Baltimore, MD: Johns Hopkins University Press, 2000); Ingrid Farreras, C. Hannaway, and V. A. Harden, *Mind, Brain, Body and Behavior: Foundations of Neuroscience and Behavioral Research at the National Institutes of Health* (Amsterdam: IOS Press, 2004).

45. L. J. Friedman, "The 'Golden Years' of Psychoanalytic Psychiatry in America: Emergence of the Menninger School of Psychiatry," *Psychohistory Review* 19 (1990): 5–40.

46. J. H. Scully, C. B. Robinowitz, and J. H. Shore, "Psychiatric Education after World War II," in *American Psychiatry after World War II*, ed. R. W. Menninger and J. C. Nemiah (Washington, DC: American Psychiatric Press, 2000), 124–51.

47. Rebecca Plant, "William Menninger and American Psychoanalysis, 1946–48," *History of Psychiatry* 16 (2005): 181–202.

48. Nathan Hale Jr., *The Rise and Crisis of Psychoanalysis in the United States* (Oxford: Oxford University Press, 1995), 246

49. Hale, *Rise and Crisis of Psychoanalysis*, 246–48, 253–56; J. MacIver and F. C. Redlich, "Patterns of Psychiatric Practice," *American Journal of Psychiatry* 115 (1959): 692–97.

50. Ellen Herman, *The Romance of American Psychology* (Berkeley: University of California Press, 1995), 84, 92, 94.

51. K. Danziger, *Constructing the Subject: Historical Origins of Psychological Research* (Cambridge: Cambridge University Press, 1990).

52. C. Hannaway and V. A. Harden, *Mind, Brain, Body and Behavior: Foundations of Neuroscience and Behavioral Research at the National Institutes of Health* (Amsterdam: IOS Press, 2004); Gerald Grob, *From Asylum to Community: Mental Health Policy in Modern America* (Princeton, NJ: Princeton University Press. 1991), 107–8.

53. D. B. Baker and L. T. Benjamin Jr., "The Affirmation of the Scientist-Practitioner: A Look Back at Boulder," *American Psychologist* 55 (2000): 241–47; Ingrid Farreras, "The Historical Context for National Institute of Mental Health

Support of American Psychological Association Training and Accreditation Efforts," in *Psychology and the National Institute of Mental Health*, ed. W. E. Pickren and S. Schneider (Washington, DC: American Psychological Association, 2005), 153–79.

54. J. L. Brand and P. Sapir, eds., "An Historical Perspective on the National Institute of Mental Health" (unpublished mimeograph, 1964).

55. R. E. Fox, P. H. Leon, R. Newman, M. Sammons, D. Dunivin, and D. Backer, "Prescriptive Authority and Psychology: A Status Report," *American Psychologist* 64 (2009): 257–68.

56. G. T. Sawrer-Foner, ed., *The Dynamics of Psychiatric Drug Therapy: A Conference on the Psychodynamic, Psychoanalytic and Sociologic Aspects of the Neuroleptic Drugs in Psychiatry* (Springfield, IL: Thomas, 1960).

57. Karl Menninger, *The Vital Balance: The Life Process in Mental Health and Illness* (New York: Penguin Books, 1963).

58. A. T. Beck, "The Reliability of Psychiatric Diagnoses: A Critique of Systematic Studies," *American Journal of Psychiatry* 119 (1962): 210–16; A. T. Beck, C. H. Ward, M. Mendelson, J. Mock, and J. K. Erbaugh, "Reliability of Psychiatric Diagnoses: A Study of Consistency of Clinical Judgments and Ratings," *American Journal of Psychiatry* 119 (1962): 351–57.

59. J. E. Cooper, R. E. Kendell, and B. J. Gurland, *Psychiatric Diagnosis in New York and London: A Comparative Study of Mental Hospital Admissions* (London: Oxford University Press, 1972).

60. David Rosenhan, "On Being Sane in Insane Places," *Science* 179 (1973): 250–258.

61. Susannah Cahalan, *The Great Pretender* (New York: Grand Central Publishers, 2019).

62. B. Ennis and T. Litwack, "Psychiatry and the Presumption of Expertise: Flipping Coins in the Courtroom," *California Law Review* 62 (1974): 693–752.

63. Edward Shorter, *Before Prozac: The Troubled History of Mood Disorders in Psychiatry* (Oxford: Oxford University Press, 2009), 154.

64. For an extended discussion of the various versions of the *DSM*, see chapter 17.

65. "Presidential Proclamation: The Decade of the Brain, 1990–1999," *Federal Register* 55 (July 17, 1990): 29553.

66. David Healy, *Mania: A Short History of Bipolar Disorder* (Baltimore MD: Johns Hopkins University Press, 2008), 198–244.

67. Ken Silverstein, "Prozac.org," *Mother Jones*, November/December 1999, 22–23.

68. A. Johnson, "Under Criticism, Drug Maker Lilly Discloses Funding," *Wall Street Journal*, May 1, 2007. For a more general discussion of this issue, see David Healy, *Let Them Eat Prozac* (New York: New York University Press, 2004), chap. 4.

69. R. J. Baldessarini, "American Biological Psychiatry and Psychopharmacology, 1944–1994," in *American Psychiatry after World War II,* ed. R. W. Menninger and J. C. Nemiah (Washington DC: American Psychiatric Press, 2000): 396–97, 398.

70. Shorter, *Before Prozac,* 198–99.

71. Tanya Lurhmann, *Of Two Minds: The Growing Disorder in American Psychiatry* (New York: Knopf, 2000).

72. Philip Rieff, *The Triumph of the Therapeutic: Uses of Faith after Freud* (New York: Harper and Row, 1966).

73. George Crane, "Clinical Psychopharmacology in Its Twentieth Year," *Science* 181 (July 13, 1973): 124–28.

74. Peter Tyrer and Tim Kendall, "The Spurious Advance of Antipsychotic Drug Therapy," *Lancet* 373 (2009): 4–5.

75. C. D. DeAngelis and P. D. Fontanarosa, "Impugning the Integrity of Medical Science: The Adverse Effects of Industry Influence," *Journal of the American Medical Association* 299 (2008): 1833–35. See, for example, E. H. Turner, A. M. Matthews, E. Linardatos, R. Tell, and R. Rosenthal, "Selective Publication of Antidepressant Trials and Its Influence on Apparent Efficacy," *New England Journal of Medicine* 358 (2008): 252–60.

76. David Healy, *Pharmageddon* (Berkeley: University of California Press, 2012), 104–113; S. Sismondo, "Ghost Management: How Much of the Medical Literature is Shaped behind the Scenes by the Pharmaceutical Industry?" *PLoS Medicine* 4 (2007): e286.

77. C. S. Landerfeld and M. A. Steinman, "The Neurotonin Legacy: Marketing through Misinformation and Manipulation," *New England Journal of Medicine* 360 (2009): 103–6.

78. See Glen Spielmans and Peter Parry, "From Evidence-Based Medicine to Marketing-Based Medicine: Evidence from Internal Industry Documents," *Bioethical Inquiry* 7 (2010): 713–29. This article looks at what could be learned by mining these data to document drug company behavior. One of the documents they reproduce is a Pfizer communication to its sales force about how to market sertraline (Zoloft) that is at once blunt and chilling: headed "Data Ownership and Transfer," it asserts that "Pfizer-sponsored studies belong to Pfizer, not to any individual." As for the "science" they contain, the "purpose of data is to support, directly or indirectly, marketing of our product. . . . Therefore commercial marketing/medical need to be involved in all data dissemination efforts." It explicitly references the way "publications can be used to support off-label data dissemination." These are, needless to say, standard industry practices. An Eli Lilly document regarding Zyprexa, an antipsychotic, for example, lays out its plans to "mine existing data to generate and publish findings that support the reasons to believe the brand promise."

79. Healy, *Pharmageddon;* Spielmans and Parry, "Evidence-Based Medicine." Spielmans and Parry dryly comment about the issue of drug companies

suppressing data they own and don't like: "Drug manufacturers are under no obligation to publish negative results [but rather] to maximize return to shareholders, it makes no sense at all to publish results that cast a drug in a negative light" (15). "Data suppression," they conclude, "is part of the industry's standard operating procedure" (16).

80. T. Barnes and C. Paton, "Antipsychotic Polypharmacy in Schizophrenia: Benefits and Risks," *CNS Drugs* 25 (2011): 383–99.

81. Su Ling Young, Mark Taylor, and Stephen M. Lawrie, "'First Do No Harm': A Systematic Review of the Prevalence and Management of Antipsychotic Adverse Effects," *Journal of Psychopharmacology* 29 (2014): 353–62.

82. Allan Horwitz and Jerome Wakefield, *All We Have to Fear: Psychiatry's Transformation of Natural Anxiety into Mental Disorder* (Oxford: Oxford University Press, 2012).

83. J.C. Blader and G.A. Carlson, "Increased Rates of Bipolar Disorder Diagnoses among US Child, Adolescent, and Adult Inpatients, 1996–2004," *Biological Psychiatry* 62 (2006): 107–14; I. Harpaz-Rotem and R. Rosencheck, "Changes in Out-Patient Diagnosis in Privately Insured Children and Adolescents from 1995 to 2000," *Child Psychiatry and Human Development* 34 (2004): 339–40; C. Moreno, G. Laje, C. Blanco, H. Jiang, A. B. Schmitdt, and M. Olfson, "National Trends in Outpatient Diagnosis and Treatment of Bipolar Disorder in Youth," *Archives of General Psychiatry* 64 (2007): 1032–39.

13. TRAUMA

This chapter is a modified version of "Shooting Magical Bullets at PTSD," my review of *The Evil Hours: A Biography of Post-Traumatic Stress Disorder*, by David J. Morris (Boston: Houghton Mifflin, 2015), originally published in the *Los Angeles Review of Books* on February 26, 2015.

1. Morris, *Evil Hours*, 22.

2. Ibid., 30.

3. Ibid., 248, 249.

4. Ibid., 89.

5. Quoted in ibid., 155.

6. Ibid., 157.

7. Ibid., 227.

8. Ibid., 160.

9. Ibid., 230.

10. Ibid., 169.

11. Ibid., 173.

12. Ibid., 181.

13. Ibid., 188.
14. Ibid., 203.
15. Ibid., 204.
16. Ibid., 263.
17. Ibid., 25.
18. Ibid., 5–6.
19. Ibid., 271.

14. EMPATHY

This chapter draws from two of my previously published essays: "What Is Empathy?" *Times Literary Supplement,* April 10, 2018; and "Blood Flow," *Times Literary Supplement,* February 17, 2012.

1. Peter Bazalgette, *The Empathy Instinct: How to Create a More Civil Society* (London: John Murray, 2017), 6.
2. Ibid, 6.
3. Ibid, 17.
4. Ibid, 6.
5. Ibid, 21.
6. Simon Baron-Cohen, *Zero Degrees of Empathy: A New Theory of Human Cruelty* (London: Allen Lane, 2011), 88.
7. Simon Baron-Cohen, *The Essential Difference: Men, Women and the Extreme Male Brain* (New York: Basic Books, 2003).
8. Baron-Cohen, *Zero Degrees of Empathy,* xi. On its face, to suggest that "evil" should be replaced by "empathy" seems nonsensical. The kindest interpretation one can give to this proposal is that Baron-Cohen meant to say that one could use "lack of empathy" in place of "evil."
9. Ibid, 27.
10. Ibid, 4.
11. Ibid, 14, 129–39.
12. Ibid., 102, italics in the original.
13. Ibid., italics in the original.
14. Ibid., 16.
15. Ibid., 116.
16. Ibid., 15.
17. Ibid., 54.
18. Ibid., 94.
19. Ibid.
20. Ibid., 127.
21. Ibid., 125–26.

338 NOTES TO PAGES 239–249

22. Ibid., 127.

23. Paul Bloom, *Against Empathy: The Case for Rational Compassion* (London: Bodley Head, 2016), 159.

24. Adam Smith, *The Theory of Moral Sentiments* (Lawrence, KS: Digireads. com, 2010), 9.

25. Siep Stuurman, *The Invention of Humanity: Equality and Cultural Difference in World History* (Cambridge, MA: Harvard University Press, 2017), 1.

26. Bloom, *Against Empathy*, 31.

27. Ibid., 36.

28. Stuurman, *Invention of Humanity*, 5.

29. Ibid., 1.

30. Ibid., 260.

31. Ibid., 546.

15. MIND, BRAIN, LAW, AND CULTURE

This chapter is a modified version of "Mind, Brain, Law and Culture," my review of *Law and the Brain,* a collection of papers edited by Semir Zeki and Oliver Goodenough (Oxford: Oxford University Press, 2006), and *Brain and Culture: Neurobiology, Ideology, and Social Change,* by Bruce E. Wexler (Cambridge, MA: MIT Press, 2006), originally published in *Brain* 130 (2007): 585–91.

1. Zeki and Goodenough, *Law and the Brain,* xii.

2. Ibid., xiii.

3. Ibid., xii–xiv.

4. Ibid., xiv.

5. Joshua Greene and Jonathan Cohen, "For the Law, Neuroscience Changes Nothing and Everything," in Zeki and Goodenough, *Law and the Brain,* 217.

6. Ibid.

7. Ibid., 218.

8. Ibid.

9. Zeki and Goodenough, *Law and the Brain,* xiv.

10. Morris Hoffman, "The Neuroeconomic Path of the Law," in Zeki and Goodenough, *Law and the Brain,* 15.

11. Ibid.

12. Ibid., 4.

13. Jeffrey Stake, "The Property 'Instinct,'" in Zeki and Goodenough, *Law and the Brain,* 185.

14. Ibid., 186.

15. Hoffman, "Neuroeconomic Path of the Law," 15.

16. Robert Hinde, "Law and the Sources of Morality," in Zeki and Goodenough, *Law and the Brain,* 43.

17. Owen Jones, "Law, Evolution and the Brain: Applications and Open Questions," in Zeki and Goodenough, *Law and the Brain*, 59.

18. Hinde, "Law and the Sources of Morality," 45.

19. Pierre Cabanis, "Rapports du physique et du moral de l'homme," in *Œuvres complètes* (Paris: Bossange Frères, 1802), 1823–25.

20. Julian La Mettrie, *L'Homme Machine* (Leyden: Luzac, 1748).

21. William Lawrence, *An Introduction to Comparative Anatomy and Physiology* (London: Callow, 1816); and William Lawrence, *Lectures on Physiology, Zoology, and the Natural History of Man* (London: Smith, 1823), quote on p. 79.

22. Charles Rosenberg and Carroll Smith-Rosenberg, "The Female Animal: Medical and Biological Views of Woman and Her Role in Nineteenth-Century America," *Journal of American History* 60 (1973): 334.

23. C. D. Meigs, *Lecture on Some of the Distinctive Characteristics of the Female* (Philadelphia: Collins, 1847), quoted in Rosenberg and Smith-Rosenberg, "The Female Animal," 334.

24. George Man Burrows, *Commentaries on the Cause, Forms, Symptoms, and Treatment, Medical and Moral, of Insanity* (London: Underwood, 1828), 146.

25. Henry Maudsley, *The Physiology and Pathology of Mind* (London: Macmillan, 1867).

26. Henry Maudsley, "Sex in Mind and Education," *Fortnightly Review*, n.s., 15 (April 1874): 466.

27. Ibid.

28. Ibid,. 468, 479.

29. S. A. K. Strahan, "The Propagation of Insanity and Allied Neuroses," *Journal of Mental Science* 36 (1890): 334.

30. Buck v. Bell, 247 US 200 (1927).

31. Strahan, "Propagation of Insanity," 331.

32. Quoted in Harry Brunius, *Better for All the World: The Secret History of Forced Sterilization and America's Quest for Racial Purity* (New York: Knopf, 2006), 270, 265.

33. Jones, "Law, Evolution and the Brain," 63.

34. Zeki and Goodenough, *Law and the Brain*, xv.

35. Ibid.

36. Hinde, "Law and the Sources of Morality," 39; Stake, "The Property 'Instinct,'" 190; Hinde, "Law and the Sources of Morality," 44; Terence Chorvat and Kevine McCable, "The Brain and the Law," in Zeki and Goodenough, *Law and the Brain*, 120; Chorvat and McCable, "Brain and the Law," 126.

37. Greene and Cohen, "Neuroscience Changes Nothing and Everything," 208.

38. Terrence Chorvat and Kevin McCabe, "The Brain and the Law," in Zeki and Goodenough, *Law and the Brain*, 134.

39. Paul Zak, "Neuroeconomics," in Zeki and Goodenough, *Law and the Brain*, 144.

40. Sean Spence, M. Hunter, T. Farrow, R. Green, D. Leung, C. Hughes, and V. Ganesan, "A Cognitive Neurobiological Account of Deception: Evidence from Functional Neuroimaging," in Zeki and Goodenough, *Law and the Brain*, 169–182.

41. Bruce E. Wexler, *Brain and Culture: Neurobiology, Ideology, and Social Change* (Cambridge, MA: MIT Press, 2006), 3.

42. Ibid., 13.

43. Ibid., 8.

44. Ibid., 16.

45. Ibid.

46. Ibid., 32.

47. Ibid., 82.

48. Ibid., 3–4.

49. Ibid., 1.

50. Ibid., 212.

51. Ibid.

52. Ibid.

16. LEFT BRAIN, RIGHT BRAIN, ONE BRAIN, TWO BRAINS

This chapter is a modified version of "Left Brain, Right Brain: One Brain, Two Brains," my review of *The Master and His Emissary: The Divided Brain and the Making of the Western World*, by Iain McGilchrist (London: Yale University Press, 2009), originally published in *Brain* 133 (2012): 3153–56.

1. Arthur Wigan, *New View of Insanity: The Duality of Mind Proved by the Structure, Functions and Diseases of the Brain, and by the Phenomena of Mental Derangement and Shown to be Essential to Moral Responsibility* (London: Longman, Brown, Green, and Longmans, 1844), 26.

2. Xavier Bichat, *Physiological Researchers on Life and Death*, translated by F. Gold (Boston: Richardson and Lord, 1827), 25.

3. A. Harrington, *Medicine, Mind, and the Double Brain* (Princeton, NJ: Princeton University Press, 1987); see also Douwe Draaisma, *Disturbances of the Mind* (Cambridge: Cambridge University Press, 2009), 97–125.

4. Sam Dillon, "Harvard Chief Defends His Talk on Women," *New York Times*, January 18, 2005.

5. S. Henshen, "On the Function of the Right Hemisphere of the Brain in Relation to the Left in Speech, Music, and Calculation," *Brain* 49 (1926): 110–23.

6. M. Gazzinga, "Brain and Conscious Experience," *Advances in Neurology* 77 (1998): 181–92; Gazzinga, "Right Hemisphere Language Following Brain Bisection: A Twenty Year Perspective," *American Psychologist* 38, no. 5 (1983): 525–37.

7. McGilchrist, *Master and His Emissary,* 92.

8. Ibid., 2.

9. Ibid., 14.

10. Ibid., 93.

11. Ibid., 127.

12. Ibid., 285.

13. Ibid.

17. DELUSIONS OF PROGRESS

This chapter is based on "Delusions of Progress: Psychiatry's Diagnostic Manual," my review of *Hippocrates Cried: The Decline of American Psychiatry,* by Michael Alan Taylor (Oxford: Oxford University Press, 2013), and *The Book of Woe: The* DSM *and the Unmaking of Psychiatry,* by Gary Greenberg (New York: Blue Rider Press, 2013), originally published in the *Los Angeles Review of Books* on May 19, 2013. I have extensively revised and extended this critique here to allow me to consider the phenomenon that is the *DSM* at greater length.

1. John Haslam, quoted in W. A. F. Browne, *What Asylums Were, Are, and Ought to Be* (Edinburgh: Black, 1837), 7.

2. For another historian's perspective on the precursors of *DSM III* and the impact of its reconstruction of the diagnostic process, see Edward Shorter, "The History of Nosology and the Rise of the Diagnostic and Statistical Manual of Mental Disorders," *Dialogues in Clinical Neuroscience* 17 (2015): 59–67.

3. Pat Bracken, Philip Thomas, Sami Timimi, Eia Asen, Graham Behr, Carl Beuster, Seth Bhunnoo, Ivor Browne, Navjuoat Chhina, Duncan Double, Simon Downer, Chris Eveans, Suman Feernando, Malcolm Garland, William Hopkins, Rhodri Huws, Bob Johnson, Briant Martindaale, Hugh Middleton, Daniel Moldavsky, Joanna Moncreiff, Simon Mullins, Julia Nelki, Matteo Pizzo, James Rodger, Marcellino Smyth, Derek Summerfied, Jeremy Wallace, and David Yeomans, "Psychiatry beyond the Current Paradigm," *British Journal of Psychiatry* 201 (2012) 430–34.

4. Taylor, *Hippocrates Cried,* 10.

5. Sidney Bloch and Peter Reddaway, *Russia's Political Hospitals: The Abuse of Psychiatry in the Soviet Union* (London: Gollancz, 1977); Zores Medvedev and Roj Medvedev, *A Question of Madness: Repression by Psychiatry in the Soviet Union* (London: Macmillan, 1971).

6. Thomas Szsasz, *The Myth of Mental Illness: Foundations of a Theory of Personal Conduct* (New York: Hoeber-Harper, 1961).

7. Aaron T. Beck, "Reliability of Psychiatric Diagnoses: I. A Critique of Systematic Studies," *American Journal of Psychiatry* 119 (1962): 210–16; Aaron T. Beck, C. H. Ward, M. Mendelson, J. Mock, , and J. K Erbaugh, "Reliability of Psychiatric Diagnoses: 2. A Study of Consistency of Clinical Judgments and Ratings," *American Journal of Psychiatry* 119 (1962): 351–57; Robert Spitzer, J. Cohen, J. Fleiss, and J. Endicott, "Quantification of Agreement in Psychiatric Diagnosis," *Archives of General Psychiatry* 17 (1967): 83–87; M. G. Sandifer, C. Pettus, and D. Quade, "A Study of Psychiatric Diagnosis," *Journal of Nervous and Mental Disease* 139 (1964): 350–56; Benjamin Pasaminick, S. Dinitz, and M. Lefton, "Psychiatric Orientation in Relation to Diagnosis and Treatment in a Mental Hospital," *American Journal of Psychiatry* 116 (1959): 127–32.

8. John Cooper, Robert Kendall, and Barry Gurland, *Psychiatric Diagnosis in New York and London: A Comparative Study of Mental Hospital Admissions* (Oxford: Oxford University Press, 1962).

9. Bruce J. Ennis and Thomas R. Litwack, "Psychiatry and the Presumption of Expertise: Flipping Coins in the Courtroom," *California Law Review* 62 (1974): 693–752.

10. Judith P. Swazey, *Chlorpromazine in Psychiatry* (Cambridge MA: MIT Press, 1974).

11. For an excellent source on these issues, see David Healy, *The Anti-Depressant Era* (Cambridge MA: Harvard University Press, 1999).

12. David Rosenhan, "On Being Sane in Insane Places," *Science* 179 (January 19, 1973): 250–58

13. Susannah Cahalan, *The Great Pretender* (New York: Grand Central Publishers, 2019).

14. Andrew Scull to Monica Bradford, March 16, 2016.

15. Rosenhan to Spitzer, January 15, 1975; Spitzer to Rosenhan, April 30, 1975, Rosenhan Papers, Stanford University. I am grateful to Susannah Cahalan for sharing her notes on these files. In response to Spitzer's request, Rosenhan claimed, "Merely deleting institutional names and duplicating the materials is not a sufficient solution. . . . These matters are too sensitive to the reputations of the treatment centers and psychiatrists to permit their free circulation. I have asked researchers who desire raw data on our observations and/or others' observations of us to wait until I have completed analyzing them for a book I am preparing." The book never appeared, nor did the raw data, which Rosenhan claimed to have in his files. No trace of the data appears there today.

16. Monica Bradford to Andrew Scull, March 30, 2016.

17. See, for example, Gina Kolata, "A Cloning Scandal Rocks a Pillar of Science Publishing," *New York Times,* December 20, 2005.

18. Allen Frances, "DSM-5 Badly Flunks the Writing Test," *Psychiatric Times,* June 11, 2013; Frances, "Psychosis Risk Syndrome is Back," *Psychiatric Times,* November 26, 2013.

19. Allan Horwitz and Jerome Wakefield, *The Loss of Sadness: How Psychiatry Transformed Normal Sorrow in Depressive Disorder* (Oxford: Oxford University Press, 2007).

20. Steven Sharfstein, "Big Pharma and Psychiatry: The Good, the Bad, and the Ugly," *Psychiatric News*, August 19, 2005, https://psychnews.psychiatryonline.org/doi/10.1176/pn.40.16.00400003.

21. Benedict Carey, "New Definition of Autism Will Exclude Many, Study Suggests," *New York Times*, January 19, 2012; Kristin Barker and Tasha Galardi, "Diagnostic Domain Defense: Autism Spectrum Disorder and the *DSM-5*," *Social Problems* 62 (2015): 120–40.

22. See, for example, Allen Frances, "Wither DSM-V?" *British Journal of Psychiatry* 195 (2009): 391–92; Frances, "Opening Pandora's Box: The 19 Worst Suggestions for DSM-5," *Psychiatric Times*, January 1, 2010; Robert Spitzer, "DSM-V Transparency: Fact or Rhetoric?" *Psychiatric Times*, March 7, 2009, www.psychiatrictimes.com/diagnostic-and-statistical-manual-mental-disorders/dsm-v-transparency-fact-or-rhetoric.

23. Alan Schatzberg, James Scully Jr., David Kupfer, and Darrel Regier, "Setting the Record Straight: A Response to Frances [*sic*] Commentary on DSM-V," *Psychiatric Times*, July 1, 2009.

24. Taylor, *Hippocrates Cried*, 29.

25. Ibid.

26. Ibid., 60–61.

27. Ibid., 64.

28. Charles Ornstein and Kate Thomas, "What These Medical Journals Don't Reveal: Top Doctors' Ties to Industry," *New York Times*, December 8, 2018.

29. See, for example, Joel Lexchin, Lisa Bero, Benjamin Djulbegovich, and Otavio Clark, "Pharmaceutical Industry Sponsorship and Research Outcome and Quality: A Systematic Review," *British Medical Journal* 326 (2003): 1167–70; Gisela Schott, Henry Pachl, Ulrich Limbach, Ursula Gundert-Remy, Wolf-Dieter Ludwig, and Klaus Lieb, "The Financing of Drug Trials by Pharmaceutical Companies and Its Consequences," *Deutsches Arzteblatt International* 107 (2010): 279–85; and Andreas Lundh, Joel Lexchin, Barbara Mintzes, Jeppe Schroll, and Lisa Bero, "Industry Sponsorship and Research Outcome," Cochrane Database of Systematic Reviews, February 16, 2017, http://cochranelibrary-wiley.com/doi/10.1002/14651858.MR000033.pub3/abstract.

30. Taylor, *Hippocrates Cried*, 65.

31. Gardiner Harris and Benedict Carey, "Researchers Fail to Reveal Full Drug Pay," *New York Times*, June 8, 2008; Gardiner Harris, "Research Center Tied to Drug Company," *New York Times*, November 24, 2008. See also Jocelyn Kaiser, "Senate Probe of Research Psychiatrists," *Science* 325 (2009): 30.

32. An internal email from a Johnson & Johnson marketing executive reveals how Biederman reacted when one of his requests for money ($3,000 as a

speaking fee) was turned down: "I have never seen someone so angry. Since that time, our business has become non-existant [*sic*] in his area of control." If the money was not forthcoming, he warned, "I am truly afraid of the consequences." Quoted in Greenberg, *Book of Woe*, 87.

33. Quoted in Greenberg, *Book of Woe*, 147.

34. For some reason, I am reminded of Bob Dylan's song "The Lonesome Death of Hattie Carroll."

35. Gardiner Harris, "Top Psychiatrist Didn't Report Drug Makers' Pay," *New York Times*, October 3, 2008.

36. J. Wislar, A. Flanagin, P. Fontanarosa, and C. DeAngelis, "Honorary and Ghost Authorship in High Impact Biomedical Journals," *British Medical Journal* 343 (2011): d6128, www.bmj.com/content/343/bmj.d6128.

37. Recent Supreme Court decisions sharply restricting the ability of plaintiffs to secure class action status may curtail further revelations of this sort. See, for example, Epic Systems Corporation v. Lewis, a 5–4 decision announced in May 2018.

38. David Healy, *Pharmaggedon* (Berkeley: University of California Press, 2012).

39. See Alex Berenson, Gardiner Harris, Barry Meier, and Andrew Pollack, "Despite Warnings, Drug Giant Took Long Path to Vioxx Recall," *New York Times*, November 14, 2004; Jim Giles, "Drug Giant Merck Accused of Deaths Cover-Up," *New Scientist*, April 15, 2008. Jose Baselga, the chief medical officer at Sloan Kettering, routinely "failed to disclose millions of dollars in payments from drug and health care companies in recent years, omitting his financial ties from dozens of research articles in prestigious publications like *The New England Journal of Medicine* and *The Lancet*." His clear violations of written and widely publicized policies designed to reveal conflicts of interest included putting "a positive spin on the results of two Roche-sponsored clinical trials that many others considered disappointing, without disclosing [that] . . . he has received more than $3 million from Roche in consulting fees and for his stake in a company it acquired." Charles Ornstein and Katie Thomas, "Top Cancer Researcher Fails to Disclose Corporate Financial Ties in Major Research Journals," New York Times, September 8, 2018. After trying initially to dismiss the criticisms and claiming that the omissions were "inadvertent," Baselga resigned his post on September 13, 2018. Medical center personnel, it would appear, are not as insulated as tenured professors from the effects of public exposure of wrongdoing.

40. Katie Thomas and Michael Schmidt, "Glaxo Agrees to Pay $3 Billion in Fraud Settlement," *New York Times*, July 2, 2012.

41. Tracy Staton, "Pfizer Adds Another $325M to Neurontin Settlement. Total? $945M," *Fierce Pharma*, June 2, 2014.

42. Denise Lavoie and Associated Press, "Bristol-Myers Squibb to pay $515M settlement," *ABC News*, accessed June 26, 2018, https://abcnews.go.com/Business/story?id=3670595.

43. Katie Thomas, "J.&J. to Pay $2.2 Billion in Risperdal Settlement," *New York Times,* November 4, 2013.

44. Juan-Carlos Martinez-Aguayo, Marcelo Arancibia, Sebastian Concha, and Eva Madrid, "Ten Years After the FDA Black Box Warning for Antidepressant Drugs: A Critical Narrative Review," *Archives of Clinical Psychiatry* 43 (2016): 60–66.

45. Greenberg, *Book of Woe,* 110.

46. Thomas Insel quit NIMH two years later, in 2015, and Steven Hyman, former provost of Harvard University, remains director of its Staley Center for Psychiatric Research. Their comments appear in Pam Belluck and Benedict Carey, "Psychiatry's Guide is Out of Touch with Science, Experts Say," *New York Times,* May 6, 2013.

47. Quoted in Gary Greenberg, *The Book of Woe.*

48. Greenberg, *Book of Woe,* 352.

Index

Abbott, Andrew, 18
Abilify (antipsychotic), 294
Abu Ghraib, 228
Adler, Alfred, 93
Alexander, Franz, and Chicago Psychoanalytic Institute, 155–156, 157
Alienists, 7, 11, 18, 44, 54, 64–66. *See also* Maudsley, Henry; Psychiatry
Alleged Lunatics' Friend Society, 62
Alzheimer's disease, 23, 49
American Journal of Insanity, 178, 188
American Medical Association, founding of, 189
American Medico-Psychological Association, 48, 188–189. *See also* American Psychiatric Association
American Psychiatric Association, 102, 147, 169, 198; and *DSM*, 205, 274–275, 276, 282, 295; and income from pharmaceutical industry, 295; vote on homosexuality as mental illness, 222
American Psychological Association, 201
Angel at My Table, An (film), 67
Anna O. *See* Pap penheim, Bertha
Annese, Jacopo, 140–141
Antidepressants, 291; as blockbuster drugs, 209, 284, 293; side effects of, 211, 212, 226, 294, 297

Antipsychiatry, 47, 52
Antipsychotic medications, 82, 207–208, 293; atypical or second generation drugs, 175, 176, 291, 294; limitations of, 174, 176, 211; long-term use of, 213; side effects of, 174, 175, 176, 211, 212, 226, 294, 297
Aphasia, 263
Armenian genocide, 232, 234, 239
Asperger's syndrome, 235, 284, 289
Assault on Truth, The (Masson), 89
AstraZeneca Pharmaceuticals, 292
Asylums, 7; and birth of psychiatry, 19, 55–56, 142, 186–187, 189; conscientious objectors in, 51–52; creation in nineteenth century, 44, 187, 271; as death camps, 51; decay of, 52–53, 187–188, 190–191, 287; declining cure rates, 45; reputation of, 45, 189; rising population of, 42–43, 45, 47, 48–49, 50–51, 187; utopian visions of, 9–10, 45, 187
Attention deficit hyperactivity disorder (ADHD), 69, 214, 275, 297
Autism, 21, 69, 70, 82, 214, 284–285, 297
Autism spectrum disorder, 235, 290
Avicenna, 39

Bacteriological revolution, 15; and psychiatry, 192, 193

Cooper, John E., and diagnosis in Britain and US, 203
Corkin, Suzanne: and Luke Dittrich, 140; and Patient H.M., 139–140, 141
Cornell University, and psychiatry, 155
Cotton, Henry: and focal sepsis, 118, 119, 193, 194; and Phyllis Greenacre, 119, 120; and Adolf Meyer, 117, 119
Crews, Frederick: early career of, 13; and Sigmund Freud's failings, 83, 85–90, 91, 92, 93–94
Cruden, Alexander, 59
Cruise, Tom, 70, 286

Dana, Charles, 75
Davenport, Charles, 253
Dax, Marc, 263
Decade of the brain, 206, 248, 275
Deep sleep therapy, 51
Defoe, Daniel, 60
Degeneration/degenerates, 46, 49–50, 187–188, 222, 252
Deinstitutionalization, 2, 52–53, 186
Dementia praecox, 150, 192, 272. See also Schizophrenia
Depression, 69; and drug treatments, 207–208; and genetics, 233; myth of chemical origins of, 223; questions about, 71, 296, 298
Derrida, Jacques, 31
Descartes, René, 33, 180, 262
Description of the Retreat (Tuke), 35
Deutsch, Helene, 133
Dewey, John, 98, 145
Distress'd Orphan, The (Haywood), 57–58
Dittrich, Luke: and Patient H.M., 136–139; and William Beecher Scoville, 138
Dix, Dorothea, 44, 187
Dopamine, 83, 207–208
Dora. See Bauer, Ida
Draper, George, 155,
DSM (Diagnostic and Statistical Manual), 55, 272; continual expansion of, 207, 213–214, 275, 283, 288, 297; early editions of, 203, 273; and PTSD, 20; ramshackle foundations of, 210, 213–214, 222, 277, 288, 295; worldwide influence of, 210
DSM III (third ed., 1980), 23, 55, 69, 272; acceptance of, 205; creation of, 205–206, 282–283; flaws of, 206, 282; and homosexuality, 222; and hostility to psychoanalysis; 83, 172, 184, 205–206, 275; and

reorientation of psychiatry, 206, 275–276, 282, 283
DSM III R (third ed., revised, 1987), 214, 277
DSM IV (fourth ed., 1994), 55, 70, 71, 275, 286, 291; and loosening of diagnostic criteria, 284, 297; and pharmaceutical industry, 289
DSM IV TR (text revision, 2000), 214, 273
DSM 5 (fifth ed., 2013) 70, 173; attempt to link diagnosis to etiology, 285; criticism of, 70–71, 184, 272, 276–277, 285–286, 296, 297; new diagnoses in, 283, 289; and pharmaceutical industry, 289, 290; publication of, 276; value to the American Psychiatric Association, 71, 273, 276, 286
Dubois, Paul, 12
Dürer, Albrecht, 180
Dutch asylums, 40

Ebaugh, Franklin, 144–145
Eckstein, Emma, 93
Eddy, Mary Baker, 12, 73, 74, 75, 77
Eden, Frederick Morton, 35
Edsall, David, views of psychiatry, 149–150, 152
Electro-convulsive therapy (ECT), 51, 67, 82, 138–139, 159, 195; and transorbital lobotomy, 136
Eli Lilly, 292
Emmanuel Movement, 12, 75, 76
Emory University, and ethical violations of faculty, 291, 292, 293
Empathy, 21, 267; deficit of, 240; definition of, 240; degrees of, 235–236, 237; empathy quotient (EQ), 235–236, 237; genetics of, 233; as instinct, 230, 231, 232; problems with, 240–242; and publishers, 242
Enlightenment, The, 9–10, 27, 29, 31, 243, 244, 249, 250, 268
Ennis, Bruce, 279
Epilepsy, 127, 180, 182, 252, 265; drug treatment of, 202; and psychopathology, 183
Erhard Seminars Training (EST), 76
Erikson, Erik, 92, 127
Esalen, 76
Esquirol, J. E. D., 44
Eugenics, 46

Fairbank, Ruth, 110
Falret, Jules, 47–48
Federal government: and clinical psychology, 199, 200; and mental illness, 148, 198; and universities, 200, 209
"Fight to a Finish" (Sassoon), 229

Harvard University: and ethical violations of faculty, 290, 292, 293; and psychiatry, 153, 154
Haslam, John, 270
Haywood, Eliza, 57–58
Healy, David, 169, 294
Henderson, David, 102
Henschen, Saloman, 263
Hill, Charles, 48
Hill, Robert Gardiner, 63
Hinkle, Beatrice, 125
Hippocrates Cried (Taylor), 276
Hippocratic medicine, 39, 56–57, 180
Hogarth, William, 43
Hollywood, 5, 82–83
Holmes, Oliver Wendell, 252
Homelessness, 4
Homer, 268
Homosexuality, and psychiatry, 222, 233
Hooke, Robert, 34, 41
Horney, Karen, 133, 156
Hoskins, W. G., 150
Howard, Richard, 10, 28, 31, 32
Hubbard, L. Ron, 77
Human Potential Movement, 76
Human rights, 240, 242; Universal Declaration of, 245
Huntington, Samuel, 245
Huntington's disease, 23
Hutchins, Robert, 155
Hydrotherapy, 138
Hyman, Steven: and critique of *DSM V*, 71, 173, 295; and lack of progress in psychiatry, 176
Hypnosis, 88, 182
Hysteria, 4, 17, 47, 83, 180, 183, 275; and American neurology, 143; and Jean-Martin Charcot, 87, 182; disappearance of, 205; and Sigmund Freud, 88–89, 91

Improper confinement of mental patients, 57–59, 60, 61, 62–65
Insel, Thomas, 55; critique of *DSM 5*, 71, 173, 295–296
Institute of Living, 134, 138–139, 199. *See also* Hartford Retreat
Institute of Psychiatry (London), 50
Insulin coma therapy, 51, 67, 138, 159, 171, 195
Insurance industry, and mental illness, 206, 207–208
International Classification of Diseases, ninth edition (*ICD 9*), 205

Interpretation of Dreams, The (Freud), 87
Islam, and hospitals, 38–40

Jackson, John Hughlings, 96, 182
Jacobson, Edith, 125
James, William, 181; and Emmanuel Movement, 75–76; reaction to Sigmund Freud, 84; and pragmatism, 98, 145, 146
Janet, Pierre, 12
Jansen Pharmaceuticals, 292
Jelliffe, Smith Ely, 12; and Adolf Meyer, 102
Johns Hopkins University, 13–14, 15, 50; and focal sepsis, 194; prominence of medical school, 101–102; and psychiatry, 152, 153, 154
Johnson & Johnson, 292; fines paid, 294–295
Jones, Ernest, 84
Jones, Owen, 254
Joyce, James, 181
Jung, Carl, 93
Juvenile bipolar disorder, 214, 290, 297

Kanner, Leo, 153
Katherina. *See* Kronick, Aurelia
Kellogg, John Harvey, 46, 74, 75
Kelly, Howard, 102
Kendall, Tim, 176
Kesey, Ken, 67
Kraepelin, Emil: and Sigmund Freud, 203; and nosology, 192, 193, 272; and Rockefeller Foundation, 154; and toxic origins of dementia praecox, 193
Kraft-Ebbing, Richard, 92
Kronick, Aurelia, 90
Ku Klux Klan, 220

Laing, R. D., 27–28, 30, 36, 54, 68
Lambert, Robert A., 154, 157
La Mettrie, Julian, 249
Lawn House Asylum, 66
Lawrence, William, 249
Lennon, John, 239
Leonard, E. M., 35
Leprosy, 32, 33, 35
Lewis, Aubrey, 50; and Adolf Meyer, 102
Lieberman, Jeffrey, 17, 169; on *DSM III*, 171–174; on Sigmund Freud, 170; and psychopharmacology, 175; on wonders of contemporary psychiatry, 174
Life chart, 98, 130–131, 132, 144–145
Lifton, Robert J., 220, 221, 223
Lindner, Robert, 5
Litwack, Thomas, 279